FIFTH EDITION

HEALTH CARE FINANCE

FINANCE

Basic Tools For Nonfinancial Managers

JUDITH J. BAKER, PhD, CPA

R.W. BAKER, JD

NEIL R. DWORKIN, PhD

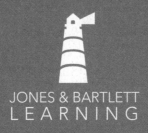

World Headquarters
Jones & Bartlett Learning
5 Wall Street
Burlington, MA 01803
978-443-5000
info@jblearning.com
www.jblearning.com

Jones & Bartlett Learning books and products are available through most bookstores and online booksellers. To contact Jones & Bartlett Learning directly, call 800-832-0034, fax 978-443-8000, or visit our website, www.jblearning.com.

Substantial discounts on bulk quantities of Jones & Bartlett Learning publications are available to corporations, professional associations, and other qualified organizations. For details and specific discount information, contact the special sales department at Jones & Bartlett Learning via the above contact information or send an email to specialsales@jblearning.com.

11835-3

Production Credits

VP, Executive Publisher: David D. Cella
Publisher: Michael Brown
Associate Editor: Danielle Bessette
Associate Production Editor: Rebekah Linga
Senior Marketing Manager: Sophie Fleck Teague
Manufacturing and Inventory Control Supervisor: Amy Bacus
Composition: Integra Software Services Pvt. Ltd.
Cover Design: Theresa Manley
Rights & Media Specialist: Merideth Tumasz
Media Development Editor: Shannon Sheehan
Cover Image: © LFor/Shutterstock
Printing and Binding: Edwards Brothers Malloy
Cover Printing: Edwards Brothers Malloy

Library of Congress Cataloging-in-Publication Data
Names: Baker, Judith J., author. | Baker, R. W., author. | Dworkin, Neil R., author.
Title: Health care finance : basic tools for nonfinancial managers / Judith Baker, R.W. Baker, and Neil R. Dworkin.
Description: Fifth edition. | Burlington, Massachusetts : Jones & Bartlett Learning, [2018] | Includes bibliographical references and index.
Identifiers: LCCN 2016054734 | ISBN 9781284118216 (pbk.)
Subjects: | MESH: Financial Management | Health Facilities–economics | Health Facility Administration | United States
Classification: LCC RA971.3 | NLM W 80 | DDC 362.1068/1–dc23
LC record available at https://lccn.loc.gov/2016054734

6048

Printed in the United States of America
21 20 19 18 17   10 9 8 7 6 5 4 3 2 1

Table of Contents

New to This Edition

The *Fifth Edition* continues to provide practical information, with examples taken from real life in the healthcare finance world. For example, we have added the following:

NEW MATERIAL IN THE 5TH EDITION:

- Chapter 3 "The Digital Age: Changing the Landscape of Healthcare Finance"—This new chapter is about understanding the impact of data analytics and big data, along with other important trends in the changing landscape of healthcare finance. It is important to recognize that digital advancements in health care are the drivers that enable innovation.
- Chapter 26 "Understanding Strategic Relationships: Health Delivery Systems, Finance and Reimbursement"—This new chapter focuses upon describing the strategic relationships between and among health delivery systems, finance, and reimbursement. This chapter assists a manager in recognizing both differences and interrelationships and in applying this recognition to their own organization's structure.
- Chapter 27 "Understanding Value-Based Health Care and Its Financial and Digital Outcomes"—Value-based performance, the subject of this new chapter, is particularly important because it is the key to both improving patient care and reforming payment systems. Healthcare organizations should define what value means and make sure that definition is shared across the entire entity.
- Chapter 28 "New Payment Methods and Measures: MIPS and APMs for Eligible Professionals"—This new chapter highlights significant legislation and regulations that change payment methods and performance measures for physicians and other eligible professionals. The new payment method for physicians hinges upon proper reporting of new performance measures. The new system is a true reform, as it replaces a physician payment system that has been in effect for decades.
- Appendix 28-A "Meaningful Use: Modified and Streamlined with a New Name"—This new appendix describes the evolution of meaningful use before and after its transition into the new physician performance measures that are described in Chapter 28.
- Chapter 29 "Standardizing Measures and Payment in Post-Acute Care: New Requirements"—This new chapter is about important legislation and regulations that standardize measures and require studies about payment reform for post-acute care. This means performance measures for skilled nursing facilities, home health agencies, inpatient rehabilitation facilities, and long-term care hospitals are being standardized. Models for a patient-centered payment system that cuts across all four care settings are also being created.
- Chapter 30 "ICD-10 Implementation Continues: Finance and Strategic Challenges for the Manager"—This updated chapter focuses upon challenges for the manager within ICD-10 implementation. An all-new section introduces useful Key Performance Indicators that are used to assess an organization's ICD-10 implementation progress.

Other new material in this edition includes the following:

- Chapter 9 "Understanding Inventory and Depreciation Concepts"—A new section about drug distribution systems in use in hospitals has been added to this chapter.
- Chapter 10 "Staffing: Methods, Operations, and Regulation"—A new section has been added describing legislation that requires reporting "verifiable and auditable" payroll information for the "Nursing Compare" website, along with information about existing Certificate of Need regulations.

- Appendix 16-A "Creating A DRG Budget for Respiratory Care: The Resource Consumption Approach"—This new appendix sets out a step-by-step DRG budget methodology.
- Appendix 16-B "Reviewing a Comparative Operating Budget Report"—This new appendix describes the review of a section from an actual operating budget report.
- Chapter 21 "Understanding Investment and Statistical Terms Used in Finance"—This chapter was originally only about investment terms; it now has a new section about understanding statistical terms.
- Chapter 31 "Case Study: The Doctor's Dilemma"—This new case study is about a physician deciding whether or not to sell his practice to a health delivery system.

MATERIAL OMITTED FROM THIS EDITION

- Two *Fourth Edition* chapters and a *Fourth Edition* appendix have been omitted because they are becoming outdated. This includes the following: Chapter 24 "Information Technology and EHR: Adoption Requirements, Initiatives, and Management Decisions" has been replaced with the new value-based chapter.
- Appendix 24-A Accordingly, the e-Prescribing (eRx) appendix has also been omitted because the incentive program is ending.
- Chapter 25 "Electronic Health Records Framework: Incentives, Standards, Measures, and Meaningful Use" has been omitted because the incentives are ending.
- Relevant additions and deletions have been made to the "Examples and Exercises" section.

To summarize: A fundamental theme in the *Fifth Edition* is that healthcare financing is embracing the digital age. This is manifested by its coverage of electronic health records (EHRs), data analytics, value-based health care, and social media, among other topics. In this era of population health and the resulting need for clinical integration, data-driven collaboration has the potential to improve outcomes and lower costs, as well as more effectively engage the patient. The upshot: Everything is connected.

Preface

Our world of work is divided into three parts: the healthcare consultant, the instructor, and the writer. Over the years, we have taught managers in seminars, academic settings, and corporate conference rooms. Most of the managers were mid-career adults, working in all types of healthcare disciplines. We taught them and they taught us. One of the things they taught us was this: A nonfinancial manager pushed into dealing with the world of finance often feels a dislocation and a change of perspective, and that experience can be both difficult and exciting. We have listened to their questions and concerns as these managers grapple with this new world. This book is the result of their experiences, and ours.

The book is designed for use by a manager (or future manager) who does not have an educational background in financial management. It has long been our philosophy that if you can truly understand how a thing works—whatever it is—then you own it. This book is created around that philosophy. In other words, we intend to make financial management transparent by showing how it works and how a manager can use it.

USING THE BOOK

All our examples are drawn from the healthcare industry. Thus users will find examples and exercises covering many types of healthcare settings and providers, including hospitals, clinics, physician practices, long-term care facilities, and home health agencies.

Standard Elements

Each chapter within these parts contains the following four elements:

- "Progress Notes" set out learning objectives at the beginning of each chapter.
- An "Information Checkpoint" segment at the end of each chapter tells the user three things: information needed, where this information can be obtained, and how this information can be used.
- A "Key Terms" section follows the "Information Checkpoint." Every Key Term is defined in the Glossary; it is also bold faced the first time it appears in the text.
- The "Discussion Questions" segment inquires about practical uses of chapter material and encourages responses based upon experience.

Structure and Topics

The book is structured in 12 parts, as follows.

Part I: Healthcare Finance Overview [Three chapters; one is new]
Part II: Record Financial Operations [Four chapters]
Part III: Tools To Analyze and Understand Financial Operations [Three chapters plus appendix; new text added to two chapters]
Part IV: Report and Measure Financial Results [Three chapters plus three appendices]
Part V: Tools to Review and Manage Comparative Data [Two chapters]
Part VI: Construct and Evaluate Budgets [Two chapters plus two new appendices]
Part VII: Tools to Plan, Monitor, and Control Financial Status [Three chapters; one is new]
Part VIII: Financial Terms, Costs, and Choices [Three chapters; one entire new section]

Part IX: Strategic Planning: A Powerful Tool [Three chapters plus one appendix; one chapter is new]

Part X: Information Technology As A Financial and Strategic Tool [Four chapters plus two appendices; three chapters and one appendix are all new and the fourth chapter has been substantially revised. In addition, two previous chapters and a previous appendix that have become outdated have been omitted and replaced in the *Fifth Edition*.]

Part XI: Case Studies [One new case study about the doctor's dilemma, one case study about strategic financial planning in long-term care, and a group of four interrelated case studies about the Metropolis Health System]

Part XII: Mini-Case Studies [Two mini-case studies; one concerns resource misallocation in a public health clinic and the other is about automating admissions processes]

More About the Metropolis Health System Case Studies

A group of four case studies about the Metropolis Health System (MHS) represents a comprehensive suite of information. This section includes the major case study about the system, followed by an appendix containing an MHS financial statement and excerpts from notes. A second case study appendix shows how one MHS hospital was turned around using comparative analysis of benchmarks and statistical data. A third case study appendix describes a detailed proposal to add a retail pharmacy to another of the MHS hospitals. The Metropolis grouping thus provides an interactive suite of case study material.

Supplemental Resources

At the back of the book you will find additional resources as follows, all of which have been updated for the *Fifth Edition*:

- An Appendix containing Checklists
- A Glossary
- Examples and Exercises, with Solutions
- Other Supplemental Materials

Acknowledgments

With this edition we welcome Dr. Neil R. Dworkin as our coauthor. Neil brings a formidable combination of both educational and practical on-the-ground experience in health care. He also brings fresh viewpoints that are as valuable as his career achievements.

The *Fifth Edition* has evolved with the help of numerous instructors and students who give us feedback; we listen. We owe a great debt of thanks to Mike Brown, our long-suffering and understanding publisher. And we thank our *Fifth Edition* first readers, including Teresa Schroder, AuD, CCC-A, along with others who prefer to be anonymous; you know who you are. The continuing support and suggestions of Janet Feldman, PhD, RN, Vice President, Qualitas Associates, along with certain continuing technical support provided by Colleene McMurphy, CPA, of McMurphy and Associates, are also appreciated.

The input from finance sessions we taught as Adjunct Faculty at Texas Woman's University in Dallas also contributed to shaping the content of the *Fifth Edition*. Our continued gratitude goes to Craig Sheagren, Senior Vice President/CFO, McDonough District Hospital, Macomb, Illinois; and Nancy M. Borkowski, PhD, Professor, Department of Professional Management/Health Management, St. Thomas University, Miami, Florida, for their encouragement, information, suggestions, and assistance with the original concept of the book. We also thank John Brocketti, Chief Financial Officer, SUMA Health System, Akron, Ohio; Christine Pierce, Partner, The Resource Group, Cleveland, Ohio; and Dr. Frank Welsh, Cincinnati, Ohio, for their ongoing information and suggestions.

Many others also contributed suggestions, recommendations, and information to help shape and refine the initial concept. We continue to acknowledge these individuals, listed below, including their original affiliations:

Ian G. Worden, CPA, Regional Vice President of Finance/CFO, PeaceHealth, Eugene, Oregon

Carol A. Robinson, Medical Records Director, Titus Regional Medical Center, Mt. Pleasant, Texas

John Congelli, Vice President of Finance, Genesee Memorial Hospital, Batavia, New York

Charles A. Keil, Cost Accountant, Genesee Memorial Hospital, Batavia, New York

George O. Kimbro, CPA, CFO, Hunt Memorial Hospital District, Greenville, Texas

Bob Gault, Laboratory Director, Hunt Memorial Hospital District, Greenville, Texas

Ted J. Stuart, Jr., MD, MBA, Northwest Family Physicians, Glendale, Arizona

Mark Potter, EMS Director, Hopkins County Memorial Hospital, Sulphur Springs, Texas

Leonard H. Friedman, PhD, Assistant Professor, Coordinator, Health Care Administration Program, Oregon State University, Corvallis, Oregon

Patricia Chiverton, EdD, RN, Dean, University of Rochester School of Nursing, Rochester, New York

Donna M. Tortoretti, RNC, Chief Operating Officer, Community Nursing Center, University of Rochester School of Nursing, Rochester, New York

Billie Ann Brotman, PhD, Professor of Finance, Department of Economics and Finance, Kennesaw State University, Kennesaw, Georgia

About the Authors

Judith J. Baker, PhD, CPA, has worked with healthcare systems, costing, finance, and reimbursement throughout her career. With over 40 years' experience in health care, she is a co-founder of Resource Group, Ltd., a healthcare consulting firm. As a CMS contractor, she has assisted in validation of costs for new programs and for rate setting and has also consulted on cost report design. More recently, she has provided activity-based costing, rate setting, and organizational systems expertise to national clients within the healthcare industry.

Judith's doctorate is in human and organizational systems, with a concentration in healthcare costing systems. She has served as adjunct faculty at the University of Texas at Houston and the Texas Woman's University in Dallas, as well as the University of Rochester School of Nursing and the Case Western Reserve University Francis Payne Bolton School of Nursing.

Judith has written numerous peer-reviewed articles and has served as Consulting Editor for Aspen Publishers, Inc. Her books include *Activity-Based Costing and Activity-Based Management for Health Care*, *Prospective Payment for Long-Term Care*, *Prospective Payment for Home Health Agencies*, *Management Accounting for Health Care Organizations* (with Robert Hankins) and *Essentials of Cost Accounting for Health Care Organizations* (with Steven Finkler and David Ward). She is Editor Emeritus of the quarterly *Journal of Healthcare Finance*.

R. W. Baker, JD, is also a co-founder of Resource Group, Ltd., a healthcare consulting firm. He has more than 40 years of experience in health care and has designed, directed, and administered numerous financial impact studies for healthcare providers. His early studies centered around facility-specific MDS data collection and analysis. He and his firm subcontracted to the HCFA/CMS Nursing Home Case Mix and Quality Demonstration for over nine years. More recently he has designed, implemented, and managed a series of national time studies for pharmaceutical and medical device clients.

R. W. is the editor of continuing professional education seminar manuals and training manuals for facility personnel and for research staff members. He served as a Consulting Editor with Aspen Publishers, Inc. and is co-author of *A Step-by-Step Guide to the Minimum Data Set* (with Dr. Janet Feldman).

Neil R. Dworkin, PhD, is Emeritus Associate Professor of Management at Western Connecticut State University, where he was Coordinator of the Masters in Health Administration Program and where he taught Strategic Management, Finance, Marketing, Health Policy, and Health Delivery Systems. He is presently an adjunct faculty member at Charter Oak State College, which is part of the Connecticut State University System and where he teaches Continuous Quality Improvement in Health Care and Health Care Systems and Administration.

Neil has hospital administration experience, and has been a nursing home administrator in New York and Connecticut. He has over 40 years' experience in the healthcare field. He was the lead author in a three-article series on "Managerial Socialization in Short-Term Hospitals" that was published in *Hospital Topics* and *Problems and Perspectives in Management*. Neil has also served as an editor of *The Journal of Health Administration Education*.

PART

I

Healthcare Finance Overview

Introduction to Healthcare Finance

© LFor/Shutterstock

THE HISTORY

Financial management has a long and distinguished history. Consider, for example, that Socrates wrote about the universal function of management in human endeavors in 400 B.C. and that Plato developed the concept of specialization for efficiency in 350 B.C. Evidence of sophisticated financial management exists from much earlier times: the Chinese produced a planning and control system in 1100 B.C., a minimum-wage system was developed by Hammurabi in 1800 B.C., and the Egyptians and Sumerians developed planning and record-keeping systems in 4000 B.C.[1]

Many managers in early history discovered and rediscovered managerial principles while attempting to reach their goals. Because the idea of management thought as a discipline had not yet evolved, they formulated principles of management because certain goals had to be accomplished. As management thought became codified over time, however, the building of techniques for management became more organized. Management as a discipline for educational purposes began in the United States in 1881. In that year, Joseph Wharton created the Wharton School, offering college courses in business management at the University of Pennsylvania. It was the only such school until 1898, when the Universities of Chicago and California established their business schools. Thirteen years later, in 1911, 30 such schools were in operation in the United States.[2]

Over the long span of history, managers have all sought how to make organizations work more effectively. Financial management is a vital part of organizational effectiveness. This text's goal is to provide the keys to unlock the secrets of financial management for nonfinancial managers.

Progress Notes

After completing this chapter, you should be able to

1. Discuss the three viewpoints of managers in organizations.
2. Identify the four elements of financial management.
3. Understand the differences between the two types of accounting.
4. Identify the types of organizations.
5. Understand the composition and purpose of an organization chart.

THE CONCEPT

A Method of Getting Money in and out of the Business

One of our colleagues, a nurse, talks about the area of healthcare finance as "a method of getting money in and out of the business." It is not a bad description. As we shall see, revenues represent inflow and expenses represent outflow. Thus, "getting money in" represents the inflow (revenues), whereas "getting money out" (expenses) represents the outflow. The successful manager, through planning, organizing, controlling, and decision making, is able to adjust the inflow and outflow to achieve the most beneficial outcome for the organization.

HOW DOES FINANCE WORK IN THE HEALTHCARE BUSINESS?

The purpose of this text is to show how the various elements of finance fit together: in other words, how finance works in the healthcare business. The real key to understanding finance is understanding the various pieces and their relationship to each other. If you, the manager, truly see how the elements work, then they are yours. They become your tools to achieve management success.

The healthcare industry is a service industry. It is not in the business of manufacturing, say, widgets. Instead, its essential business is the delivery of healthcare services. It may have inventories of medical supplies and drugs, but those inventories are necessary to service delivery, not to manufacturing functions. Because the business of health care is service, the explanations and illustrations within this book focus on the practice of financial management in the service industries.

VIEWPOINTS

The managers within a healthcare organization will generally have one of three views: (1) financial, (2) process, or (3) clinical. The way they manage will be influenced by which view they hold.

1. The financial view. These managers generally work with finance on a daily basis. The reporting function is part of their responsibility. They usually perform much of the strategic planning for the organization.
2. The process view. These managers generally work with the system of the organization. They may be responsible for data accumulation. They are often affiliated with the information system hierarchy in the organization.
3. The clinical view. These managers generally are responsible for service delivery. They have direct interaction with the patients and are responsible for clinical outcomes of the organization.

Managers must, of necessity, interact with one another. Thus, managers holding different views will be required to work together. Their concerns will intersect to some degree, as illustrated by **Figure 1–1**. The nonfinancial manager who understands healthcare finance will be able to interpret and negotiate successfully such interactions between and among viewpoints.

In summary, financial management is a discipline with a long and respected history. Healthcare service delivery is a business, and the concept of financial management assists in balancing the inflows and outflows that are a part of the business.

WHY MANAGE?

Business does not run itself. It requires a variety of management activities in order to operate properly.

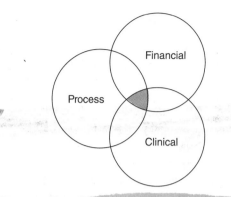

Figure 1-1 Three Views of Management Within an Organization.

THE ELEMENTS OF FINANCIAL MANAGEMENT

There are four recognized elements of financial management: (1) planning, (2) controlling, (3) organizing and directing, and (4) decision making. The four divisions are based on the purpose of each task. Some authorities stress only three elements (planning, controlling, and decision making) and consider organizing and directing as a part of the controlling element. This text recognizes organizing and directing as a separate element of financial management, primarily because such a large proportion of a manager's time is taken up with performing these duties.

1. Planning. The financial manager identifies the steps that must be taken to accomplish the organization's objectives. Thus, the purpose is to identify objectives and then to identify the steps required for accomplishing these objectives.
2. Controlling. The financial manager makes sure that each area of the organization is following the plans that have been established. One way to do this is to study current reports and compare them with reports from earlier periods. This comparison often shows where the organization may need attention because that area is not effective. The reports that the manager uses for this purpose are often called feedback. The purpose of controlling is to ensure that plans are being followed.
3. Organizing and directing. When organizing, the financial manager decides how to use the resources of the organization to most effectively carry out the plans that have been established. When directing, the manager works on a day-to-day basis to keep the results of the organizing running efficiently. The purpose is to ensure effective resource use and provide daily supervision.
4. Decision making. The financial manager makes choices among available alternatives. Decision making actually occurs parallel to planning, organizing, and controlling. All types of decision making rely on information, and the primary tasks are analysis and evaluation. Thus, the purpose is to make informed choices.

THE ORGANIZATION'S STRUCTURE

The structure of an organization is an important factor in management.

Organization Types

Organizations fall into one of two basic types: profit oriented or nonprofit oriented. In the United States, these designations follow the taxable status of the organizations. The profit-oriented entities, also known as proprietary organizations, are responsible for paying income taxes. Proprietary subgroups include individuals, partnerships, and corporations. The nonprofit organizations do not pay income taxes.

There are two subgroups of nonprofit entities: voluntary and government. Voluntary nonprofits have sought tax-exempt status. In general, voluntary nonprofits are associated with churches, private schools, or foundations. Government nonprofits, on the other hand, do not pay taxes because they are government entities. Government nonprofits can be (1) federal, (2) state, (3) county, (4) city, (5) a combination of city and county, (6) a hospital taxing district (with the power to raise revenues through taxes), or (7) a state university (perhaps with a teaching hospital affiliated with the university). The organization's type may affect its structure. **Exhibit 1–1** summarizes the subgroups of both proprietary and nonprofit organizations.

Organization Charts

In a small organization, top management will be able to see what is happening. Extensive measures and indicators are not necessary because management can view overall operations. But in a large organization, top management must use the management control system to understand what is going on. In other words, to view operations, management must use measures and indicators because he or she cannot get a first-hand overall picture of the total organization.

As a rule of thumb, an informal management control system is acceptable only if the manager can stay in close contact with all aspects of the operation. Otherwise, a formal system is required. In the context of health care, therefore, a one-physician practice (**Figure 1–2**) could use an informal method, but a hospital system (**Figure 1–3**) must use a formal method of management control.

The structure of the organization will affect its financial management. Organization charts are often used to illustrate the structure of the organization. Each box on an organization chart represents a particular area of management responsibility. The lines between the boxes are lines of authority.

In the health system organization chart illustrated in Figure 1–3, the president/chief executive officer oversees seven senior vice presidents. Each senior vice president has vice presidents reporting to him or her in each

Exhibit 1–1 Types of Organizations

Profit Oriented—Proprietary
Individual
Partnership
Corporation
Other
Nonprofit—Voluntary
Church Associated
Private School Associated
Foundation Associated
Other
Nonprofit—Government
Federal
State
County
City
City–County
Hospital District
State University
Other

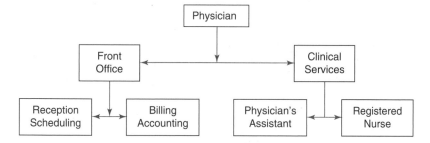

Figure 1–2 Physician's Office Organization Chart.
Courtesy of Resource Group, Ltd., Dallas, Texas.

particular area of responsibility designated on the chart. These vice presidents, in turn, have an array of other managers reporting to them at varying levels of managerial responsibility.

The organization chart also shows the degree of decentralization within the organization. Decentralization indicates the delegating of authority for decision making. The chart thus illustrates the pattern of how managers are allowed—or required—to make key decisions within the particular organization.

The purpose of an organization chart, then, is to indicate how responsibility is assigned to managers and to indicate the formal lines of communication and reporting.

TWO TYPES OF ACCOUNTING

Financial

Financial accounting is generally for outside, or third party, use. Thus, financial accounting emphasizes external reporting. External reporting to third parties in health care includes, for example, government entities (Medicare, Medicaid, and other government programs) and health plan payers. In addition, proprietary organizations may have to report to stockholders, taxing district hospitals have to report to taxpayers, and so on.

Financial reporting for external purposes must be in accordance with generally accepted accounting principles. Financial reporting is usually concerned with transactions that have already occurred: that is, it is retrospective.

Managerial

Managerial accounting is generally for inside, or internal, use. Managerial accounting, as its title implies, is used by managers. The planning and control of operations and related performance measures are common day-by-day uses of managerial accounting. Likewise, the reporting of profitability of services and the pricing of services are other common ongoing uses of managerial accounting. Strategic planning and other intermediate and long-term decision making represent an additional use of managerial accounting.[3]

Managerial accounting intended for internal use is not bound by generally accepted accounting principles. Managerial accounting deals with transactions that have already occurred, but it is also concerned with the future, in the form of projecting outcomes and preparing budgets. Thus, managerial accounting is prospective as well as retrospective.

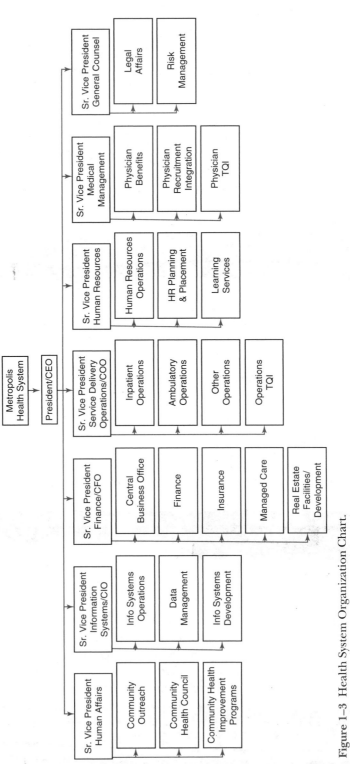

Figure 1–3 Health System Organization Chart.
Courtesy of Resource Group, Ltd., Dallas, Texas.

INFORMATION CHECKPOINT

What is needed?	Reports for management purposes.
Where is it found?	With your supervisor.
How is it used?	To manage better.
What is needed?	Organization chart.
Where is it found?	With your supervisor or in the administrative offices.
How is it used?	To better understand the structure and lines of authority in your organization.

KEY TERMS

Controlling
Decision Making
Financial Accounting
Managerial Accounting
Nonprofit Organization (also see Voluntary Organization)
Organization Chart
Organizing
Planning
Proprietary Organization (also see Profit-Oriented Organization)

DISCUSSION QUESTIONS

1. What element of financial management do you perform most often in your job?
2. Do you perform all four elements? If not, why not?
3. Of the organization types described in this chapter, what type is the one you work for?
4. Have you ever seen your company's organization chart? If so, how decentralized is it?
5. If you receive reports in the course of your work, do you believe that they are prepared for outside (third party) use or for internal (management) use? What leads you to believe this?

NOTES

1. C. S. George, Jr., *The History of Management Thought*, 2nd ed. (Englewood Cliffs, NJ: Prentice Hall, 1972), 1–27.
2. Ibid., 87.
3. S. Williamson et al., *Fundamentals of Strategic Planning for Healthcare Organizations* (New York: The Haworth Press, 1997).

Four Things the Healthcare Manager Needs to Know About Financial Management Systems

2

WHAT DOES THE MANAGER NEED TO KNOW?

Financial management is both an art and a science. You, as a manager, need to perceive the structure and reasoning that underlies management actions. To do so, you need to be able to answer the following four questions:

1. What are the four segments that make a financial management system work?
2. How does the information flow?
3. What are the basic system elements?
4. What is the annual management cycle for reporting results?

This chapter provides answers to each of these four questions. It also discusses how to communicate financial information to others. This ability is a valuable skill for a successful manager.

HOW THE SYSTEM WORKS IN HEALTH CARE

The information that you, as a manager, work with is only one part of an overall system. To understand financial management, it is essential to recognize the overall system in which your organization operates. An order exists within the system, and it is generally up to you to find that order. Watch for how the information fits together. The four segments that make a healthcare financial system work are (1) the original records, (2) the information system, (3) the accounting system, (4) and the reporting system. Generally speaking, the original records provide evidence that some event has occurred; the information system gathers this evidence; the accounting system records the evidence; and the reporting system produces reports

Progress Notes

After completing this chapter, you should be able to

1. Understand that four segments make a financial management system work.
2. Follow an information flow.
3. Recognize the basic system elements.
4. Follow the annual management cycle.

of the effect. The healthcare manager needs to know that these separate elements exist and that they work together for an end result.

THE INFORMATION FLOW

Structure of the Information System

Information systems can be simplistic or highly complex. They can be fully automated or semi-automated. Occasionally—even today—they can still be generated by hand and not by computer. (This last instance is becoming rare and can happen today only in certain small and relatively isolated healthcare organizations that are not yet required to electronically submit their billings.)

We will examine a particular information system and point out the basics that a manager should be able to recognize. **Figure 2–1** shows information system components for an ambulatory care setting. This complex system uses a clinical and financial data repository; in other words, both clinical and financial data are fed into the same system. An automated medical record is also linked to the system. These are basic facts that a manager should recognize about this ambulatory information system.

In addition, the financial information, both outpatient and any relevant inpatient, is fed into the data repository. Scheduling-system data also enter the data repository, along with any relevant inpatient care plan and nursing information. Again, all of these are basic facts that a manager should recognize about this ambulatory care information system.

These items have all been inputs. One output from the clinical and financial data repository (also shown in Figure 2–1) is insurance verification for patients through an electronic data

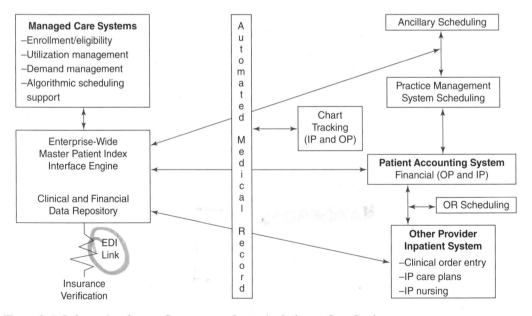

Figure 2–1 Information System Components for an Ambulatory Care Setting. OP, Outpatient; IP, Inpatient; OR, Operating Room.

information (EDI) link to insurance company databases. Insurance verification is daily operating information. Another output is decision-making information for managed care strategic planning, including support for demand, utilization, enrollment, and eligibility, plus some statistical support. The manager does not have to understand the specifics of all the inputs and outputs of this complex system, but he or she should recognize that these outputs occur when this ambulatory system is activated.

Function of Flowsheets

Flowsheets illustrate, as in this case, the flow of activities that capture information.[1] Flowsheets are useful because they portray who is responsible for what piece of information as it enters the system. The manager needs to realize the significance of such information. We give, as an example, obtaining confirmation of a patient's correct address. The manager should know that a correct address for a patient is vital to the smooth operation of the system. An incorrect address will, for example, cause the billing to be rejected. Understanding this connection between deficient data (e.g., a bad address) and the consequences (the bill will be rejected by the payer and thus not be paid) illustrates the essence of good financial management knowledge.

We can examine two examples of patient information flows. The first, shown in **Figure 2–2**, is a physician's office flowsheet for address confirmation. Four different personnel are involved, in addition to the patient. This physician has computed the cost of a bad address as $12.30 to track down each address correction. He pays close attention to the handling of this information because he knows there is a direct financial management consequence in his operation.

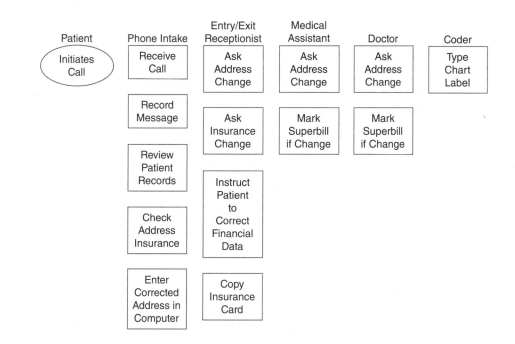

Figure 2–2 Physician's Office Flowsheet for Address Confirmation.

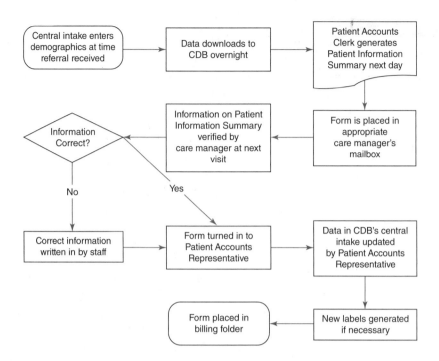

Figure 2–3 Health System Flowsheet for Verification of Patient Information.

The second example, shown in **Figure 2–3**, is a health system flowsheet for verification of patient information. This flowsheet illustrates the process for a home care system. In this case, the flow begins not with a receptionist, as in the physician office example, but with a central database. This central database downloads the information and generates a summary report to be reviewed the next day. Appropriate verification is then made in a series of steps, and any necessary corrections are made before the form goes to the billing department. The object of the flow is the same in both examples: that is, the billing department must have a correct address to receive payment. But the flow is different within two different systems. A manager must understand how the system works to understand the consequences—then good financial management can prevail.

BASIC SYSTEM ELEMENTS

To understand financial management, it is essential to decipher the reports provided to the manager. To comprehend these reports, it is helpful to understand certain basic system elements that are used to create the information contained in the reports.

Chart of Accounts—The Map

The chart of accounts is a map. It outlines the elements of your company in an organized manner. The chart of accounts maps out account titles with a method of numeric coding. It is designed to compile financial data in a uniform manner that the user can decode.

The groupings of accounts in the chart of accounts should match the groupings of the organization. In other words, the classification on the organization chart (as discussed in the previous chapter) should be compatible with the groupings on the chart of accounts. Thus, if there is a human resources department on your facility's organization chart, and if expenses are grouped by department in your facility, then we would expect to find a human resources grouping in the chart of accounts.

The manager who is working with financial data needs to be able to read and comprehend how the dollars are laid out and how they are gathered together, or assembled. This assembly happens through the guidance of the chart of accounts. That is why we compare it to a map.

Basic guidance for healthcare charts of accounts is set out in publications such as that of Seawell's *Chart of Accounts for Hospitals*.[2] However, generic guides are just that—generic. Every organization exhibits differences in its own chart of accounts that express the unique aspects of its structure. We examine three examples to illustrate these differences. Remember, we are spending time on the chart of accounts because your comprehension of detailed financial data may well depend on whether you can decipher your facility's own chart of accounts mapping in the information forwarded for your use.

The first format, shown in **Exhibit 2–1**, is a basic use, probably for a smaller organization. The exhibit is in two horizontal segments, "Structure" and "Example." There are three parts to the account number. The first part is one digit and indicates the financial statement element. Thus, our example shows "1," which is for "Asset." The second part is two digits and is the primary subclassification. Our example shows "10," which stands for "Current Asset" in this case. The third and final part is also two digits and is the secondary subclassification. Our example shows "11," which stands for "Petty Cash—Front Office" in this case. On a report, this account number would probably appear as 1-10-11.

The second format, shown in **Exhibit 2–2**, is full use and would be for a large organization. The exhibit is again in two horizontal segments, "Structure" and "Example," and there are now

Exhibit 2–1 Chart of Accounts, Format I

Structure		
X	XX	XX
Financial Statement Element	Primary Subclassification	Secondary Subclassification

Example		
1	10	11
Asset	Current Asset	Petty Cash— Front Office
(Financial Statement Element)	(Primary Subclassification)	(Secondary Subclassification)

Exhibit 2–2 Chart of Accounts, Format II

Structure				
XX	XX	X	XXXX	XX
Entity Designator	Fund Designator	Financial Statement Element	Primary Subclassification	Secondary Subclassification

Example				
10	10	4	3125	03
Hospital A	General Fund	Revenue	Lab—Microbiology	Payer: XYZ HMO
10	10	6	3125	10
Hospital A	General Fund	Expense	Lab—Microbiology	Clerical Salaries
(Entity Designator)	(Fund Designator)	(Financial Statement Element)	(Primary Subclassification)	(Secondary Subclassification)

two line items appearing in the Example section. This full-use example has five parts to the account number. The first part is two digits and indicates the entity designator number. Thus, we conclude that there is more than one entity within this system. Our example shows "10," which stands for "Hospital A." The second part is two digits and indicates the fund designator number. Thus, we conclude that there is more than one fund within this system. Our example shows "10," which stands for "General Fund."

The third part of Exhibit 2–2 is one digit and indicates the financial statement element. Thus, the first line of our example shows "4," which is for "Revenue," and the second line of our example shows "6," which is for "Expense." (The third part of this example is the first part of the simpler example shown in Exhibit 2–1.) The fourth part is four digits and is the primary subclassification. Our example shows 3125, which stands for "Lab—Microbiology." The number 3125 appears on both lines of this example, indicating that both the revenue and the expense belong to Lab—Microbiology. (The fourth part of this example is the second part of the simpler example shown in Exhibit 2–1. The simpler example used only two digits for this part, but this full-use example uses four digits.) The fifth and final part is two digits and is the secondary subclassification. Our example shows "03" on the first line, the revenue line, which stands for "Payer: XYZ HMO" and indicates the source of the revenue. On the second line, the expense line, our example shows "10," which stands for "Clerical Salaries." Therefore, we understand that these are the clerical salaries belonging to Lab—Microbiology in Hospital A. (The fifth part of this example is the third and final part of the simpler example shown in Exhibit 2–1.) On a report, these account numbers might appear as 10-10-4-3125-03 and 10-10-6-3125-10. Another optional use that is easier to read at a glance is 10104-3125-03 and 10106-3125-10.

Because every organization is unique and because the chart of accounts reflects that uniqueness, the third format, shown in **Exhibit 2–3**, illustrates a customized use of the chart of accounts. This example is adapted from a large hospital system. There are four parts to its chart of accounts number. The first part is an entity designator and designates a company within the hospital system. The fund designator two-digit part, as traditionally used (see Exhibit 2–2), is missing here. The financial statement element one-digit part, as traditionally used (see Exhibit 2–2), is also missing here. Instead, the second part of Exhibit 2–3 represents the primary classification, which is shown as an expense category ("Payroll") in the example line. The third part of Exhibit 2–3 is the secondary subclassification, representing a labor subaccount expense designation ("Regular per-Visit RN"). The fourth and final part of Exhibit 2–3 is another subclassification that indicates the department within the company ("Home Health"). On a report for this organization, therefore, the account number 21-7000-2200-7151 would indicate the home care services company's payroll for regular per-visit registered nurses (RNs) in the home health department. Finally, remember that time spent understanding your own facility's chart of accounts will be time well spent.

Books and Records—Capture Transactions

The books and records of the financial information system for the organization serve to capture transactions. **Figure 2–4** illustrates the relationship of the books and records to each other. As a single transaction occurs, the process begins. The individual transaction is recorded in the appropriate subsidiary journal. Similar such transactions are then grouped and balanced within the subsidiary journal. At periodic intervals, the groups of transactions are gathered, summarized, and entered in the general ledger. Within the general ledger, the transaction groups

Exhibit 2–3 Chart of Accounts, Format III

Structure			
XX	XXXX	XXXX	XXXX
Company Category	Expense	Subaccount	Department
(Entity Designator)	(Primary Classification)	(Secondary Subclassification)	(Additional Subclassification)

Example			
21	7000	2200	7151
Home Care Services	Payroll	Regular per-Visit RN	Home Health
(Company)	(Expense Category)	(Subaccount)	(Department)

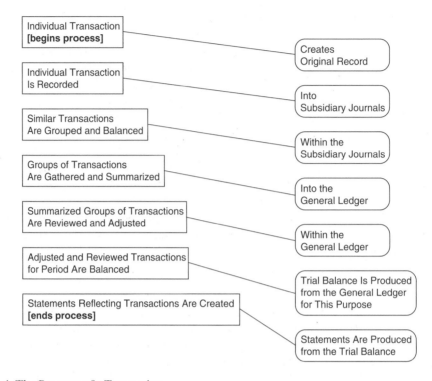

Figure 2–4 The Progress of a Transaction.
Courtesy of Resource Group, Ltd., Dallas, Texas.

are reviewed and adjusted. After such review and adjustment, the transactions for the period within the general ledger are balanced. A document known as the trial balance is used for this purpose. The final step in the process is to create statements that reflect the transactions for the period. The trial balance is used to produce the statements.

All transactions for the period reside in the general ledger. The subsidiary journals are so named because they are "subsidiary" to the general ledger: in other words, they serve to support the general ledger. **Figure 2–5** illustrates this concept. Another way to think of the subsidiary journals is to picture them as feeding the general ledger. The important point here is to understand the source and the flow of information as it is recorded.

Reports—The Product

Reports are more fully treated in a subsequent chapter of this text (see Chapter 11). It is sufficient at this point to recognize that reports are the final product of a process that commences with an original transaction.

THE ANNUAL MANAGEMENT CYCLE

The annual management cycle affects the type and status of information that the manager is expected to use. Some operating information is "raw"—that is, unadjusted. When the same information has passed further through the system and has been verified, adjusted, and

THE BOOKS

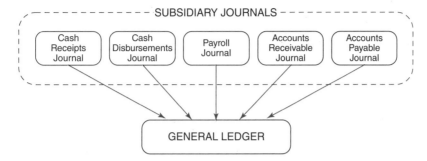

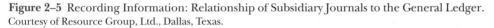

Figure 2–5 Recording Information: Relationship of Subsidiary Journals to the General Ledger. Courtesy of Resource Group, Ltd., Dallas, Texas.

balanced, it will usually vary from the initial raw data. These differences are a part of the process just described.

Daily and Weekly Operating Reports

The daily and weekly operating reports generally contain raw data, as discussed in the preceding paragraph. The purpose of such daily and weekly reports is to provide immediate operating information to use for day-to-day management purposes.

Quarterly Reports and Statistics

The quarterly reports and statistics generally have been verified, adjusted, and balanced. They are called interim reports because they have been generated some time during the reporting period of the organization and not at the end of that period. Managers often use quarterly reports as milestones. A common milestone is the quarterly budget review.

Annual Year-End Reports

Most organizations have a 12-month reporting period known as a fiscal year. A fiscal year, therefore, covers a period from the first day of a particular month (e.g., January 1) through the last day of a month that is one year, or 12 months, in the future (e.g., December 31). If we see a heading that reads, "For the year ended June 30," we know that the fiscal year began on July 1 of the previous year. Anything less than a full 12-month year is called a "stub period" and is fully spelled out in the heading. If, therefore, a company is reporting for a three-month stub period ending on December 31, the heading on the report will read, "For the three-month period ended December 31." An alternative treatment uses a heading that reads, "For the period October 1 to December 31."

Annual year-end reports cover the full 12-month reporting period or the fiscal year. Such annual year-end reports are not primarily intended for managers' use. Their primary purpose is for reporting the operations of the organization for the period to outsiders, or third parties.

Annual year-end reports represent the closing out of the information system for a specific reporting period. The recording and reporting of operations will now begin a new cycle with a new year.

COMMUNICATING FINANCIAL INFORMATION TO OTHERS

The ability to communicate financial information effectively to others is a valuable skill. It is important to

- Create a report as your method of communication.
- Use accepted terminology.
- Use standard formats that are accepted in the accounting profession.
- Begin with an executive summary.
- Organize the body of the report in a logical flow.
- Place extensive detail into an appendix.

The rest of this book will help you learn how to create such a report. Our book will also sharpen your communication skills by helping you better understand how heathcare finance works.

INFORMATION CHECKPOINT

What is needed? An explanation of how the information flow works in your unit.

Where is it found? Probably with the information system staff; perhaps in the administrative offices.

How is it used? Study the flow and relate it to the paperwork that you handle.

KEY TERMS

Accounting System
Chart of Accounts
General Ledger
Information System
Original Records
Reporting System
Subsidiary Journals
Trial Balance

DISCUSSION QUESTIONS

1. Have you ever been informed of the information flow in your unit or division?
2. If so, did you receive the information in a formal seminar or in an informal manner, one-on-one with another individual? Do you think this was the best way? Why?

3. Do you know about the chart of accounts in your organization as it pertains to information you receive?
4. If so, is it similar to one of the three formats illustrated in this chapter? If not, how is it different?
5. Do you work with daily or weekly operating reports? With quarterly reports and statistics?
6. If so, do these reports give you useful information? How do you think they could be improved?

NOTES

1. J. J. Baker, *Activity-Based Costing and Activity-Based Management for Health Care* (Gaithersburg, MD: Aspen Publishers, Inc., 1998).
2. L. V. Seawell, *Chart of Accounts for Hospitals* (Chicago: Probus Publishing Company, 1994).

The Digital Age: Changing the Landscape of Healthcare Finance

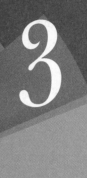

HIGH-TECH AND HIGH-TOUCH APPROACHES

Healthcare systems are using high-tech and high-touch approaches to reach patients where they are and with what they need in an attempt to meet the challenges of patient engagement. Digital platforms, including mobile apps and social networks, are changing customer interactions and expectations.

We characterize the current state of online technology as Web 2.0, which goes beyond simply letting people access information on the Internet (as was the case in the early days of the Internet). The current state is now characterized by greater user interactivity and collaboration, more pervasive network connectivity, and enhanced communication channels.[1]

Social media, such as Facebook and Twitter, are the outgrowth of Web 2.0. The challenge to a healthcare organization's marketing staff is to determine how to harness social media to reach customers and turn social media content into business value.

PATIENT ENGAGEMENT

Central to understanding the changes that are now occurring due to the variety of digital impacts and changes in health information technology is the concept of patient engagement. Technology and patient engagement go hand-in-hand. An overarching objective of the healthcare digital age is to make patient engagement more meaningful and effective.

The Engaged Patient

A truly engaged patient is one who is an active partner in his or her own health care. It stands to reason that primary care

Progress Notes

After completing this chapter, you should be able to

1. Understand what drives changes to health information technology.
2. Identify types of high-tech and high-touch digital approaches.
3. Identify the digital impact areas for patient engagement.
4. Define digital media.
5. Understand the difference between EMR and EHR.
6. Recognize how to effectively manage population health.

This chapter explores major digital age influences that are impacting healthcare finance.

would be the specialty wherein this concept can most effectively be operationalized. Patients who are punctual with their annual checkup and those with chronic diseases like diabetes who are adhering to their regimens would be considered engaged patients.

Jacqueline Fellows assembled a comprehensive list of digital impact areas under the rubric of "Patient Engagement Investments" and examined them by setting (e.g., hospital, physician organization) and by net patient revenue.[2] Among the areas that attracted the most interest were patient portals, patient access to medical records, telemedicine, remote monitoring, and telehealth to track patient health status.

The major factors driving the growth of the telehealth market appear to be the rise in aging and chronically ill population and the shortage of physicians in some areas of the country. However, there are reimbursement issues that must be overcome, which also encompass telemedicine.

Rapid Change

Mobile technology has the potential to help healthcare providers manage risk, encourage healthy behaviors, and engage with consumers. Garmin (producers of GPS programs), along with various partners, has launched new products including a wide range of "wearables" to help people reach their health and wellness goals. In one example, OffTheScale (OTS) has entered into partnership with Garmin and its innovative healthcare platform that fights against obesity and other chronic diseases. OTS provides a Garmin wearable device that measures steps taken and combines it with user data to calculate distance walked and calories burned.[3]

Leaders in performance technology such as Garmin also produce remote monitoring devices for patients with other conditions such as diabetes and heart failure. These types of mobile technology have the true potential to improve wellness and to lower healthcare costs.[4] It is essential, however, that the devices and systems that are flooding the market (including apps) be properly studied or vetted through clinical trials.

SOCIAL MEDIA

Recognizing the importance of social media is a first step in bringing a hospital, for example, into the digital world. Social media can help a hospital manage the patient experience, connect with community members and potential patients before they arrive, and manage their care transactions after they leave. Providing an alternative mode of communication can help make patient interactions more comfortable and less clinical. The intersection of health care and social media is unavoidable. Social networks, blogs, discussion forums, and other social and digital media highlight these alternative modes of communication.

Digital Media

Digital media may be defined as any type of information stored in a computer or mobile device, including data, voice, and video.[5] A common misconception related to social media is that it requires the creation of additional content. Any content that is being used for print media (newsletters, information packets, marketing materials, or other promotional items) can be repurposed for digital media. An effective social media strategy is integral to managing a healthcare organization's reputation.

What Do the Data Show?

It is estimated that between 70% and 75% of Internet users in the United States seek healthcare information on line.[6] According to a 2014 study, nearly 95% of hospitals had a Facebook page, and just over 50% had a Twitter account.[7] For all the good that may come from patients and healthcare consumers use of social media, there are also risks and challenges. For example, it can be difficult to control the quality of information that appears on patient social networks. In addition, patient privacy and security of health-related information are major concerns.

RESOURCE ALLOCATION

The types of resources needed to grow a healthcare organization's digital brand are technological and human resources-related. In addition, with the locus of responsibility for social media typically residing in a marketing and/or communications department in a healthcare organization, full-time employee staff costs dedicated to electronic media should result in additional budgetary expenses. These staff expenses are in addition to the cost of establishing and maintaining a website (purchasing a domain name, hosting fees, etc.). A website is a collection of related Web pages, images, videos, or other digital assets that are addressed with a common domain name or internet protocol (IP) address in an IP-based network.[8] That said, in today's competitive environment, it isn't enough just to have a Web presence. Instead, healthcare organizations need to have online visibility.

CHANGES IN HEALTH INFORMATION TECHNOLOGY

The changes that are occurring in health information technology are driven by health informatics, or the application of information technology to healthcare delivery. These changes include the following:

- More open, cloud-based systems that facilitate data sharing
- Mobile devices and sensors that enable increased participation by patients
- Adoption of digital or electronic health records

Still another major technology change involves data mining. Electronic records are increasingly being mined and analyzed to uncover new medical knowledge, promote evidence-based treatments, and determine the clinical and cost-effectiveness of care.[9] (For additional information on data mining, see the chapter entitled, "Understanding the Impact of Data Analytics and Big Data.")

EMRs and EHRs

At the center of the health information technology evolution is the electronic health record (EHR). A distinction has been made between the electronic medical record (EMR) and the EHR. The EMR is essentially the digital version of the traditional paper chart, the electronic record of a particular physician's office. The EHR ideally represents the total health status of the patient across all providers.[10]

Incorporating EMRs and EHRs into clinical practice will require large investments in new technology, in addition to changes in existing systems and processes. These barriers tend to slow EHR adoption rates. Moreover, in some instances, this technology may serve as a distraction during care delivery. On the other hand, the hope is that EHRs will realize their potential to improve quality, reduce medical errors, and lower administrative costs.

Interoperability

Interoperability, or the ability of two or more information systems to "talk" to each other (exchange data), is the key to the future success of EHRs as is the effectiveness of health information exchanges (HIEs). These exchanges are a key component of health informatics through which information from various electronic record systems is shared according to nationally recognized standards.

POPULATION HEALTH AND THE DIGITAL AGE: CROSSING AT THE INTERSECTION

Population health is now center stage in healthcare delivery, and it is transforming the industry. This represents an industry-wide shift in focus; while health care used to be transactional and focused on the individual, population health emphasizes outcomes—not just of a single patient, but of an entire population.

This concept is being operationalized through the advent of Accountable Care Organizations (ACOs) and their rapid growth and maturation. ACOs are groups of hospitals, doctors, and other healthcare providers who come together voluntarily to provide coordinated, high-quality care to their (primarily) Medicare patients. At the time of this writing, there are approximately 750 ACOs in operation, covering 23.5 million lives.[11]

The Challenge

To fully appreciate the challenge, one must understand what the essence of population health is. First, the provider has to define the population. Then, the care that the population is receiving must be determined. Next, identify what gaps exist when comparing the care that the population is receiving with the care that the population requires. Finally, the delivery system should be able to address the care gaps.[12] Improving the health of populations is one element of the well-regarded Institute For Healthcare Improvement's "Triple Aim," the other two being improving the patient experience and reducing the per-capita cost of health care.[13] Taken together, the three elements describe an approach to optimizing health system performance.

Assessing Information Technology Capabilities

In order to effectively engage in population health management, healthcare organizations will have to assess their information technology (IT) capabilities and address the gaps therein. Glaser[14] maintains that efficient data sharing among multiple providers will be key; hospitals working with other organizations such as provider groups, post-acute providers, and social services. That data will have to be combined to formulate a complete picture of the patient in order to determine care planning, predict utilization patterns, and assess risk.

These imperatives go beyond the functionality of EHRs and envision real-time population health management solutions that are intended to work in tandem with that certified technology.

Most assuredly, the use of big data analytics will be part of the enabling platform, as well as cloud-based applications and telemedicine.

ADDITIONAL TRENDS AND COMPLEXITIES: OTHER DELIVERY SYSTEMS

The trends and complexities related to population health and the digital age involve other delivery systems. Most notably among them are urgent care, retail medicine clinics, and behavioral health.

Urgent Care Medicine

The growth and development of urgent care medicine has not been unexpected. For many patients, there are long waits in the emergency room for nonemergent care, and there has been a concomitant shortage of primary care physicians in parts of the country. Since 2008, the number of urgent care facilities has increased from 8,000 to 9,300.[15]

Further evidence of the continuing maturation of this type of care is that many centers are now seeking accreditation. Urgent care centers offer imaging and other services not found in retail outlets. However, the challenge therein lies in the ability of the centers to share clinical data with a patient's primary care physician in a timely manner for continuity of care purposes.

Retail Medicine Clinics

Retail medicine clinics may be found in drugstores, grocery chains, and even airports. They are typically small clinics staffed by Nurse Practitioners. Retail health clinics, by definition, are clinics in which the consumer pays the provider directly at the point of sale.[16] Hospital systems are increasingly opening satellite care centers in retail locations, either partnering with chains like Walmart on in-store centers or going it alone. Many consumers of retail medicine are uninsured individuals looking for a fixed cost-of-care. There are also regulatory concerns and questions about quality of care.

Behavioral Health

Behavioral health presents a myriad of unique challenges in the digital age. The nature of behavioral health care (mental health care) makes the application of current health IT challenging. The use of EHRs in behavioral health is limited because of strict privacy concerns, which cause persistent barriers to information sharing.[17] Thus, few behavioral health organizations have formal linkages or agreements to securely share their information. A recent survey found that while 97% of U.S. hospitals and 74% of physicians have implemented interoperable EHRs, only 30% of behavioral health providers have implemented these systems.[18]

SUMMARY

Within the heathcare finance world, it is important to recognize the impact and consequences of the Digital Age. To be successful today, managers must work toward fully recognizing and understanding these significant trends.

INFORMATION CHECKPOINT

What Is Needed?	Your healthcare organization's online visibility.
Where Is It Found?	Websites, blogs, discussion forums, Facebook, Twitter, and/or LinkedIn.
How Is It Used?	The particular online visibility sources will vary depending upon your organization's media strategy.

KEY TERMS

Digital Media
Electronic Health Record (EHR)
Electronic Medical Record (EMR)
Health Information Technology
Patient Engagement
Population Health
Social Media

OTHER ACRONYMNS

ACO: Accountable Care Organization
HIE: Health Information Exchange
IP: Internet Protocol
IT: Information Technology

DISCUSSION QUESTIONS

1. Does your organization have a social media marketing plan?
2. Are you aware of how widespread the use of electronic health records (EHRs) is in your organization? Is it embraced by the medical staff?
3. Does your organization have a population health strategy?

NOTES

1. "Web 2.0," WhatIs.com, http://whatis.techtarget.com/definition/Web-20-or-Web-2, accessed January 5, 2016.
2. J. Fellows, "Meeting the Challenge of Patient Engagement," *Health Leaders*, 18, no 6 (2015): 12–26.
3. OffTheScale, www.prnewswire.com/news-releases/groundbreaking-healthcare-platform -offthescale-partners-with-Garmin-300136825.html, accessed September 2, 2015, and http://site.garmin.com/en-US/wellness, accessed September 19, 2016.

4. Ibid.

5. Society for Healthcare Strategy & Market Development, *A Hospital Leadership Guide to Digital & Social Media Engagement* (Chicago: American Hospital Association, 2015).

6. J. Glaser, "Five Reasons to 'Like' Patients Use of Social Media," *H&HN*, April 11, 2016, http://www.hhnmag.com/articles/7090-five-reasons-to-like-patients-use-of-social-media

7. Ibid.

8. C. B. Thielst, *Social Media in Healthcare: Connect, Communicate, Collaborate* (Chicago: Health Administration Press, 2010).

9. M. L. Braunstein, *Contemporary Health Informatics* (Chicago: American Health Information Management Association, 2014).

10. Ibid.

11. J. Glaser, "All Roads Lead to Population Health Management," *H&HN*, June 13, 2016, http://www.hhnmag.com/articles/7332-all-roads-lead-to-population-health-management

12. M. Zeis, "Toward Population Health," *Health Leaders*, 16, no 8 (2013): 24–28.

13. Institute for Healthcare Improvement, http://www.ihi.org/engage/tripleaim/pages/default.aspx, accessed June 18, 2016.

14. J. Glaser (Op.Cit), June 19, 2016.

15. American Academy of Urgent Care Medicine, "Future of Urgent Care," aaucm.org/about/future/default.aspx, accessed June 18, 2016.

16. "How Retail Medicine Lost its Way," *Managed Healthcare Executive*, June 17, 2015, managedhealthcareexecutive.modernmedicine.com/managed-healthcare-executive/news/how-retail-medicine-lost-its-way

17. P. A. Ranallo, A. M. Kilbourne, A. S. Whatley, and H. A. Pincus, "Behavioral Health Information Technology: From Chaos to Clarity," *Health Affairs*, 35, no 6 (2016): 1106–1113.

18. Ibid.

PART

II

Record Financial Operations

Assets, Liabilities, and Net Worth

4

OVERVIEW

Assets, liabilities, and net worth are part of the language of finance. As such, it is important to understand both their composition and how they fit together. Short definitions appear below, followed by examples.

Assets

Assets are economic resources that have expected future benefits to the business. In other words, assets are what the organization owns and/or controls.

Liabilities

Liabilities are "outsider claims" consisting of economic obligations, or debts, payable to outsiders. Thus, liabilities are what the organization owes, and the outsiders to whom the debts are due are creditors of the business.

Net Worth

"Insider claims" are also known as owner's equity, or net worth. These are claims held by the owners of the business. An owner has a claim to the entity's assets because he or she has invested in the business. No matter what term is used, the sum of these claims reflects what the business is worth, net of liabilities—thus "net worth."

The Three-Part Equation

An accounting equation reflects a relationship among assets, liabilities, and net worth as follows: assets equal

Progress Notes

After completing this chapter, you should be able to

1. Recognize typical assets.
2. Recognize typical liabilities.
3. Understand net worth terminology.
4. See how assets, liabilities, and net worth fit together.

liabilities plus net worth. The three pieces must always balance among themselves because this is how they fit together. The equation is as follows:

$$\text{Assets} = \text{Liabilities} + \text{Net Worth}$$

WHAT ARE EXAMPLES OF ASSETS?

All of the following are typical business assets.

Examples of Assets

Cash, accounts receivable, notes receivable, and inventory are all assets. If the Great Lakes Home Health Agency (HHA) has cash in its bank account, that is an economic resource—an asset. The HHA is owed money for services rendered; these accounts receivable are also an economic resource—an asset. If certain patients have signed a formal agreement to pay the HHA, then these notes receivable are likewise economic resources—assets. All types of business receivables are assets. The Great Lakes HHA also has an inventory of medical supplies (dressings, syringes, IV tubing, etc.) that are used in its day-to-day operations. This inventory on hand is an economic resource—an asset. Land, buildings, and equipment are also assets. **Exhibit 4–1** summarizes asset examples.

Short-Term Versus Long-Term Assets

Assets are often labeled either "current" or "long-term" assets. Current is another word for "short-term." If an asset can be turned into cash within a 12-month period, it is current, or short term. If, on the other hand, an asset cannot be converted into cash within a 12-month period, it is considered long term. In our Great Lakes HHA example, accounts receivable should be collected within 1 year and thus should be current assets. Likewise, the inventory should be converted to business use within 1 year; thus, it too is considered short term.

Classification of the note receivable depends on the length of time that payment is promised. If the entire note receivable will be paid within 1 year, it is a short-term asset. Consider, however, what would happen if the note is to be paid over 3 years. A portion of the note—that amount to be paid in the coming 12 months—will be classified as short-term, or current, and the rest of the note—that amount to be paid further in the future—will be classified as long-term.

The land, building, and equipment will generally be classified as long-term because these assets will not be converted into cash in the coming 12 months. Buildings and equipment are also generally stated at a net figure called book value, which reduces their historical cost by any accumulated depreciation. (The concept of depreciation is discussed in Chapter 8.)

Exhibit 4–1 Asset Examples

Cash
Accounts receivable
Notes receivable
Inventory
Land
Buildings
Equipment

WHAT ARE EXAMPLES OF LIABILITIES?

All of the following are typical business liabilities.

Examples of Liabilities

Accounts payable, payroll taxes due, notes payable, and mortgages payable are all liabilities. The Great Lakes HHA owes vendors for medical supplies it has purchased. The amount owed to the vendors is recognized as accounts payable. When the HHA paid its employees, it withheld payroll taxes, as required by the government. The payroll taxes withheld are due to be paid to the government and thus are also a liability. The HHA has borrowed money and signed a formal agreement and thus the amount due is a liability. The HHA also has a mortgage on its building. This mortgage is likewise a liability. In other words, debts are liabilities. **Exhibit 4–2** summarizes liability examples.

Short-Term Versus Long-Term Liabilities

Liabilities are also usually labeled as either "current" (short-term) or "long-term" liabilities. In this case, if a liability is expected to be paid within a 12-month period, it is current, or short-term. If, however, the liability cannot reasonably be expected to be paid within a 12-month period, it is considered long-term. In our Great Lakes HHA example, accounts payable and payroll taxes due should be paid within 1 year and thus should be labeled as current liabilities.

Classification of the note payable depends on the length of time that payment is promised. If the HHA is going to pay the entire note payable within 1 year, it is a short-term liability. But consider what would happen if the note is to be paid over 3 years. A portion of the note—that amount to be paid in the coming 12 months—will be classified as short-term, or current, and the rest of the note—that amount to be paid further in the future—will be classified as long-term. The mortgage will be treated slightly differently. That portion to be paid within the coming 12 months will be classified as a short-term liability, while the remaining mortgage balance will be labeled as long-term.

WHAT ARE THE DIFFERENT FORMS OF NET WORTH?

Net worth—the third part of the accounting equation—is labeled differently, depending on the type of organization. For-profit organizations will have equity accounts with which to report their net worth. (Equity is the ownership right in property or the money value of property.) For example, a sole proprietorship or a partnership's net worth may simply be labeled as "Owners' Equity." A corporation, on the other hand, will generally report two types of equity accounts: "Capital Stock" and "Retained Earnings." Capital stock represents the owners' investment in the company, indicated by their purchase of stock. Retained earnings, as the name implies, represents undistributed company income that has been left in the business.

Exhibit 4–2 Liability Examples

Accounts payable
Payroll taxes due
Notes payable
Mortgage payable
Bonds payable

Not-for-profit organizations will generally use a different term such as "Fund Balance" to report the difference between assets and liabilities in their report. This is presumably because nonprofits should not, by definition, have equity. Governmental entities in the United States may also use the term "Fund Balance" in their reports. **Exhibit 4–3** summarizes terminology examples for net worth as just discussed.

Exhibit 4–3 Net Worth Terminology Examples

For-profit sole proprietors or partnerships:
  Owners' Equity
For-profit corporations:
  Capital Stock
  Retained Earnings
Not-for-profit (nonprofit) companies:
  Fund Balance

 INFORMATION CHECKPOINT

What is needed?	A report that shows the balance sheet for your organization.
Where is it found?	Probably with your supervisor.
How is it used?	Study the balance sheet to find the assets and liabilities. Check the equity section to see whether equity is listed as net worth or as fund balance.

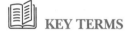 **KEY TERMS**

Assets
Equity
Fund Balance
Liabilities
Net Worth

DISCUSSION QUESTIONS

1. Do you ever work with balance sheets in your current position?
2. If so, is the balance sheet you receive for your department only or for the entire organization? Do you know why this reporting method (departmental versus entire organization) was chosen by management?
3. If you receive a copy of the balance sheet, is one distributed to you once a month, once a year, or on some other more irregular basis? What are you supposed to do with it upon receipt?
4. Do you think the balance sheet report you receive gives you useful information? How do you think it could be improved?

Revenues (Inflow)

OVERVIEW

Revenue represents amounts earned by an organization: that is, actual or expected cash inflows due to the organization's major business. In the case of health care, revenue is mostly earned by rendering services to patients. Revenue flows into the organization and is sometimes referred to as the revenue stream.

Revenue is generally defined as the value of services rendered, expressed at the facility's full established rates. For example, hospital A's full established rate for a certain procedure is $100, but Giant Health Plan has negotiated a managed care contract whereby the plan pays only $90 for that procedure. The revenue figure—the full established rate—is $100. Revenues can be received in the form of cash or credit. Most, but not all, healthcare revenues are received in the form of credit.

RECEIVING REVENUE FOR SERVICES

One way that revenue is classified is by whether payment is received before or after the service is delivered. The amount of revenue received for services is often influenced by this classification.

Payment After Service Is Delivered

The traditional payment method in health care is that of payment after service is delivered. Two basic types of payment after service is delivered are discussed in this section: fee for service and discounted fee for service. One evolved from the other.

Progress Notes

After completing this chapter, you should be able to

1. Understand how receiving revenue for services is a revenue stream.
2. Recognize contractual allowances and discounts and their impact on revenue.
3. Understand the differences in sources of healthcare revenue.
4. See how to group revenue for planning and control.

1. **Fee for service.** The truly traditional U.S. method of receiving revenue for services is fee for service. The provider of services is paid according to the service performed. Before the 1970s, with very few exceptions, fee for service was the dominant method of payment for health services in the United States.[1]
2. **Discounted fee for service.** In this variation on the original fee for service, a contracted discount is agreed upon. The organization providing the services then receives a payment that is discounted in accordance with the contract. Sometimes the contract contains fee schedules. A large provider of services can have many different contracts, all with different discounted contractual arrangements. Many variations are therefore possible.

Payment Before Service Is Delivered

Traditional payment methods in the United States have begun to give way to payment before service is delivered. There are multiple names and definitions for such payment. We have chosen to use a general descriptive term for payment received before service is delivered: predetermined per-person payment. The payment method itself and its rate-setting variations are discussed in this section.

1. Predetermined per-person payment. Payment received before service is delivered is generally at an agreed-upon predetermined rate. Payment, therefore, consists of the predetermined rate for each person covered under the agreement. Thus, the amount received is a per-head or per-person count at a particular point in time.
2. Rate-setting differences. Different agreements can use varying assumptions about the group to be served, and these variations will affect the rate-setting process. Numerous variations are therefore possible.

Contractual Allowances and Other Deductions from Revenue

Revenues are recorded at the organization's full established rates, as previously discussed. Those amounts estimated to be uncollectible are considered to be deductions from revenues and are recorded as such on the books of the organization. (For purposes of the external financial statements released for third-party use, reported revenue must represent the amounts that payers [or patients] are obligated to pay. Therefore, the terms gross revenue and deductions from revenue will not be seen on external statements. The discussion that follows, however, pertains to the books and records that are used for internal management, where these classifications will be used.)

Contractual allowances are the difference between the full established rate and the agreed-upon contractual rate that will be paid. Contractual allowances are often for composite services. Take the case of hospital A as an example. As discussed in the overview to this chapter, hospital A's full established rate for a certain procedure is $100, but Giant Health Plan has negotiated a managed care contract whereby the plan pays only $90 for that procedure. The $10 difference between the revenue figure ($100) and the contracted amount that the plan pays ($90) represents the contractual allowance.

It is not uncommon for different plans to pay different contractual rates for the same service. This practice is illustrated in **Table 5–1**, which shows contractual rates to be paid for visit codes 99213 and 99214 for 10 different health plans. Note the variations in rates.

The second major deduction from revenue classification is an allowance for bad debts, also known as a provision for doubtful accounts. (Again, for purposes of the external financial statements released for third-party use, the provision for doubtful reports must be reported separately as an expense item. The discussion that follows, however, still pertains to the books and records that are used for internal management, where the classification of deductions from revenue will be used.) The allowance for bad debts is charged with the amount of services received on credit (recorded as accounts receivable) that are estimated to result in credit losses.

Beyond contractual allowances and a provision for bad debts, the third major deduction from revenue classification is charity service. Charity service is generally defined as services provided to financially indigent patients.

Table 5–1 Variations in Physician Office Revenue for Two Visit Codes

| | Visit Codes | |
Payer	99213	99214
FHP	$25.35	$35.70
HPHP	42.45	58.85
MC	39.05	54.90
UND	39.90	60.40
CCN	44.00	70.20
MAYO	45.75	70.75
CGN	10.00	10.00
PRU	39.05	54.90
PHCS	45.00	50.00
ANA	38.25	45.00

Rates for illustration only.

SOURCES OF HEALTHCARE REVENUE

Healthcare revenue in the United States comes from a variety of public programs (governmental sources) and private payers. The sources of healthcare revenue are generally termed payers. Payer mix—the proportion of revenues realized from the different types of payers—is a measure that is often included in the profile of a healthcare organization. For example, "Hospital A has a payer mix that includes 40% Medicare and 33% Medicaid" might be part of the profile.

Governmental Sources

The Medicare Program

Title XVIII of the Social Security Act is commonly known as Medicare. Actually entitled "Health Insurance for the Aged and Disabled," Medicare legislation established a health insurance program for the aged in 1965. The program was intended to complement other benefits (such as retirement, survivors', and disability insurance benefits) under other titles within the Social Security Act.

The Medicare program currently has four parts. The first part, known as Part A, is hospital insurance (HI) and is funded primarily by a mandatory payroll tax. The second part, known as Part B, is called supplementary medical insurance (SMI). SMI is voluntary and is funded primarily by insurance premiums (usually deducted from monthly Social Security benefit checks of those enrolled) supplemented by federal general revenue funds. Guidelines determine both the services to be covered and the eligibility of the individual to receive the services under the Medicare program. Medicare claims (billings) are processed by fiscal agents who act on behalf of the federal government. These fiscal agents, known as Medicare Administrative Contractors (MACs), process both Part A (HI) and Part B (SMI) Medicare claims.

Medicare's third part, Part C, is known as "Medicare Advantage." Medicare Advantage consists of managed care plans, private fee-for-service plans, preferred provider organization plans, and specialty plans. Although Medicare Advantage is offered as an alternative to traditional Medicare, coverage must never be less than what Part A and Part B (traditional Medicare) would offer the beneficiary.

Medicare's fourth part, Part D, is the prescription drug benefit, effective as of January 1, 2006. The prescription drug benefit represents expanded coverage. It is a voluntary program that requires payment of a separate premium and contains cost-sharing provisions.

The Medicare program covers approximately 95% of the U.S. aged population along with certain eligible individuals receiving Social Security disability benefits.[2] Medicare is an important source of healthcare revenue to most healthcare organizations.

The Medicaid Program

Title XIX of the Social Security Act is commonly known as Medicaid. Medicaid legislation established a federal and state matching entitlement program in 1965. The program was intended to provide medical assistance to eligible needy individuals and families.

The Medicaid program is state specific. The federal government has established broad national guidelines. Each state has the power to set eligibility, service restrictions, and payment rates for services within that state. In doing so, each state is bound only by the broad national guidelines. Medicaid policies are complex, and considerable variation exists among states. The federal government is responsible for a certain percentage of each state's Medicaid expenditures; the specific amount due is calculated by an annual formula. The state pays the providers of Medicaid services directly. Thus, the source of Medicaid revenue to a healthcare organization is considered to be the state government's Medicaid program representative.

The Medicaid program is the largest U.S. government program providing funds for medical and health-related services for the poor.[3] Therefore, although the proportion of Medicaid services within the payer mix may vary, Medicaid is a source of healthcare revenue in almost every healthcare organization.

Other Programs

There are numerous other sources of federal, state, and local revenues for healthcare organizations. Generally speaking, for most organizations, none of the other revenue sources will exceed the Title XVIII and Title XIX programs just discussed. Other programs include the Department of Veterans' Affairs health programs, workers' compensation programs, and state-only general assistance programs (versus the federal-and-state jointly funded Medicaid program). Still other public programs are school health programs, public health clinics, maternal and child health services, migrant healthcare services, certain mental health and drug and alcohol services, and special programs such as Native American healthcare services.

Managed Care Sources

In the 1970s, managed care began to appear in healthcare models in the United States. An all-purpose definition of managed care is: managed care is a means of providing healthcare services within a network of healthcare providers. The responsibility to manage and provide high-quality and cost-effective health care is delegated to this defined network of providers.[4] A central concept of managed care is the coordination of all healthcare services for an individual. In general, managed care plans receive a predetermined amount per member in premiums.

Types of Plans

The most prevalent type of managed care plan today is the health maintenance organization (HMO). Members enroll in the HMO. They prepay a fixed monthly amount; in return, they receive comprehensive health services. The members must use the providers who are designated by the HMO; if they go outside the designated providers, they must pay all or a large part of the cost themselves. The designated providers of services in turn contract with the HMO to provide services at agreed-upon rates. Several different forms of HMOs have evolved over time.

The preferred provider organization (PPO) is a type of plan found across the United States. It consists of a group of providers called a panel. The panel members are an approved group of various types of providers, including hospitals and physicians. The panel is limited in size and generally has utilization review powers. If the patients in a PPO use health providers who are not within the PPO itself, they must pay a higher amount in deductibles and coinsurance.

Types of Contracts

In the case of an HMO, the designated providers of health services contract with the HMO to provide services at agreed-upon rates. The different types of HMOs—including the staff model, the group model, the network model, the point-of-service model, and the individual practice association (IPA) model—have various methods of arriving at these rates. A PPO contracts with its selected group, who are all participating payers, to buy services for its eligible beneficiaries on the basis of discounted fee for service. A large healthcare facility will have one or more individuals responsible for managed care contracting.[5]

Other Revenue Sources

A considerable amount of healthcare revenue is still realized from sources other than Title XVIII, Title XIX, and managed care:

- Commercial insurers. Generally speaking, conventional indemnity insurers, or commercial insurers, simply pay for the eligible health services used by those individuals who pay premiums for healthcare insurance. They do not tend to have a say in how those health services are administered.
- Private pay. This is payment by patients themselves or by the families of patients. Private pay is more prevalent in nursing facilities and in assisted-living facilities than in hospital settings. Physicians' offices also receive a certain amount of private pay revenue.
- Other. Additional sources of revenue for healthcare facilities include donations received by voluntary nonprofit organization, tax revenues levied by governmental nonprofit organizations, and grant funding.

Healthcare revenue is often reported to managers by source of the revenue. **Table 5–2** presents such a revenue summary. This example covers all types of sources discussed in this section. Both dollar totals and proportionate percentages by source are reported.

Table 5–2 Sample Monthly Statement of Revenue by Source

Summary	Year to Date	%
Private revenue	$100,000	2.9
HMO revenue	560,000	16.7
Medicare revenue	1,420,000	42.4
Medicaid revenue	820,000	24.5
Commercial revenue	400,000	12.0
Other revenue	50,000	1.5
Total	$3,350,000	100.0%

GROUPING REVENUE FOR PLANNING AND CONTROL

Grouping revenue by different classifications is an effective method for managers to use the information to plan and to control. In the preceding paragraphs, we have seen revenue reported by source. Other classification examples are now discussed.

Revenue Centers

A revenue center classification is one form of a responsibility center. In a responsibility center, the manager is responsible, as the name implies, for a particular set of activities. In the case of a revenue center, a particular unit of the organization is given responsibility for generating revenues to meet a certain target. Actually, the responsibility in the healthcare setting is more for generating volume than for generating a specific revenue dollar amount. (The implication is that the volume will, in turn, generate the dollars.) Revenue centers tend to occur most often in special programs where volume is critical to survival of the program.

Care Settings

Grouping revenue by care setting recognizes the different sites at which services are delivered. The most basic grouping by care settings is inpatient versus ambulatory services. **Exhibit 5–1**, however, illustrates a six-way classification of care setting revenues within a health system. In this case, hospital inpatient, hospital outpatient, off-site clinic, skilled nursing facility, home health agency, and hospice are all accounted for. A percentage is shown for each. This type of classification is useful for a brochure or a report that profiles the different types of healthcare services offered by the organization.

Exhibit 5–1 Revenues by Care Setting

42% Hospital Inpatient	38% Hospital Outpatient	4% Off-Site Clinic
8% Skilled Nursing Facility	6% Home Health Agency	2% Hospice

Service Lines

In traditional cost accounting circles, a product line is a grouping of similar products.[6] In the healthcare field, many organizations opt instead for "service line" terminology. A service line is a grouping of similar services. Strategic planning sometimes sets out service lines.

Hospitals

A number of hospitals have adopted the major diagnostic categories (MDCs) as service lines. One advantage of MDCs is that they are a universal designation in the United States. MDCs also have the advantage of possessing a standard definition. In another approach to service line classification, a hospital recently updated its strategic plan and settled on five service lines: (1) medical, (2) surgical, (3) women and children, (4) mental health, and (5) rehabilitation (neuro-ortho rehab) (**Figure 5–1**).[7]

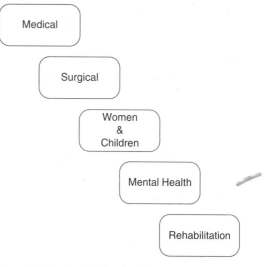

Figure 5–1 Hospital Service Lines.
Courtesy of Resource Group, Ltd., Dallas, Texas.

Long-Term Care

A continuing care retirement community (CCRC) can use its various levels of care as a starting point. Thus, the CCRC usually has four service lines, listed in the descending order of resident acuity: (1) skilled nursing facility, (2) nursing facility, (3) assisted living, and (4) independent living. The skilled nursing facility provides services for the highest level of resident acuity, and the independent living provides services for the lowest level of resident acuity. One adjustment to this approach includes isolating subacute services from the remainder of skilled nursing facility services. Another adjustment involves splitting independent living into two categories, one for Housing and Urban Development (HUD)–subsidized independent housing and the other for private-pay independent housing. **Figure 5–2** illustrates CCRC service lines by acuity level.

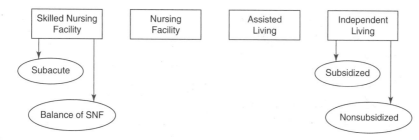

Figure 5–2 Long-Term Care Service Lines.
Courtesy of Resource Group, Ltd., Dallas, Texas.

Home Care

Numerous categories of service delivery can be considered "home care." A practical approach was taken by one home care entity—part of a health system—that defined its "key functions." Key functions can in turn be converted to service lines (**Figure 5–3**).

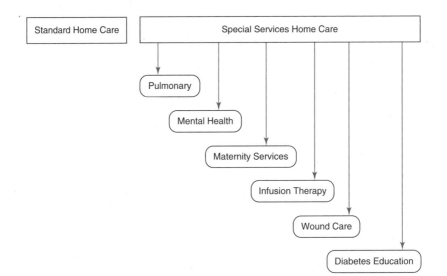

Figure 5–3 Home Care Service Lines.
Courtesy of Resource Group, Ltd., Dallas, Texas.

Physician Groups

Service delivery for physician groups will vary, of course, with the nature of the group itself. A generic set of service lines is presented in **Figure 5–4**.

Other Service Designations

Other classifications may meet the needs of particular organizations. Columbia/HCA is now reported to classify its services in a disease management approach. The classification consists of eight disease management areas: (1) cancer, (2) cardiology, (3) diabetes, (4) behavioral health, (5) workers' compensation, (6) women's services, (7) senior care, and (8) emergency services.[8]

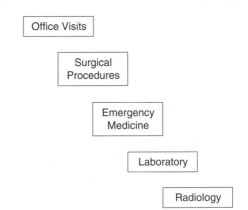

Figure 5–4 Physician's Group Service Lines.
Courtesy of Resource Group, Ltd., Dallas, Texas.

Other Types of Revenue Groupings

Other healthcare organizations may have revenue groupings that are not service lines. An entity that provides services is able to choose service lines as a method of grouping its revenue. But if the entity sells or makes a product (rather than providing services), its revenue will have to be classified differently. Two examples within the healthcare industry follow: a retail pharmacy and a pharmaceutical manufacturer.

Retail Pharmacy

A retail pharmacy's revenue primarily comes from sales. A typical retail pharmacy may group revenues into three major categories of sales: Prescription Drugs, Nonprescription (Over-the-Counter, or OTC) Drugs, and Other Merchandise. (The major category of "Other Merchandise" would then have subcategories such as Cosmetics, Greeting Cards, Gifts, etc.)

Pharmaceutical Manufacturer

A pharmaceutical manufacturer's revenue groupings would likewise be specific to its type of healthcare business. These organizations are producing a product rather than providing a service. Its major categories of revenues will probably be by type of drug manufactured. The next subcategory might then either be national versus international revenues, or perhaps a classification of revenues by U.S. geographic region.

In summary, the entity's revenue classification system, whatever it may be, must be consistent with the current structure and purpose of the organization.

INFORMATION CHECKPOINT

What is needed?	A report that shows revenue in your organization.
Where is it found?	With your supervisor.
How is it used?	Examine the report to find various revenue sources; look for how the contractual allowances and discounts are handled on the report.
What is needed?	A report that groups revenue by some type of classification.
Where is it found?	With your supervisor, or in the information services division.
How is it used?	Examine the report to discover the methods that are used for grouping. You will probably find that these groupings are used for performance measures. They can also be used for control and planning.

KEY TERMS

Discounted Fee for Service
Fee for Service
Managed Care
Medicaid Program
Medicare Program
Payer Mix
Revenue

DISCUSSION QUESTIONS

1. Does your organization receive revenue mainly in the form of payment after service is delivered or payment before service is delivered?

2. Why do you think this is so?
3. What do you believe the proportion of revenues from different sources is for your organization?
4. Do you believe that this proportion (payer mix) will change in the future? Why?
5. What grouping of revenue do you believe your organization uses (revenue centers, care settings, service lines, other)?
6. From your perspective, would there be a better grouping possible? If so, why do you think it is not used?

NOTES

1. Texas Medical Association, American Medical Association, Texas Medical Foundation, and Texas Osteopathic Medical Association, *A Guide to Forming Physician-Directed Managed Care Networks* (Austin, TX: Texas Medical Association, 1994), 3.
2. Health Care Financing Administration, *Health Care Financing Review: Medicare and Medicaid Statistical Supplement* (Baltimore, MD: U.S. Department of Health and Human Services, 1997), 8.
3. Ibid., 9.
4. D. I. Samuels, *Capitation: New Opportunities in Healthcare Delivery* (Chicago: Irwin Professional Publishing, 1996), 20–21.
5. D. E. Goldstein, *Alliances: Strategies for Building Integrated Delivery Systems* (Gaithersburg, MD: Aspen Publishers, Inc., 1995), 283; and Texas Medical Association, American Medical Association, Texas Medical Foundation, and Texas Osteopathic Medical Association, *A Guide to Forming Physician-Directed Managed Care Networks* (Austin, TX: Texas Medical Association, 1994), 4–6.
6. C. Horngren et al., *Cost Accounting: A Managerial Emphasis*, 9th ed. (Englewood Cliffs, NJ: Prentice Hall, 1998), 116.
7. When ICD-10 is fully implemented, it is possible that the term "major diagnostic categories" (MDCs) may have to be replaced with some other universal designation. Whether these hospitals will change the names of their service line designations to match the new titles is unknown at this point. We do know it will take time to decide upon such a change and then additional time to implement the change.
8. A. Sharpe and G. Jaffe, "Columbia/HCA Plans for More Big Changes in Health-Care World," *Wall Street Journal*, 28 May, 1997, A8.

Expenses (Outflow)

OVERVIEW

Expenses are the costs that relate to the earning of revenue. Another way to think of expenses is as the costs of doing business. Just as revenues represent the inflow into the organization, so do expenses represent the outflow—a stream of expenditures flowing out of the organization. Examples of expenses include salary expense for labor performed, payroll tax expense for taxes paid on the salary, utility expense for electricity, and interest expense for the use of money.

In fact, expenses are expired costs—costs that have been used up, or consumed, while carrying on business. Revenues and expenses affect the equity of the business. The inflow of revenues increases equity, whereas the outflow of expenses decreases equity. In nonprofit organizations, the term is fund balance rather than equity. This is because a nonprofit organization, by its nature, is not in business to make a profit. Thus, it should not have equity. However, the principle of inflow and outflow remains the same. In the case of nonprofits, the inflow of revenues increases fund balance, and the outflow of expenses decreases fund balance.

Many managers use the terms expense and cost interchangeably. Expense in its broadest sense includes every expired (used up) cost that is deductible from revenue. A narrower interpretation groups expenses into categories such as operating expenses, administrative expenses, and so on. Cost is the amount of cash expended (or property transferred, services performed, or liability incurred) in consideration of goods or services received or to be received. As we have already said, costs can be either expired or unexpired. Expired costs are used up in the current period and are thus matched against current revenues. Unexpired costs are not yet used up and will be matched against future revenues.[1]

Progress Notes

After completing this chapter, you should be able to

1. Understand the distinction between expense and cost.
2. Understand how disbursements for services represent an expense stream (an outflow).
3. Follow how expenses are grouped in different ways for planning and control.
4. Recognize why cost reports have influenced expense formats.

47

For example, an electric bill for $500 is recorded in the books of the clinic as an expense. The administrator sees the $500 as the cost of electricity for that month in the clinic. And the administrator is actually correct in seeing the $500 as a cost because it has been used up (expired) within the month.

Confusion also exists in healthcare reporting over the term cost versus the term charges. Charges are revenue, or inflow. Costs are expenses, or outflow. Charges add; costs take away. Because the two are inherently different, they should never be intermingled.

DISBURSEMENTS FOR SERVICES

There are two types of disbursements for services:

1. Payment when expense is incurred. If an expense is paid for at the point where it is incurred, it does not enter the accounts payable account. In large organizations, it is relatively rare to see payments when expenses are incurred. The only place where this usually occurs is the petty cash fund.
2. Payment after expense is incurred. In most healthcare organizations, expenses are paid at a later time and not at the point when the expense is incurred. If this is the case, the expense is recorded in the accounts payable account. It is cleared from accounts payable when payment is made. One measurement of operations is "days in accounts payable," whereby the operating expenses for the organization are reduced to a rate per day and compared with the amount in accounts payable.

GROUPING EXPENSES FOR PLANNING AND CONTROL

Cost Centers

A cost center is one form of a responsibility center. In a responsibility center, the manager is responsible, as the name implies, for a particular set of activities. In the case of a cost center, a particular unit of the organization is given responsibility for controlling costs of the operations over which it holds authority. The medical records division is an example of a cost center. The billing and collection office might be another example. A cost center might be a division, an office, or an entire department, depending on how the organization is structured.

In healthcare organizations, it is common to find departments as cost centers. This is often a logical way to designate a cost center because the lines of authority are generally organized by department. Cost centers can then be grouped into larger groups that have something in common. Within this method of grouping, the manager of a cost center may receive his or her own reports and figures, but not those of the entire group. The director or officer that is in charge of all of those particular departments receives the larger report that contains multiple cost centers. The chief executive officer receives a total report because he or she is ultimately responsible for overseeing the operations of all of the cost centers involved in that segment of the organization.

Exhibit 6–1 illustrates this concept. It contains 20 different cost centers, all of which are revenue producing. The 20 cost centers are divided into two groups: nursing services and other professional services. There are five cost centers in the nursing services group, ranging from operating room to obstetrics–nursery. There are 15 cost centers in the other professional services group. In the hospital that uses the grouping shown in Exhibit 6–1, however, not all of the 20 cost centers are departments. Some are divisions within departments. For example, EKG and EEG operate out of the same department but are two separate cost centers.

Exhibit 6–2 shows 11 different cost centers that are not directly revenue producing. (The dietary department yields some cafeteria revenue, but that revenue is not central to the major business of the organization, which is to provide healthcare services.) The 11 cost centers are divided into two groups: general services and support services. The 6 cost centers in the general services group happen to all be departments in this hospital. (Other hospitals might not have security as a separate department. The other cost centers— dietary, maintenance, laundry, housekeeping, and medical records—would be separate departments.) The 5 cost centers in the support services group include a "general" cost center that contains administrative costs; the remaining 4 are related to employee salaries and wages. These 4 are insurance, Social Security taxes, employee welfare, and pension cost centers, all of which will probably be in the same department. It is the prerogative of management to set up cost centers specific to the organization's own needs and preferences. It is the responsibility of management to make the cost centers match the proper lines of authority.

Exhibit 6–2 illustrates two categories of healthcare expense: general services and support. A third related category is operations expense. An operations expense provides service directly related to patient care. Examples are radiology expense and drug expense. A general services expense provides services necessary to maintain the patient, but the service is not directly related to patient care. Examples are laundry and dietary. Support services expenses, on the other hand, provide support to both general services expenses and operations expenses. A support service expense is necessary for support, but it is neither directly related to patient care nor is it a service necessary to maintain the patient. Examples of support services are insurance and payroll taxes.

Exhibit 6–1 Nursing Services and Other Professional Services Cost Centers

Nursing Services Cost Center	
Routine Medical-Surgical	$390,000
Operating Room	30,000
Intensive Care Units	40,000
OB–Nursery	15,000
Other	35,000
Total	$510,000

Other Professional Services Cost Center	
Laboratory	$220,000
Radiology	139,000
CT Scanner	18,000
Pharmacy	128,000
Emergency Service	89,000
Medical and Surgical Supply	168,000
Operating Rooms and Anesthesia	142,000
Respiratory Therapy	48,000
Physical Therapy	64,000
EKG	16,000
EEG	1,000
Ambulance Service	7,000
Substance Abuse	43,000
Home Health and Hospice	120,000
Other	12,000
Total	$1,215,000

Diagnoses and Procedures

It is common to group expenses by diagnoses and procedures for purposes of planning and control. This grouping is beneficial because it matches costs against common classifications

Exhibit 6–2 General Services and Support Services Cost Centers

General Services Cost Center	
Dietary	$97,000
Maintenance	92,000
Laundry	27,000
Housekeeping	43,000
Security	5,000
Medical Records	30,000
Total	$294,000

Support Services Cost Center	
General	$455,000
Insurance	24,000
Social Security Taxes	112,000
Employee Welfare	188,000
Pension	43,000
Total	$822,000

of revenues. Much of the revenue in many healthcare organizations is designated by either diagnoses or procedures. One prevalent method groups costs into cost centers by major diagnostic categories (MDCs). The 23 MDCs serve as the basic classification system for diagnosis-related groups (DRGs). (Each DRG represents a category of patients. This category contains patients whose resource consumption, on statistical average, is equivalent. DRGs are part of the prospective payment reimbursement methodology.) **Exhibit 6–3** provides a listing of the 23 MDCs.[2] (The number of MDCs may increase when ICD-10 coding is fully implemented.)

How does the hospital use the MDC grouping? **Exhibit 6–4** shows a departmental and cost center grouping in actual use. This hospital uses 27 cost center codes: the 23 MDCs plus 4 other codes ("Special Drugs," "HIV," "Unassigned," and "Outpatient"). The special drugs and HIV cost centers represent high-cost elements that management wants to track separately. Unassigned is a default category and should have little assigned to it. Outpatient is a separate cost center at the preference of management.

Exhibit 6–5 illustrates the grouping of costs for MDC 18 (Infectious Diseases). The hospital's departmental code is 18, per Exhibit 6–4. The DRG classification, ranging from 415 to 423, appears in the next column. The description of the particular DRG appears in the third column, and the related cost appears in the fourth and final column. These costs can now be readily matched to equivalent revenues.

Outpatient services in particular are generally designated by procedure codes. Procedure codes, known as Current Procedural Terminology (CPT) codes, are commonly used to group cost centers for outpatient services. (CPT codes represent a listing of descriptive terms and identifying codes for identifying medical services and procedures performed.) However, procedures can be—and are—also used for purposes of grouping inpatient costs, generally within a certain cost center. A hospital example of reporting radiology department costs by procedure code appears in **Table 6–1**. In this example, the procedure code is in the left column, the description of the procedure is in the middle column, and the departmental cost for the particular procedure appears in the right column. These costs can now be readily matched to equivalent revenue.

Care Settings and Service Lines

Expenses can be grouped by care setting, which recognizes the different sites at which services are delivered. "Inpatient" versus "outpatient" is a basic type of care setting grouping. Or expenses can be classified by service lines, a method that groups similar services.[3]

Exhibit 6–3 Major Diagnostic Categories

MDC 1	Diseases and Disorders of the Nervous System
MDC 2	Eye
MDC 3	Ear, Nose, Mouth, and Throat
MDC 4	Respiratory System
MDC 5	Circulatory System
MDC 6	Digestive System
MDC 7	Hepatobiliary System and Pancreas
MDC 8	Musculoskeletal System and Connective Tissue
MDC 9	Skin, Subcutaneous Tissue, and Breast
MDC 10	Endocrine, Nutritional, and Metabolic
MDC 11	Kidney and Urinary Tract
MDC 12	Male Reproductive System
MDC 13	Female Reproductive System
MDC 14	Pregnancy, Childbirth, and the Puerperium
MDC 15	Newborns and Other Neonates with Conditions Originating in the Perinatal Period
MDC 16	Blood and Blood-Forming Organs and Immunological Disorders
MDC 17	Myeloproliferative and Poorly and Differentiated Neoplasms
MDC 18	Infections and Parasitic Diseases (Systemic or Unspecified Sites)
MDC 19	Mental Diseases and Disorders
MDC 20	Alcohol/Drug Use and Alcohol/Drug-Induced Organic Mental Disorders
MDC 21	Injuries, Poisoning, and Toxic Effect of Drugs
MDC 22	Burns
MDC 23	Factors Influencing Health Status and Other Contacts with Health Services

Exhibit 6–4 Hospital Departmental Code List Based on Major Diagnostic Categories

1	Nervous System
2	Eye
3	Ear, Nose, Mouth, and Throat
4	Respiratory System
5	Circulatory System
6	Digestive System
7	Hepatobiliary System
8	Musculoskeletal System and Connective Tissue
9	Skin, Subcutaneous Tissue, and Breast
10	Endocrine, Nutritional, and Metabolic
11	Kidney and Urinary Tract
12	Male Reproductive System
13	Female Reproductive System
14	Obstetrics
15	Newborns
16	Immunology
17	Oncology
18	Infectious Diseases
19	Mental Diseases
20	Substance Use
21	Injury, Poison, and Toxin
22	Burns
23	Other Health Services
24	Special Drugs
25	HIV
26	Unassigned
59	Outpatient

If revenues are grouped by care setting or by service line, as discussed in the previous chapter, then expenses should also be grouped by these categories. In that way, matching of revenues and expenses can readily occur. A more detailed discussion of care settings and service lines, with examples, was presented in the preceding chapter.

Programs

A program can be defined as a project that has its own objectives and its own program

Exhibit 6–5 Example of Hospital Departmental Costs Classified by Diagnoses, MDC, and DRG

Hospital Departmental Code	DRG	Description	Cost
18 INFECTIOUS DISEASES	415	O/R—INFECT/PARASITIC DIS	$4,000
18 INFECTIOUS DISEASES	416	SEPTICEMIA 17	10,000
18 INFECTIOUS DISEASES	417	SEPTICEMIA 0–17	20,000
18 INFECTIOUS DISEASES	418	POSTOP/POSTTRAUMA INFECT	2,000
18 INFECTIOUS DISEASES	419	FEVER—UKN ORIG 17W/C	3,000
18 INFECTIOUS DISEASES	420	FEVER—UKN ORIG 17W/OC	6,000
18 INFECTIOUS DISEASES	421	VIRAL ILLNESS 17	4,000
18 INFECTIOUS DISEASES	422	VIR ILL/FEVER UNK 0–17	1,000
18 INFECTIOUS DISEASES	423	OT/INFECT/PARASITIC DX	3,000

Table 6–1 Example of Radiology Department Costs Classified by Procedure Code

Procedure Code	Procedure Description	Department Cost
557210	Ribs, Unilateral	$ 60,000
557230	Spine Cervical Routine	125,000
557280	Pelvis	33,000
557320	Limb—Shoulder	55,000
557360	Limb—Wrist	69,000
557400	Limb—Hip, Unilateral	42,000
557410	Limb—Hip, Bilateral	14,000
557430	Limb—Knee Only	62,000
	Total	$460,000

Exhibit 6–6 Program Cost Center: Southside Homeless Intake Center

Program:	Southside Homeless Intake Center
Department:	Feeding Ministry
For the Month of:	January 2XXX
Raw Food	$14,050
Dietary Supplies	200
Paper Supplies	300
Minor Equipment	50
Consultant Dietitian	50
Utilities	300
Telephone	50
Program Total	$15,000

indicators. Within management's functions of planning, controlling, and decision making, the program must stand on its own. A program is often funded separately and for finite periods of time. For example, funds from a grant might fund a specific project for—as an example—three years. Often programs—especially those funded separately from the revenue stream of the main organization—have to arrange their expenses in a special format that is specified by the entity that provides the grant funds.

Program expenses should be grouped in such a way that they are distinguishable. Also, if such programs have been specially funded, the reporting of their expenses should not be commingled. An example of a program cost center is given in **Exhibit 6–6**. This cost center example has received special funds and must be reported separately, as shown.

COST REPORTS AS INFLUENCERS OF EXPENSE FORMATS

Cost reports are required by both the Medicare program (Title XVIII) and the Medicaid program (Title XIX). Every provider participating in the program is required to file an annual cost report. A selection of providers who must file cost reports is illustrated in **Table 6–2**. The arrangement of expense headings on the cost reports has been primarily consistent since the advent of such reports

Table 6–2 Selected Cost Report Forms

Type	Form
Hospital and Hospital Healthcare Complex	CMS 2552-10
Skilled Nursing Facility and Skilled Nursing Facility Complex	CMS 2540-10
Home Health Agencies	CMS 1728-94

in 1966. Therefore, this standard and traditional arrangement has strongly influenced the arrangement of expenses in many healthcare information systems.

The cost report uses a method of cost finding. Its focus is what is called a cost center. The concept is not the same as the type of responsibility center "cost center" that has been discussed earlier in this chapter. Instead, the cost-finding "cost center" is, broadly speaking, a type of cost pool used in the cost-finding process. The primary purpose of the cost pool/cost center in cost finding is to assist in allocating overhead.

The central worksheets for cost finding are Worksheet A, Worksheet B, and Worksheet B-1. Worksheet A contains the basic trial balance of all expenses for the facility. (Trial balances are discussed in a preceding chapter.) The beginning trial balance is reflected in the first three columns:

$$[\text{Column 1}] \quad [\text{Column 2}] \quad\quad\quad [\text{Column 3}]$$
$$\text{"Salaries"} \quad + \quad \text{"Other"} \quad = \quad \text{"Total"}$$
$$\text{(all other expenses)}$$

The trial balance is grouped at the outset into cost center categories. The placement of these categories and their respective line items on the page stay constant throughout the flow of Worksheets A, B, and B-1. The cost centers are grouped into seven categories:

1. General service
2. Inpatient routine service
3. Ancillary service
4. Outpatient service
5. Other reimbursable
6. Special purpose
7. Nonreimbursable

The line items within these seven categories represent the long-lived traditional arrangement that has strongly influenced the arrangement of expenses in so many healthcare information systems.

 INFORMATION CHECKPOINT

What is needed?	A report that shows expense in your organization.
Where is it found?	With your supervisor.
How is it used?	Examine the report to find various types of expenses; look for how the expense flow is handled on the report.

What is needed?	A report that groups expenses by some type of classification.
Where is it found?	With your supervisor or in the information services division.
How is it used?	Examine the report to discover the methods that are used for grouping. You will probably find that these groupings are used for performance measures. They can also be used for control and planning.

KEY TERMS

Cost
Diagnoses
Expenses
Expired Costs
General Services Expenses
Support Services Expenses
Operations Expenses
Procedures
Unexpired Costs

DISCUSSION QUESTIONS

1. Have you worked with cost centers in your duties? If so, how have you been exposed to them?
2. Have you had to manage from a cost center type of report? If so, how was it categorized?
3. Do you believe that grouping expenses by diagnoses and procedures (based on type of services provided) is better to use for control and planning than grouping expenses by care setting (based on location of service provided)?
4. If so, why?
5. What grouping of expenses do you believe your organization uses (traditional cost centers, diagnoses/procedures, care settings, other)?
6. From your perspective, would there be a better grouping possible? If so, why do you think it is not used?

NOTES

1. S. A. Finkler, *Essentials of Cost Accounting for Health Care Organizations*, 2nd ed. (Gaithersburg, MD: Aspen Publishers, Inc., 1999).
2. At the time of this writing, 23 major diagnostic categories (MDCs) serve as the basic classification system for diagnosis-related groups (DRGs). When ICD-10 is fully implemented, it is probable that the number of MDCs will be increased. It is also possible that the terminology itself (MDCs) may be changed to some other designation.
3. G. F. Longshore, "Service-line Management/Bottom-line Management for Health Care," *Journal of Health Care Finance*, 24, no. 4 (1998): 72–79.

Cost Classifications

© LFor/Shutterstock

DISTINCTION BETWEEN DIRECT AND INDIRECT COSTS

Direct costs can be specifically associated with a particular unit or department or patient. The critical distinction for the manager is that the cost is directly attributable. Whatever the manager is responsible for—that is, the unit, the department, or the patient—is known as a *cost object*.

The somewhat vague definition of a cost object is any unit for which a separate cost measurement is desired. It might help the manager to think of a *cost object* as a *cost objective* instead.[1] The important thing is that direct costs can be traced. Indirect costs, on the other hand, cannot be specifically associated with a particular cost object. The controller's office is an example of indirect cost. The controller's office is essential to the overall organization itself, but its cost is not specifically or directly associated with providing healthcare services. The critical distinction for the manager is that indirect costs usually cannot be traced, but instead must be allocated or apportioned in some manner.[2] **Figure 7–1** illustrates the direct–indirect cost distinction.

To summarize, it is helpful to recognize that direct costs are incurred for the sole benefit of a particular operating unit—a department, for example. As a rule of thumb, if the answer to the following question is "yes," then the cost is a direct cost: "If the operating unit (such as a department) did not exist, would this cost not be in existence?"

Indirect costs, in contrast, are incurred for the overall operation and not for any one unit. Because they are shared, indirect costs are sometimes called joint costs or common costs. As a rule of thumb, if the answer to the following question is "yes," then the cost is an indirect cost: "Must this cost be allocated in order to be assigned to the unit (such as a department)?"

Progress Notes

After completing this chapter, you should be able to

1. Distinguish between direct and indirect costs.
2. Understand why the difference is important to management.
3. Understand the composition and purpose of responsibility centers.
4. Distinguish between product and period costs.

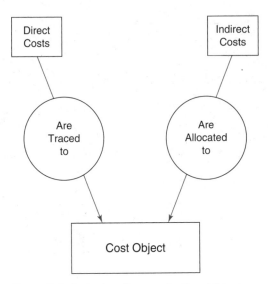

Figure 7–1 Assigning Costs to the Cost Object.

EXAMPLES OF DIRECT COST AND INDIRECT COST

It is important for managers to recognize direct and indirect costs and how they are treated on reports. Two sets of examples illustrate the reporting of direct and indirect costs. The first example concerns a rehab cost center; the second concerns an ambulance service center.

Table 7–1 represents a report of both direct cost and indirect cost for a rehab cost center. The report concerns three types of therapy— physical, occupational, and speech therapy— and a total. In this report, the manager can observe the proportionate differences between direct and indirect costs and can also see the differences among the three types of therapies.

Greater detail is provided to the manager in **Table 7–2**, which presents the method of allocating indirect costs and the result of such allocation. Managers should notice that the "Total Indirect Costs" in Table 7–2 carry forward and become the "Indirect Costs" in Table 7–1. Thus, this report showing allocation of indirect costs is considered a subsidiary report because it is supporting, or subsidiary to, the preceding main report. This use of one or more supporting reports to reveal details behind the main report is quite common in managerial reports. The allocation of indirect costs subsidiary report contains quite a lot of information. It shows what particular expenses (clerical salaries, administrative salaries, computer services) are contained in the $185,000 total. It also shows how each of these expenses are allocated across the three separate types of therapy. And the report also shows how each item was allocated; see the Allocation Key containing codes A, B, and C. The basis for allocation is presented in the Key (A = number of visits; B = proportion of direct costs, by percentage; C = number of computers in service) and the computation detail by therapy type is also noted. This set of tables is worthy of further study by the manager.

Table 7–1 Examples of Rehab Cost Center Direct and Indirect Cost Totals

Rehab Cost Centers	Direct Cost	Indirect Cost	Total
Physical Therapy (PT)	$410,000	$107,500	$517,500
Occupational Therapy (OT)	190,000	44,000	234,000
Speech Therapy (ST)	120,000	33,500	153,500
Total	$720,000	$185,000	$905,000

Note: Direct Cost proportions, rounded, are as follows:

PT = 57%/OT = 26%/ST = 17%/Total = 100%

Courtesy of J. J. Baker and R. W. Baker, Dallas, Texas.

Table 7–2 Example of Indirect Costs Allocated to Rehab Cost Center

	Clerical Salaries	Administrative Salaries	Computer Services	Total Indirect Cost
Allocation Basis:	A	B	C	
Indirect Cost to Be Allocated	$60,000	$50,000	$75,000	$185,000
Allocated to:				
Physical Therapy (PT)	34,000	28,500	45,000	107,500
Occupational Therapy (OT)	16,000	13,000	15,000	44,000
Speech Therapy (ST)	10,000	8,500	15,000	33,500
Proof Total	$60,000	$50,000	$75,000	$185,000

Allocation Key:
A = # Visits (Volume): PT = 8500/OT = 4000/ST = 2500/Total = 15,000 (15,000 x $4.00 = $60,000)
B = Proportion of Direct Costs: PT = 57%/OT = 26%/ST = 17%/Total = 100% (% x $50,000)
C = # Computers in Service: PT = 9/OT = 3/ST = 3/Total = 15 (15 x $5,000 each = $75,000)

Courtesy of J. J. Baker and R. W. Baker, Dallas, Texas.

Exhibit 7–1 sets out the direct costs for an ambulance service center. These costs, as direct costs, are what the organization's managers believe can be traced to the specific operation of the freestanding center. **Exhibit 7–2** sets out the indirect costs for a freestanding ambulance service center. These costs are what the organization's managers believe are not directly attributable to the specific operation of the freestanding center. The decisions about what will and what will not be considered direct or indirect costs will almost always have been made for the manager.[3] What is important is that the manager understand two things: first, why this is so, and second, how the relationship between the two works. Remember the rule of thumb discussed earlier in this chapter. If the answer to the following question is "yes," then the cost is a direct cost: "If the operating unit (such as a department) did not exist, would this cost not be in existence?"

Exhibit 7–1 Example of Ambulance Direct Costs

Ambulance salaries & benefits	$32,500
RN salaries & benefits	9,600
Vehicle expense	21,300
Supplies	5,000
Uniforms	1,200
Employee education	3,900
Purchased services	1,900
Purchased maintenance	2,600
Utilities & telephone	5,000
Vehicle depreciation	15,000
Miscellaneous expense	2,000
Total direct costs	$100,000

Exhibit 7–2 Example of Ambulance Indirect Costs

Administrative costs	$12,000
Facility costs	8,000
Total indirect costs	$20,000

RESPONSIBILITY CENTERS

We previously discussed revenue centers, whereby managers are responsible for generating revenue (or volume). We also previously discussed cost centers, whereby managers are

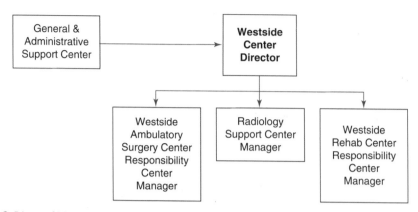

Figure 7–2 Lines of Managerial Responsibility at Westside Center.
Courtesy of Resource Group, Ltd., Dallas, Texas.

responsible for managing and controlling cost. The responsibility center (R/C) makes a manager responsible for both the revenue/volume (inflow) side and the expense (outflow) side of a department, division, unit, or program. In other words, the manager is responsible for generating revenue/volume and for controlling costs. Another term for responsibility center is *profit center*.

We will examine the type of information a manager receives about his or her own responsibility center by reviewing the Westside Center operations. Westside Center offers two basic types of services: an ambulatory surgery center (ASC) and a rehabilitation center. The management of Westside is overseen by Bill, the director. Joe manages the ambulatory surgery center. Bonnie manages the rehabilitation center. Denise, a part-time radiologist, provides radiology services on an as-needed basis. Joe, Bonnie, and Denise, the managers, all report to Bill, the director. **Figure 7–2** illustrates the managerial relationships.

To restate the relationships shown in Figure 7–2, Joe manages a responsibility center for ambulatory surgery services. Bonnie manages a responsibility center for rehabilitation services. These services represent the business of Westside Center. Denise manages the radiology services, but this is not a responsibility center in the Westside organization. Instead, it is a support center. Bill, the director, manages a bigger responsibility center that includes all of the functions just described, plus the general and administrative support center.

Bill, the director, receives a managerial report, shown in **Exhibit 7–3**. Bill's "Director's Summary" contains the data for the entire Westside operation.

Figure 7–3 illustrates the reports received by each manager at Westside. Joe's report for the ambulatory surgery center is at the top right of Figure 7–3. His report shows the controllable revenues he is responsible for ($225,000), less the controllable expenses he is responsible for ($155,000). The difference is labeled "ASC Responsibility Center Surplus" on his report. The surplus amounts to $70,000 ($225,000 minus $155,000).

Exhibit 7–3 Director's Summary of Westside ASC and Rehab Responsibility Center

ASC R/C Surplus	$70,000.00
Rehab R/C Surplus	85,000.00
Less G&A Support Ctr	(80,000.00)
Less Radiology Support Ctr	(20,000.00)
Net Surplus	$55,000.00

Courtesy of Resource Group, Ltd., Dallas, Texas.

Westside ASC Responsibility Center Medical/Surgical Manager		
Controllable revenues:		
Patient fees		$225,000.00
Controllable expenses:		
Wages	100,000.00	
Payroll taxes, other fringes	25,000.00	
Billable supplies	20,000.00	
Medical supplies	10,000.00	
Total expenses		155,000.00
ASC R/C surplus		$70,000.00

Westside ASC Responsibility Center Therapy Manager		
Controllable revenues:		
Patient fees		$300,000.00
Controllable expenses:		
Wages	120,000.00	
Payroll taxes, other fringes	30,000.00	
Billable supplies	50,000.00	
Medical supplies	10,000.00	
Continuing education	3,000.00	
Licenses and permits	2,000.00	
Total expenses		215,000.00
Rehab R/C surplus		$85,000.00

Director's Summary of Westside ASC & Rehab Center	
ASC R/C Surplus	$70,000.00
Rehab R/C Surplus	85,000.00
Less G&A Support Ctr	(80,000.00)
Less Radiology Support Ctr	(20,000.00)
Net Surplus	$55,000.00

General & Administrative Support Center	
Salaries	$40,000.00
Payroll taxes, other fringes	10,000.00
Office supplies	1,200.00
Telephone	2,400.00
Rent	10,800.00
Utilities	4,800.00
Insurance	1,200.00
Depreciation	9,600.00
Total expenses	$80,000.00

Radiology Support Center Radiology Manager	
Salaries	$12,000.00
Payroll taxes, other fringes	3,000.00
Radiology supplies	5,000.00
Total expenses	$20,000.00

Figure 7–3 Westside Costs by Responsibility Center.
Courtesy of Resource Group, Ltd., Dallas, Texas.

Bonnie's report for the rehabilitation center is the second report on the right of Figure 7–3. Her report shows the controllable revenues she is responsible for ($300,000), less the controllable expenses she is responsible for ($215,000). The difference is labeled "Rehab Responsibility Center Surplus" on her report. The surplus amounts to $85,000 ($300,000 minus $215,000).

Denise's report for radiology services is at the bottom right of Figure 7–3. Her report shows the controllable expenses she is responsible for, which amount to $20,000. Her report shows only expenses because it is a support center, not a responsibility center. Therefore, Denise is responsible for expenses but not for revenue/volume.

Bill, the director, receives a report for the general and administrative (G&A) expenses, as shown second from the bottom on the right of Figure 7–3. This report shows the G&A controllable expenses that Bill himself is responsible for at Westside, which amount to $80,000. The G&A report shows only expenses because it also is a support center, not a responsibility center. Therefore, Bill is responsible for expenses but not for revenue/volume in the case of G&A.

However, Bill is also responsible for the entire Westside operation. That is, the overall Westside operation is his responsibility center. Therefore, Bill's director's summary, reproduced on the left side of Figure 7–3, contains the results of both responsibility centers and both support centers. The surplus figures from Joe and Bonnie's reports are positive figures of $70,000 and $85,000, respectively. The expense-only figures from Bill's G&A support center report and from Denise's radiology support center report are negative figures of $80,000 and $20,000, respectively. Therefore, to find the result of operations for Bill's entire Westside operation, the $80,000 and the $20,000 expense figures are subtracted from the surplus figures to arrive at a net surplus for Westside of $55,000.

Although the lines of managerial responsibility will vary in other organizations, the relationships between and among responsibility centers, support centers, and overall supervision will remain as shown in this example.

DISTINCTION BETWEEN PRODUCT AND PERIOD COSTS

Product costs is a term that was originally associated with manufacturing rather than with services. The concept of product costs assumes that a product has been manufactured and placed into inventory while waiting to be sold. Then, whenever that product is sold, the product is matched with revenue and recognized as a cost. Thus, *cost of sales* is the common usage for manufacturing firms. (The concept of matching revenues and expenses has been discussed in a preceding chapter.)

Period costs, in the original manufacturing interpretation, are not connected with the manufacturing process. They are matched with revenue on the basis of the period during which the cost is incurred (thus *period costs*). The term comes from the span of time in which matching occurs, known as *time period*.

Service organizations have no manufacturing process as such. The business of healthcare service organizations is service delivery, not the manufacturing of products. Although the overall concept of product versus period cost is not as vital to service delivery, the distinction remains important for managers in health care to know.

In healthcare organizations, product cost can be viewed as traceable to the cost object of the department, division, or unit. A period cost is not traceable in this manner. Another way to view this distinction is to think of product costs as those costs necessary to actually deliver the service, whereas period costs are costs necessary to support the existence of the organization itself.

Finally, medical supply and pharmacy departments do have inventories on hand. In their case, a product is purchased (rather than manufactured) and placed into inventory while waiting to be dispensed. Then, whenever that product is dispensed, the product is matched with revenue and recognized as a cost of providing the service to the patient. Therefore, the product cost concept is important to managers of departments that hold a significant amount of inventory.

☝ INFORMATION CHECKPOINT

What is needed?	Example of a management report that uses direct/indirect cost.
Where is it found?	With your supervisor, in administration, or in information services.
How is it used?	To track operations directly associated with the unit.
What is needed?	Example of a management report that uses responsibility centers.
Where is it found?	With your supervisor, in administration, or in information services.
How is it used?	To reflect operations that a manager is specifically responsible for and to measure those operations for planning and control.

📖 KEY TERMS

Cost Object
Direct Cost
Indirect Cost
Joint Cost
Responsibility Centers

❓ DISCUSSION QUESTIONS

1. In your own workplace, can you give a good example of a direct cost? An indirect cost?
2. What is the difference?
3. Does your organization use responsibility centers?
4. If not, do you think they should? Why?
5. If so, do you believe the responsibility centers operate properly? Would you make changes? Why?

NOTES

1. C. Horngren et al., *Cost Accounting: A Managerial Emphasis*, 9th ed. (Englewood Cliffs, NJ: Prentice Hall, 1998), 70.
2. J. J. Baker, *Activity-Based Costing and Activity-Based Management for Health Care* (Gaithersburg, MD: Aspen Publishers, Inc., 1998).
3. D. A. West, T. D. West, and P. J. Malone, "Managing Capital and Administrative (indirect) Costs to Achieve Strategic Objectives: The Dialysis Clinic versus the Outpatient Clinic," *Journal of Health Care Finance*, 25, no. 2 (1998): 20–24.

PART

III

Tools to Analyze and Understand Financial Operations

Cost Behavior and Break-Even Analysis

DISTINCTIONS AMONG FIXED, VARIABLE, AND SEMIVARIABLE COSTS

This chapter emphasizes the distinctions among fixed, variable, and semivariable costs because this knowledge is a basic working tool in financial management. The manager needs to know the difference between fixed and variable costs to compute contribution margins and break-even points. The manager also needs to know about semivariable costs to make good decisions about how to treat these costs.

Fixed costs are costs that do not vary in total when activity levels (or volume) of operations change. This concept is illustrated in **Figure 8–1**. The horizontal axis of the graph shows number of residents in the Jones Group Home, and the vertical axis shows total monthly fixed cost in dollars. In this graph, the total monthly fixed cost for the group home is $3,000, and that amount does not change, whether the number of residents (the activity level or volume) is low or high. A good example of a fixed cost is rent expense. Rent would not vary whether the home was almost full or almost empty; thus, rent is a fixed cost.

Variable costs, on the other hand, are costs that vary in direct proportion to changes in activity levels (or volume) of operations. This concept is illustrated in **Figure 8–2**. The horizontal axis of the graph shows number of residents in the Jones Group Home, and the vertical axis shows total monthly variable cost in dollars. In this graph, the monthly variable cost for the group home changes proportionately with the number of residents (the activity level or volume) in the home. A good example of a variable cost is food for the group home residents. Food would vary directly, depending on the number of individuals in residence; thus, food is a variable cost.

Progress Notes

After completing this chapter, you should be able to

1. Understand the distinctions among fixed, variable, and semivariable costs.
2. Be able to analyze mixed costs by two methods.
3. Understand the computation of a contribution margin.
4. Be able to compute the cost-volume-profit (CVP) ratio.
5. Be able to compute the profit-volume (PV) ratio.

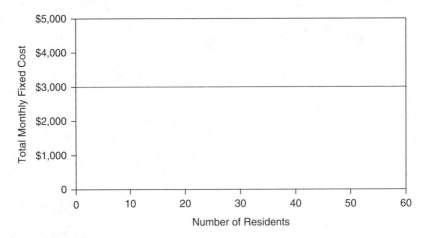

Figure 8–1 Fixed Costs—Jones Group Home.

Semivariable costs vary when the activity levels (or volume) of operations change, but not in direct proportion. The most frequent pattern of semivariable costs is the step pattern, where the semivariable cost rises, flattens out for a bit, and then rises again. The step pattern of semi-variable costs is illustrated in **Figure 8–3**. The horizontal axis of the graph shows number of residents in the Jones Group Home, and the vertical axis shows total monthly semivariable cost. In this graph, the behavior of the cost line resembles stair steps: thus, the "step pattern" name for this configuration. The most common example of a semivariable expense in health care is supervisors' salaries. A single supervisor, for example, can perform adequately over a range of rises in activity levels (or volume). When another supervisor has to be added, the rise in the step pattern occurs.

It is important to know, however, that there are two ways to think about fixed cost. The usual view is the flat line illustrated on the graph in Figure 8–1. That flat line represents total monthly cost for the group home. However, another perception is presented in **Figure 8–4**. The top view of fixed costs in Figure 8–4 is the usual flat line just discussed. The bottom view is fixed cost per resident. Think about the figure for a moment: the top view is dollars in total for the home for

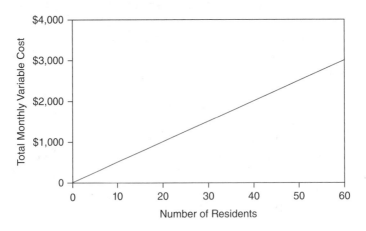

Figure 8–2 Variable Cost—Jones Group Home.

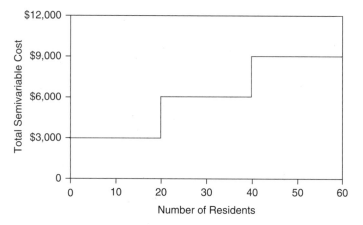

Figure 8–3 Semivariable Cost—Jones Group Home.

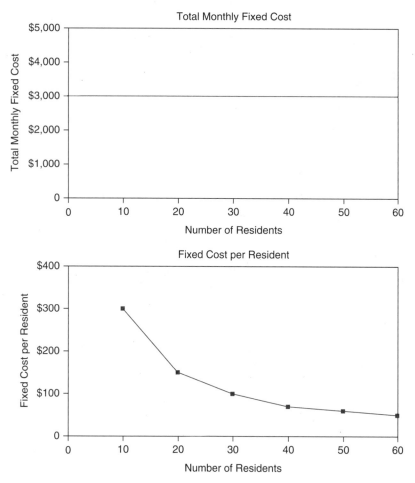

Figure 8–4 Two Views of Fixed Costs.

the month, and the bottom view is fixed-cost dollars by number of residents. The line is no longer flat but declines because this view of cost declines with each additional resident.

We can also think about variable cost in two ways. The usual view of variable cost is the diagonal line rising from the bottom of the graph to the top, as illustrated in Figure 8–2. That steep diagonal line represents monthly cost varying in direct proportion with number of residents in the home. However, another perception is presented in **Figure 8–5**. The top view of variable costs in Figure 8–5 represents total monthly variable cost and is the usual diagonal line just discussed. The bottom view is variable cost per resident. Think about this figure for a moment: the top view is dollars in total for the home for the month, and the bottom view is variable-cost dollars by number of residents. The line is no longer diagonal but is now flat because this view of variable cost stays the same proportionately for each resident. A good way to think about Figures 8–4 and 8–5 is to realize that they are close to being mirror images of each other.

Semifixed costs are sometimes used in healthcare organizations, especially in regard to staffing. Semifixed costs are the reverse of semivariable costs: that is, they stay fixed for a time as activity levels (or volume) of operations change, but then they will rise; then they will plateau; then they will rise. Thus, semifixed costs can exhibit a step pattern similar to that of variable costs.[1] However, the semifixed cost "steps" tend to be longer between rises in cost. In

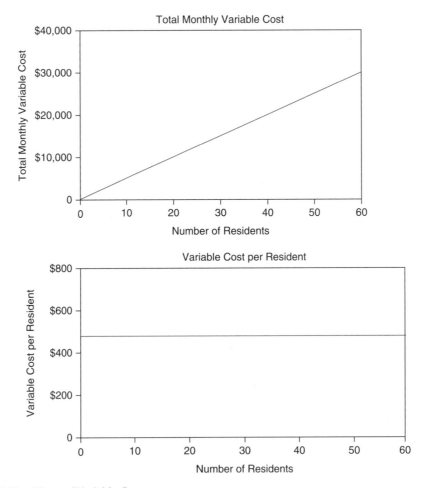

Figure 8–5 Two Views of Variable Costs.

summary, both semifixed and semivariable costs have mixed elements of fixed and variable costs. Thus, both semivariable and semifixed costs are called mixed costs.

EXAMPLES OF VARIABLE AND FIXED COSTS

Studying examples of expenses that are designated as variable and fixed helps to understand the differences between them. It should also be mentioned that some expenses can be variable to one organization and fixed to another because they are handled differently by the two organizations. Operating room fixed and variable costs are illustrated in **Table 8–1**.

Table 8–1 Operating Room Fixed and Variable Costs

Account	Total	Variable	Fixed	Equipment
Social Security	$ 60,517	$ 60,517	$	$
Pension	20,675	20,675		
Health Insurance	8,422	8,422		
Child Care	4,564	4,564		
Patient Accounting	155,356	155,356		
Admitting	110,254	110,254		
Medical Records	91,718	91,718		
Dietary	27,526	27,526		
Medical Waste	2,377	2,377		
Sterile Procedures	78,720	78,720		
Laundry	40,693	40,693		
Depreciation—Equipment	87,378			87,378
Depreciation—Building	41,377		41,377	
Amortization—Interest	(5,819)		(5,819)	
Insurance	4,216		4,216	
Administration	57,966		57,966	
Medical Staff	1,722		1,722	
Community Relations	49,813		49,813	
Materials Management	64,573		64,573	
Human Resources	31,066		31,066	
Nursing Administration	82,471		82,471	
Data Processing	17,815		17,815	
Fiscal	17,700		17,700	
Telephone	2,839		2,839	
Utilities	26,406		26,406	
Plant	77,597		77,597	
Environmental Services	32,874		32,874	
Safety	2,016		2,016	
Quality Management	10,016		10,016	
Medical Staff	9,444		9,444	
Continuous Quality Improvement	4,895		4,895	
EE Health	569		569	
Total Allocated	$1,217,756	$600,822	$529,556	$87,378

Table 8–2 Operating Room Semivariable and Fixed Staffing

Job Positions	Total No. of FTEs	Semivariable	Fixed
Supervisor	2.2		2.2
Techs	3.0	3.0	
RNs	7.7	7.7	
LPNs	1.2	1.2	
Aides, orderlies	1.0		1.0
Clerical	1.2		1.2
Totals	16.3	11.9	4.4

Thirty-two expense accounts are listed in Table 8–1: 11 are variable, 20 are designated as fixed by this hospital, and 1, equipment depreciation, is listed separately.[2] (The separate listing is because of the way this hospital's accounting system handles equipment depreciation.)

Another example of semivariable and fixed staffing is presented in **Table 8–2**. The costs are expressed as full-time equivalent staff (FTEs). Each line-item FTE will be multiplied times the appropriate wage or salary to obtain the semivariable and fixed costs for the operating room. (The further use of FTEs for staffing purposes is fully discussed in the chapter on staffing.) The supervisor position is fixed, which indicates that this is the minimum staffing that can be allowed. The single aide/orderly and the clerical position are also indicated as fixed. All the other positions—technicians, RNs, and LPNs—are listed as semivariable, which indicates that they are probably used in the semivariable step pattern that has been previously discussed in this chapter. This table is a good example of how to show clearly which costs will be designated as semivariable and which costs will be designated as fixed.

Another example illustrates the behavior of a single variable cost in a doctor's office. In **Table 8–3**, we see an array of costs for the procedure code 99214 office visit type. Nine costs are listed. The first cost is variable and is discussed momentarily. The other eight costs are all shown at the same level for a 99214 office visit: supplies, for example, is the same amount in all four columns. The single figure that varies is the top line, which is "report of lab tests," meaning laboratory reports. This cost directly varies with the proportion of activity or volume, as variable cost has been defined. Here we see a variable cost at work: the first column on the left has no lab report, and the cost is zero; the second column has one lab report, and the cost is $3.82; the third column has two lab reports, and the cost is $7.64; and the fourth column has three lab reports, and

Table 8–3 Office Visit with Variable Cost of Tests

Service Code	99214 No Test	99214 1 Test	99214 2 Tests	99214 3 Tests
Report of lab tests	$0.00	$3.82	$7.64	$11.46
Fixed overhead	$31.00	$31.00	$31.00	$31.00
Physician	11.36	11.36	11.36	11.36
Medical assistant	1.43	1.43	1.43	1.43
Bill	0.45	0.45	0.45	0.45
Checkout	1.00	1.00	1.00	1.00
Receptionist	1.28	1.28	1.28	1.28
Collection	0.91	0.91	0.91	0.91
Supplies	0.31	0.31	0.31	0.31
Total visit cost	$47.74	$51.56	$55.38	$59.20

the cost is $11.46. The total cost rises by the same proportionate increase as the increase in the first line.

ANALYZING MIXED COSTS

It is important for planning purposes for the manager to know how to deal with mixed costs because they occur so often. For example, telephone, maintenance, repairs, and utilities are all actually mixed costs. The fixed portion of the cost is that portion representing having the service (such as telephone) ready to use, and the variable portion of the cost represents a portion of the charge for actual consumption of the service. We briefly discuss two very simple methods of analyzing mixed costs, then we examine the high–low method and the scatter graph method.

Predominant Characteristics and Step Methods

Both the predominant characteristics and the step method of analyzing mixed costs are quite simple. In the predominant characteristic method, the manager judges whether the cost is more fixed or more variable and acts on that judgment. In the step method, the manager examines the "steps" in the step pattern of mixed cost and decides whether the cost appears to be more fixed or more variable. Both methods are subjective.

High–Low Method

As the name implies, the high–low method of analyzing mixed costs requires that the cost be examined at its high level and at its low level. To compute the amount of variable cost involved, the difference in cost between high and low levels is obtained and is divided by the amount of change in the activity (or volume). Two examples are examined.

The first example is for an employee cafeteria. **Table 8–4** contains the basic data required for the high–low computation. With the formula described in the preceding paragraph, the following steps are performed:

1. Find the highest volume of 45,000 meals at a cost of $165,000 in September (see Table 8–4) and the lowest volume of 20,000 meals at a cost of $95,000 in March.
2. Compute the variable rate per meal:

	No. of Meals	Cafeteria Cost
Highest volume	45,000	$165,000
Lowest volume	20,000	95,000
Difference	25,000	70,000

3. Divide the difference in cost ($70,000) by the difference in number of meals (25,000) to arrive at the variable cost rate:

$70,000 divided by 25,000 meals = $2.80 per meal

Table 8–4 Employee Cafeteria Number of Meals and Cost by Month

Month	No. of Meals	Employee Cafeteria Cost ($)
July	40,000	164,000
August	43,000	167,000
September	45,000	165,000
October	41,000	162,000
November	37,000	164,000
December	33,000	146,000
January	28,000	123,000
February	22,000	91,800
March	20,000	95,000
April	25,000	106,800
May	30,000	130,200
June	35,000	153,000

4. Compute the fixed overhead rate as follows:

   a. At the highest level:

Total cost	$165,000
Less: variable portion	
[45,000 meals × $2.80 @]	(126,000)
Fixed portion of cost	$ 39,000

   b. At the lowest level

Total cost	$ 95,000
Less: variable portion	
[20,000 meals × $2.80 @]	(56,000)
Fixed portion of cost	$ 39,000

   c. Proof totals: $39,000 fixed portion at both levels

The manager should recognize that large or small dollar amounts can be adapted to this method. A second example concerns drug samples and their cost. In this example, a supervisor of marketing is concerned about the number of drug samples used by the various members of the marketing staff. She uses the high–low method to determine the portion of fixed cost. **Table 8–5** contains the basic data required for the high–low computation. Using the formula previously described, the following steps are performed:

1. Find the highest volume of 1,000 samples at a cost of $5,000 (see Table 8–5) and the lowest volume of 750 samples at a cost of $4,200.

2. Compute the variable rate per sample:

	No. of Samples	Cost
Highest volume	1,000	$5,000
Lowest volume	750	4,200
Difference	250	$ 800

3. Divide the difference in cost ($800) by the difference in number of samples (250) to arrive at the variable cost rate:

$800 divided by 250 samples = $3.20 per sample

Table 8–5 Number of Drug Samples and Cost for November

Rep.	No. of Samples	Cost ($)
J. Smith	1,000	5,000
A. Jones	900	4,300
B. Baker	850	4,600
G. Black	975	4,500
T. Potter	875	4,750
D. Conner	750	4,200

4. Compute the fixed overhead rate as follows:

   a. At the highest level:

Total cost	$5,000
Less: variable portion	
[1,000 samples × $3.20 @]	(3,200)
Fixed portion of cost	$1,800

  b. At the lowest level

Total cost	$4,200
Less: variable portion	
[750 samples × $3.20 @]	(2,400)
Fixed portion of cost	$1,800

  c. Proof totals: $1,800 fixed portion at both levels

The high–low method is an approximation that is based on the relationship between the highest and the lowest levels, and the computation assumes a straight-line relationship. The advantage of this method is its convenience in the computation method.

CONTRIBUTION MARGIN, COST-VOLUME-PROFIT, AND PROFIT-VOLUME RATIOS

The manager should know how to analyze the relationship of cost, volume, and profit. This important information assists the manager in properly understanding and controlling operations. The first step in such analysis is the computation of the contribution margin.

Contribution Margin

The contribution margin is calculated in this way:

		% of Revenue
Revenues (net)	$500,000	100%
Less: variable cost	(350,000)	70%
Contribution margin	$150,000	30%
Less: fixed cost	(120,000)	
Operating income	$30,000	

The contribution margin of $150,000 or 30%, in this example, represents variable cost deducted from net revenues. The answer represents the contribution margin, so called because it contributes to fixed costs and to profits.

The importance of dividing costs into fixed and variable becomes apparent now, for a contribution margin computation demands either fixed or variable cost classifications; no mixed costs are recognized in this calculation.

Cost-Volume-Profit (CVP) Ratio or Break Even

The break-even point is the point when the contribution margin (i.e., net revenues less variable costs) equals the fixed costs. When operations exceed this break-even point, an excess of revenues over expenses (income) is realized. But if operations does not reach the break-even point, there will be an excess of expenses over revenues, and a loss will be realized.

The manager must recognize there are two ways of expressing the break-even point: either by an amount per unit or as a percentage of net revenues. If the contribution margin is expressed as a percentage of net revenues, it is often called the profit-volume (PV) ratio. A PV ratio example follows this cost-volume-profit (CVP) computation.

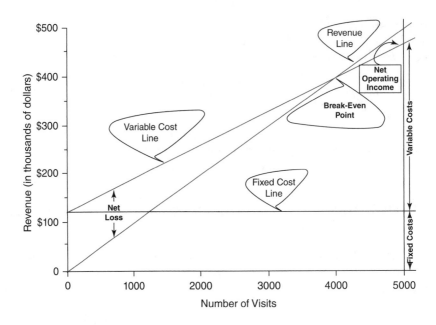

Figure 8–6 Cost-Volume-Profit (CVP) Chart for a Wellness Clinic.
Courtesy of Resource Group, Ltd., Dallas, Texas.

The CVP example is given in **Figure 8–6**. The data points for the chart come from the contribution margin as already computed:

		% of Revenue
Revenues (net)	$500,000	100%
Less: variable cost	(350,000)	70%
Contribution margin	$150,000	30%
Less: fixed cost	(120,000)	
Operating income	$30,000	

Three lines were first drawn to create the chart. They were total fixed costs of $120,000, total revenue of $500,000, and variable costs of $350,000. (All three are labeled on the chart.) The break-even point appears at the point where the total cost line intersects the revenue line. Because this point is indeed the break-even point, the organization will have no profit and no loss but will break even. The wedge shape to the left of the break-even point is potential net loss, whereas the narrower wedge to the right is potential net income (both are labeled on the chart).

CVP charts allow a visual illustration of the relationships that is very effective for the manager.

Profit-Volume (PV) Ratio

Remember that the second method of expressing the break-even point is as a percentage of net revenues and that if the contribution margin is expressed as a percentage of net revenues, it is called the profit-volume (PV) ratio. **Figure 8–7** illustrates the method. The basic data points used for the chart were as follows:

Revenue per visit	$100.00	100%
Less variable cost per visit	(70.00)	70%
Contribution margin per visit	$ 30.00	30%
Fixed costs per period	$120,000	

$30.00 contribution margin per visit divided by $100 price per visit = 30% PV Ratio

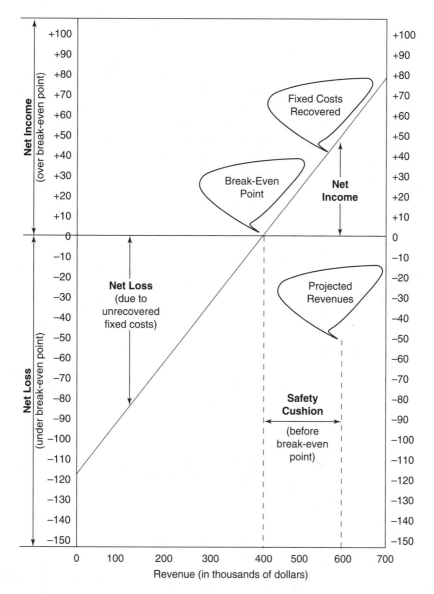

Figure 8–7 Profit-Volume (PV) Chart for a Wellness Clinic.
Courtesy of Resource Group, Ltd., Dallas, Texas.

On our chart, the profit pattern is illustrated by a line drawn from the beginning level of fixed costs to be recovered ($120,000 in our case). Another line has been drawn straight across the chart at the break-even point. When the diagonal line begins at $120,000, its intersection with the break-even or zero line is at $400,000 in revenue (see left-hand dotted line on chart). We can prove out the $120,000 versus $400,000 relationship as follows. Each dollar of revenue reduces the potential of loss by $0.30 (or 30% × $1.00). Fixed costs are fully recovered at a revenue level of $400,000, proved out as $120,000 divided by .30 = $400,000. This can be written as follows:

$$.30R = \$120,000$$
$$R = \$400,000 \ [120,000 \text{ divided by } .30 = 400,000]$$

The PV chart is very effective in planning meetings because only two lines are necessary to show the effect of changes in volume. Both PV and CVP are useful when working with the effects of changes in break-even points and revenue volume assumptions.

Contribution margins are also useful for showing profitability in other ways. An example appears in **Figure 8–8**, which shows the profitability of various DRGs, using contribution margins as the measure of profitability. Case volume (the number of cases of each DRG) is on the vertical axis of the matrix, and the dollar amount of contribution margin per case is on the horizontal axis of the matrix.[3]

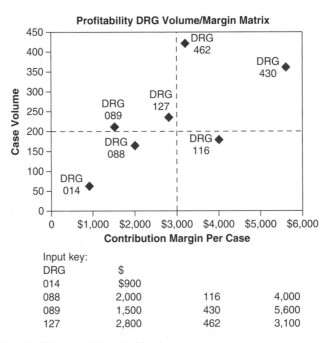

Figure 8–8 Profitability DRG Volume/Margin Matrix.
Modified from R. Hankins and J. J. Baker, *Management Accounting for Health Care Organizations* (Sudbury, MA: Jones & Bartlett, 2004), 189.

Scatter Graph Method

In performing a mixed-cost analysis, the manager is attempting to find the mixed cost's average rate of variability. The scatter graph method is more accurate than the high–low method previously described. It uses a graph to plot all points of data, rather than the highest and lowest figures used by the high–low method. Generally, cost will be on the vertical axis of the graph, and volume will be on the horizontal axis. All points are plotted, each point being placed where cost and volume intersect for that line item. A regression line is then fitted to the plotted points. The regression line basically represents the average—or a line of averages. The average total fixed cost is found at the point where the regression line intersects with the cost axis.

Two examples are examined. They match the high–low examples previously calculated. **Figure 8–9** presents the cafeteria data. The costs for cafeteria meals have been plotted on the graph, and the regression line has been fitted to the plotted data points. The regression line strikes the cost axis at a certain point; that amount represents the fixed cost portion of the mixed cost. The balance (or the total less the fixed cost portion) represents the variable portion.

The second example also matches the high–low example previously calculated. **Figure 8–10** presents the drug sample data. The costs for drug samples have been plotted on the graph, and the regression line has been fitted to the plotted data points. The regression line again strikes the cost axis at the point representing the fixed-cost portion of the mixed cost. The balance (the total less the fixed cost portion) represents the variable portion. Further discussions of this method can be found in Examples and Exercises at the back of this book.

The examples presented here have regression lines fitted visually. However, computer programs are available that will place the regression line through statistical analysis as a function of the program. This method is called the least-squares method. Least squares means that the sum of the squares of the deviations from plotted points to regression line is smaller than would occur from any other way the line could be fitted to the data: in other words, it is the best fit. This method is, of course, more accurate than fitting the regression line visually.

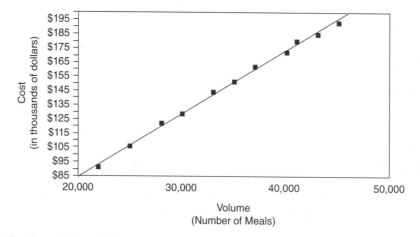

Figure 8–9 Employee Cafeteria Scatter Graph.

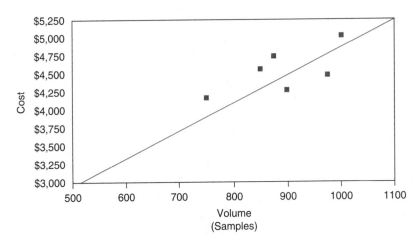

Figure 8–10 Drug Sample Scatter Graph for November.

 INFORMATION CHECKPOINT

What is needed?	Revenues, variable cost, and fixed cost for a unit, division, DRG, and so on.
Where is it found?	In operating reports.
How is it used?	Use the multiple-step calculations in this chapter to compute the CPV or the PV ratio; use to plan and control operations.

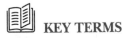 **KEY TERMS**

Break-Even Analysis
Cost-Profit-Volume
Contribution Margin
Fixed Cost
Mixed Cost
Profit-Volume Ratio
Semifixed Cost
Semivariable Cost
Variable Cost

DISCUSSION QUESTIONS

1. Have you seen reports in your workplace that set out the contribution margin?
2. Do you believe that contribution margins can help you manage in your present work? In the future? How?
3. Have you encountered break-even analysis in your work?

4. If so, how was it used (or presented)?
5. How do you think you would use break-even analysis?
6. Do you believe your organization could use these analysis tools more often than is now happening? What do you believe the benefits would be?

NOTES

1. C. Horngren et al., *Cost Accounting: A Managerial Emphasis*, 9th ed. (Englewood Cliffs, NJ: Prentice Hall, 1998).
2. J. J. Baker, *Activity-Based Costing and Activity-Based Management for Health Care* (Gaithersburg, MD: Aspen Publishers, Inc., 1998).
3. It is possible that the term "diagnosis-related groups" (DRGs) may be changed to some new terminology as a consequence of ICD-10 implementation.

Understanding Inventory and Depreciation Concepts

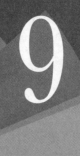

OVERVIEW: THE INVENTORY CONCEPT

This overview concerns both the inventory concept and types of inventories.

Concept of Inventory in Healthcare Organizations

"Inventory" includes all the items (goods) that an organization has for sale in the normal course of its business. Inventory is an asset, owned by the company. It appears on the balance sheet as a current asset, because the individual items that compose the inventory are expected to be "used" (sold) within a 12-month period.

Types of Inventory in Healthcare Organizations

Various healthcare organizations (or departments within organizations) deal with inventory and must account for it. The hospital gift shop and the cafeteria, for example, own inventory and must account for it. All pharmacies (hospital-based, retail brick-and-mortar, or mail order pharmacies) own inventory in the normal course of their business.

In manufacturing companies, inventory typically consists of three parts: raw materials, work in progress, and the finished goods that are for sale. We might think that most inventory items for sale in a healthcare organization are not manufactured, but are finished goods instead. However, consider this example: the hospital cafeteria purchases flour, eggs, butter, and so on (raw materials), mixes the ingredients (work in progress), and produces a cake (finished goods) that is for sale. (Another example might be a pharmacy that compounds drugs.)

Progress Notes

After completing this chapter, you should be able to

1. Understand the interrelationship between inventory and cost of goods sold.
2. Understand the difference between LIFO and FIFO inventory methods.
3. Be able to calculate inventory turnover.
4. Understand the interrelationship between depreciation expense and the reserve for depreciation.
5. Understand how to compute the net book value of a fixed asset.
6. Be able to identify the five methods of computing book depreciation.

INVENTORY AND COST OF GOODS SOLD ("GOODS" SUCH AS DRUGS)

The interrelationship between inventory and cost of goods sold is at the heart of the inventory concept.

Turning Inventory into Cost of Goods (or Drugs) Sold

The completed inventory item ("finished goods") is sold. That is how an item moves out of inventory and is recognized as cost. When the item is recognized as cost, it becomes "cost of goods sold." (Also note that different terminology may be used. In some organizations cost of goods sold is called "cost of sales.") For a business such as a retail pharmacy, the cost of inventory sold to its customers is the largest single expense of the business.

Recording Inventory and Cost of Goods (or Drugs) Sold

Recording inventory and cost of goods (or drugs) sold is a sequence of events. **Figure 9–1** illustrates the sequence as follows:

- Beginning inventory (inventory at the start of the period) is recorded.
- Purchases during the period are recorded.
- Beginning inventory plus purchases equal "cost of goods available for sale."
- Ending inventory (inventory at the end of the period) is recorded.
- Cost of goods available for sale less ending inventory equals "cost of goods sold."

Purchases added to inventory will typically include "freight in," or the shipping costs to deliver the items to you. Any discounts received on the purchases should be subtracted from the purchase cost. Thus the purchases become "net purchases"; that is, net of discounts.

Sometimes the ending inventory is estimated. An example of "Estimating the Ending Pharmacy Inventory" is shown in the chapter about estimates and benchmarking.

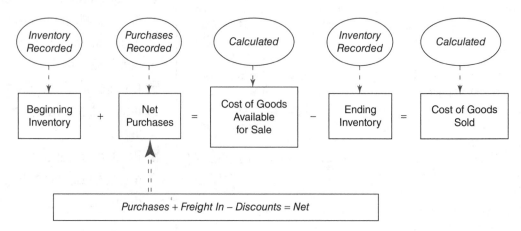

Figure 9–1 Recording Inventory in the Accounting Cycle.

Gross Margin Computation

Gross margin equals revenue from sales less the cost of goods sold. Gross margin is often expressed as a percentage. Thus, a pharmacy's gross margin might appear as follows:

Sales	100%
Cost of goods (drugs) sold	65%
Gross margin	35%

An organization's gross margin percentage can be readily compared to industry standards.

INVENTORY METHODS

How is the inventory to be valued? The two most commonly used inventory valuation methods are First-In, First-Out (FIFO) and Last-In, First-Out (LIFO). The method chosen will affect the organization's financial statements, as explained in the following sections.

First-In, First-Out (FIFO) Inventory Method

The First-In, First-Out, or FIFO inventory costing method, recognizes the first costs placed into inventory as the first costs moved out into cost of goods sold when a sale occurs. How will this method affect the organization's financial statements? Under FIFO, the ending inventory figure will be higher (because when the oldest inventory moves out first, the ending inventory will be based on the costs of the latest purchases, which we assume will have cost more). **Exhibit 9–1** illustrates this effect.

Last-In, First-Out (LIFO) Inventory Method

The Last-In, First-Out, or LIFO inventory costing method, recognizes the latest, or last, costs placed into inventory as the first costs moved out into cost of goods sold when a sale occurs. How will this method affect the organization's financial statements? Under LIFO, the ending inventory figure will be lower (because when the latest inventory moves out first, the ending inventory will be based on costs of the earliest purchases, which we assume will have cost less). **Exhibit 9–2** illustrates this effect.

Other Inventory Treatments

Two other inventory treatments deserve mention, as follows.

Weighted Average Inventory Method

This inventory costing method is based on the weighted average cost of inventory during the period. (The weighted average inventory method is also called the "average cost method.") The weighted average inventory cost is determined as follows: divide the cost of goods available for sale by the number of units available for sale.

Exhibit 9–1 FIFO Inventory Effect

	Assumptions		FIFO Inventory Effect
Sales (Revenue)	20 units @$25 =		$500
Cost of Sales:			
Beginning Inventory	10 units @$5 =	$50	
Plus: Purchases	10 units @$10 = $100 &		
	10 units @$15 = $150	250	
Subtotal		$300	
Less: Ending Inventory	10 units @$15 =	(150)	
Cost of Sales			150
Gross Profit			$350
Operating Expenses			(50)
Earnings Before Tax			$300
Income Tax			(90)
Earnings After Tax			$210

Note: Ending inventory computed as number of units in the beginning inventory plus number of units purchased less number of units sold–count oldest units sold first.

No Method: Inventory Never Recognized

This inventory costing method is no method at all. That is, inventory is never recognized. For example, a physician's office may expense all drug purchases as supplies at the time of purchase and never count such drugs as inventory. This treatment might be justified when such supplies were only a small part of the practice expenses. However, if the physician is purchasing very expensive drugs and administering them in the office (infusing expensive drugs is a good example), then not recognizing any such drugs being held as inventory on the financial statements is misleading.

INVENTORY TRACKING

The two most typical inventory-tracking systems are described as follows.

Perpetual Inventory System

With a perpetual inventory system, the healthcare organization keeps a continuous, or perpetual, record for every individual inventory item. Thus the amount of inventory on hand can

Exhibit 9–2 LIFO Inventory Effect

	Assumptions	LIFO Inventory Effect	
Sales (Revenue)	20 units @$25 =		$500
Cost of Sales:			
Beginning Inventory	10 units @$5 =	$50	
Plus: Purchases	10 units @$10 = $100 &		
	10 units @$15 = $150	250	
Subtotal		$300	
Less: Ending Inventory	10 units @$5 =	(50)	
Cost of Sales			250
Gross Profit			$250
Operating Expenses			(50)
Earnings Before Tax			$200
Income Tax			(60)
Earnings After Tax			$140

Note: Ending inventory computed as number of units purchased plus number of units in the beginning inventory less number of units sold–count newest units sold first.

be determined at any time. (A real-time system is a variation of the perpetual inventory system, whereby transactions are entered simultaneously.)

A perpetual inventory system requires, of course, a specific identification method for each inventory item. Bar coding is often used for this purpose. You are most likely to find a perpetual inventory system in the pharmacy department of a hospital.

Periodic Inventory System

With a periodic inventory system, the healthcare organization does not keep a continuous record that identifies every individual inventory item on hand. Instead, at the end of the period the organization physically counts the inventory items on hand. Then costs per item are attached to the inventory counts in order to arrive at the cost of the inventory at the end of the period (the ending inventory).

Necessary Adjustments

Certain inventory adjustments will commonly become necessary, as discussed here.

Shortages

When the periodic inventory results are compared to the inventory balance on the financial statements, it is not uncommon to find that the actual physical inventory amount is less than the amount recorded on the books. This difference, or shortage, is commonly termed "shrinkage." The inventory amount on the books must be reduced to the actual amount per the periodic inventory, and the resulting shrinkage cost must be recorded as an expense.

Obsolete Items

Most inventories will inevitably come to contain certain obsolete items. For example, the pharmacy inventory will contain drugs that have "sell by" or "use by" expiration dates. Obsolete inventory items should be discarded. Their cost must be removed from the cost of inventory on hand, and the resulting obsolescence cost must be recorded as an expense.

INVENTORY DISTRIBUTION SYSTEMS

The ability to track inventory is directly impacted by the type of documentation required for removing items from inventory. Different types of inventory require different types of distribution systems. Thus, removing an item from a particular type of inventory needs documentation that varies according to the level of permission and scrutiny required.

Distribution Using Sign-Off Forms

For example, drawing light bulbs from the Maintenance Department inventory does not require a high level of permission and/or scrutiny. In one facility's inventory distribution method, such a requisition for light bulbs must always be attached to a Maintenance Department work order. Some responsible person has signed off on this work order, and it shows the reason for the inventory request. This method not only allows for inventory tracking, but also indicates who was responsible for generating the order.

The distribution system for medical devices held in inventory typically requires a different type of requisition. (One reason: Medical devices are more expensive than light bulbs.) The inventory requisition is usually triggered by the doctor's orders, and more than one level of sign-off is typically required before the device is delivered to the operating room. Thus, tracking this inventory item may require multiple steps.

Distribution Using Robotic Technology

This discussion about technology methods of inventory distribution centers upon drug distribution within a facility.

Background

Relative to drugs or pharmaceutical inventory, it should be noted that there are some characteristics that differentiate the pharmaceutical inventory from the rest of a hospital's inventory control mechanisms. The unit-dose drug distribution system is a particular example. In unit-dose dispensing, medication is dispensed in a package that is ready to administer to the patient.

Unit-dose dispensing of medication was developed in the 1960s to support nurses in medication administration and to reduce the waste of increasingly expensive medications.[1]

Robotic Automation

Although the unit-dose system provides many safeguards and advantages in delivering medications, as a manual system it is highly labor intensive. Automation has been developed to support the patient care advantages of the system at a decreased cost, with pharmacy using robotics for the bin-filling process. Advantages of the robotic cart-filling method include improved accuracy in medication dispensing and accounting. Disadvantages include high startup costs partly resulting from needed facility renovations, high continuing support costs, significant pharmacy space requirements, and limited robot capacity.[2]

Cost/Benefit of a Robot

Capital expense or lease costs for robotic technology are high, limiting use to larger hospitals.

The decision to purchase and implement an automated bin fill system should be based on a keen and insightful analysis of the financial benefits, return on investment, and potential for demonstrated improvements in service quality and patient care. Although the cost of a robot continues to decrease, information systems and other support costs will remain high enough to make the decision to purchase or lease a robot hard to justify in many cases.

CALCULATING INVENTORY TURNOVER

Inventory turnover is a ratio that shows how fast inventory is sold, or "turns over." The computation is in two steps as follows. **Figure 9–2** illustrates the sequence.

Step 1. First compute "Average Inventory":
Beginning Inventory plus Ending Inventory divided by two equals Average Inventory

Step 2. Next compute "Inventory Turnover":
Cost of Goods Sold (or Cost of Sales) divided by Average Inventory equals Inventory Turnover

For example,
Step 1. $100,000 (beginning inventory) plus $150,000 (ending inventory) divided by 2 equals $125,000 (average inventory).

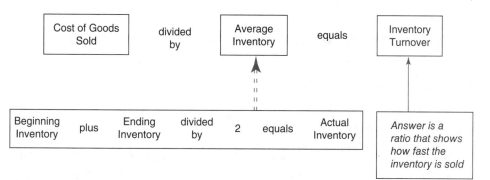

Figure 9–2 Calculating Inventory Turnover.

Step 2. $500,000 (cost of goods sold, or cost of sales) divided by $125,000 (average inventory) equals 4.0 (inventory turnover).

An organization's inventory turnover ratio can be readily compared to industry standards.

OVERVIEW: THE DEPRECIATION CONCEPT

Depreciation expense spreads, or allocates, the cost of a fixed asset over the useful life of that asset, as discussed here.

Fixed Assets and Depreciation Expense

Fixed assets, also known as long-term assets, are classified as long term and placed on the balance sheet as such because they will not be converted into cash in the coming 12 months. The purchase of a fixed asset is a capital expenditure. (Capital expenditures involve the acquisition of assets that are long lasting, such as buildings and equipment.) "Capitalizing" means recording these assets as long-term assets on the balance sheet.

We recognize the cost of owning buildings and equipment through depreciation expense. When the cost is spread, or allocated, over a period of years, each year's financial statements (for that period of years) recognize some portion of the cost, expressed as depreciation expense.

Useful Life of the Asset

The useful life determines the period over which the fixed asset's cost will be spread. For example, a piece of laboratory equipment is purchased for $20,000. It has a useful life of five years. So depreciation expense is recognized in each of the five years until the $20,000 is used up.

Salvage Value

Before depreciation expense can be calculated, we need to know whether the fixed asset will have salvage value at the end of the depreciated period. Salvage value, also known as residual value or scrap value, represents any expected cash value of the asset at the end of its useful life. If the laboratory equipment is expected to have a salvage value of $1,000 at the end of its five-year useful life, then $19,000 will be spread over the five-year life as depreciation expense, and the $1,000 will remain undepreciated at the end of that time.

BOOK VALUE OF A FIXED ASSET AND THE RESERVE FOR DEPRECIATION

This section describes important interrelationships between and among depreciation expense, the reserve for depreciation, and net book value of an asset.

The Reserve for Depreciation

Depreciation expense over the years is accumulated into the reserve for depreciation. In other words, the reserve for depreciation holds the cumulative amount of depreciation expense that has been recognized over time, beginning with the date that the fixed asset was acquired.

Another way to think about this is to view the reserve for depreciation as holding all the depreciation expense that has been recognized and recorded over the useful life of the asset.

Interrelationship of Depreciation Expense and the Reserve for Depreciation

Depreciation expense for the year is recorded in the income statement. At the same time, an equivalent amount is added to the cumulative amount that has been accumulating within the reserve for depreciation on the balance sheet. These amounts should balance each other; that is, if $25,000 is recognized as depreciation expense in the income statement, then $25,000 should be added to the reserve for depreciation on the balance sheet. This interrelationship is illustrated in **Figure 9–3**.

Net Book Value of a Fixed Asset

The net book value (also known as book value) of a fixed asset is a balance sheet figure that represents the remaining undepreciated portion of the fixed asset cost. The term derives from value recorded on the books—thus "book value."

The net book value of a fixed asset is computed as follows:

- Determine the original cost of the fixed asset on the balance sheet.
- Subtract the reserve for depreciation, which has accumulated depreciation expense as it has been recognized.
- The result equals net book value at that point in time (**Figure 9–4**).

Also note that fully depreciated fixed assets may still remain on the books if they are still in use. A fully depreciated fixed asset, of course, means that the depreciable cost has been exhausted because all the depreciation expense over the asset's useful life has already been

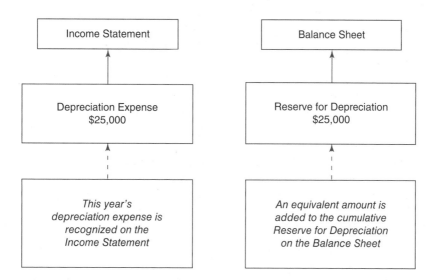

Figure 9–3 Interrelationship of Depreciation Expense and Reserve for Depreciation in the Accounting Cycle.

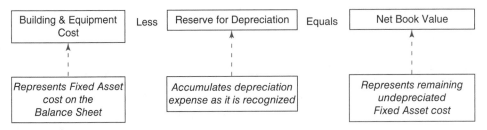

Figure 9–4 Net Book Value Computation.

recognized. Thus, the net book value would either be zero or would amount to the remaining salvage value of the asset.

Five Methods of Computing Book Depreciation

Just as "book value" means value that is recorded on the organization's books, "book depreciation" means depreciation that is recorded on the books. Book depreciation is the depreciation expense recorded in the financial accounting records and reflected on the financial statements. "Tax depreciation," on the other hand, is depreciation that is computed for tax purposes and is reflected on the applicable tax returns of the organization. Tax depreciation methods are discussed in the final section of this chapter.

You as a manager will most likely be using book depreciation in your planning, control, and decision making. Five methods of computing book depreciation are described below.

Straight-Line Depreciation Method

The straight-line depreciation method assigns an equal or even amount of depreciation expense over each year (or period) of the asset's useful life. The expense is thus spread evenly—or in a straight line—over the life of the asset. **Table 9–1** illustrates the straight-line depreciation method applied to a fixed asset costing $10,000 with a 5-year useful life and no salvage value. The depreciation expense would thus equal $2,000 for each of the 5 years ($10,000 divided by 5 equals $2,000 per year).

Table 9–2 illustrates the straight-line depreciation method applied to a fixed asset costing $10,000 with a 5-year useful life and a $1,000 salvage value. The depreciation expense would thus equal $1,800 for each year in this example, because we must leave $1,000 at the end of the asset's 5-year life ($10,000 less $1,000 equals $9,000 divided by 5 equals $1,800 per year.)

If the asset was acquired in the second half of the year, in some cases only a half-year of depreciation will be recognized in Year 1. If this is the case, the remaining half-year of depreciation will be recognized in Year 6, in order to fully depreciate the asset.

Accelerated Book Depreciation Methods

As the name would imply, accelerated book depreciation methods write off more depreciation in the first part of the asset's useful life. Thus, they "accelerate" recognizing depreciation expense. Three accelerated depreciation methods are briefly described here. Further details about the computations for each method appear in Appendix 9-A at the end of this chapter.

Table 9–1   Straight-Line Depreciation: Five-Year Life with No Salvage Value

	Cost (to Be Depreciated)	Depreciation Expense per Year*	Accumulated Depreciation (Reserve for Depreciation)
	$10,000		
Year 1		$2,000	$2,000
Year 2		2,000	4,000
Year 3		2,000	6,000
Year 4		2,000	8,000
Year 5		2,000	10,000

*$10,000 divided by 5 years = $2,000 per year.

Table 9–2   Straight-Line Depreciation: Five-Year Life with Salvage Value

	Cost (to Be Depreciated)	Depreciation Expense per Year*	Accumulated Depreciation (Reserve for Depreciation)	Net Remaining Undepreciated Cost (Net Block Value)
	$10,000			$10,000
Year 1		$1,800	$1,800	8,200
Year 2		1,800	3,600	6,400
Year 3		1,800	5,400	4,600
Year 4		1,800	7,200	2,800
Year 5		1,800	9,000	1,000**

*$9,000 divided by 5 years = $1,800 per year.
**Remaining salvage value.

Sum-of-the-Year's Digits (SYD) Method   The Sum-of-the-Year's Digits (SYD) accelerated depreciation method computes depreciation by multiplying the depreciable cost of the asset by a fraction.

Double-Declining Balance (DDB) Method   The Double-Declining Balance (DDB) accelerated depreciation method computes depreciation by multiplying the asset's net book value at the beginning of each year by a constant percentage, or factor. In the case of DDB, the constant factor is twice the straight-line rate (thus "double-declining").

150% Declining Balance (150% DB) Method   The 150% Declining Balance (150% DB) accelerated depreciation method also computes depreciation by multiplying the asset's net book value at the beginning of each year by a constant percentage, or factor. In the case of 150% DB, however, the constant factor is half again or 150% of the straight-line rate.

Units of Service or Units of Production (UOP) Depreciation Method

The Units of Service or Units of Production (UOP) method computes depreciation by assigning a fixed amount of depreciation to each unit of service or output that is produced by equipment.

"Units of Production" is a manufacturer's term for manufacturing, or producing, a product. "Units of Service" more properly describes the medical equipment providing services in healthcare organizations.

Instead of a useful life in years, equipment depreciated by the UOP method is assigned a fixed total amount of units of service. This fixed amount is the overall total for the life of the equipment. Then the number of units of service actually provided each year is depreciated.

COMPUTING TAX DEPRECIATION

The following discussion about tax depreciation is general in nature and is not to be utilized as tax advice. Any additional details about tax depreciation are beyond the scope of this text.

Overview

"Tax depreciation," as previously defined, means depreciation that is computed for tax purposes and is reflected on the applicable tax returns of the organization. The methods of tax depreciation in effect at the time of this writing fall under the Modified Accelerated Cost Recovery System as described here.

Modified Accelerated Cost Recovery System (MACRS)

The Modified Accelerated Cost Recovery System (MACRS) is currently used to depreciate most business and investment property for tax purposes. MACRS presently consists of two depreciation systems, both of which are briefly described here.

General Depreciation System (GDS)

The General Depreciation System (GDS) is the method generally used under the U.S. Internal Revenue Service rules and regulations, although there are certain exceptions. GDS provides nine property classifications for useful life, including 3-, 5-, 7-, and 10-year property, and 15-, 20-, and 25-year property, along with residential rental property and nonresidential real property. For example, computers, calculators, and copiers fall into the 5-year property classification while office furniture and fixtures such as desks, files, and safes fall into the 7-year property classification.[3]

The GDS method allows double-declining balance, 150% declining balance, and the straight-line method of depreciation, depending upon what type of property is being depreciated. For example, nonfarm 3-, 5-, 7-, and 10-year property can use any of the three methods in most (but not all) circumstances.[4]

Alternative Depreciation System (ADS)

The Alternative Depreciation System (ADS) is required for particular properties including, for example, any tax-exempt use property.[5] ADS uses fixed ADS recovery periods, along with straight-line depreciation. ADS can also be used for certain eligible property, even though the property in question could come under GDS (certain restrictions apply).[6]

The tax law changes rapidly; thus, modifications to the tax depreciation methods described in this section may have been placed into effect at any point in time. More information can be obtained from the recent Internal Revenue Service Publication 946 "How to Depreciate Property."

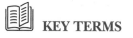

INFORMATION CHECKPOINT

What is needed?

A depreciation schedule that includes depreciation expense, reserve for depreciation, and net book value.

Where is it found?

With your supervisor or in the accounting and/or administration offices.

How is it used?

To reflect depreciation expense in order to complete the income statement.

KEY TERMS

Book Value
Depreciation
FIFO
Inventory
Inventory Turnover
LIFO
Salvage Value
Useful Life (of an asset)

DISCUSSION QUESTIONS

1. Do you or your supervisor have to deal with inventory? If so, please describe.
2. Have you ever had to count physical inventory? If so, please describe the process.
3. Do you or your supervisor have to deal with depreciation expense? If so, please describe.
4. Have you ever had to compute depreciation expense? If so, please describe the circumstances.

NOTES

1. Agency for Healthcare Research and Quality. "National Healthcare Disparities Report, 2013, Chapter 10. Access to Health Care." Content last reviewed May 2014, http://www.ahrq.gov/research/findings/nhqrdr/nhdr13/chap10.html
2. L. F. Wolper, *Health Care Administration: Managing Organized Delivery Systems* (5th ed.) (Sudbury, MA: Jones & Bartlett Publishers, 2011).
3. Department of the Treasury, Internal Revenue Service. *How to Depreciate Property*. Publication 946 (Washington, DC: U.S. Government, 2011).
4. Ibid., Table 4-1.
5. Ibid., "Required Use of ADS."
6. Ibid., "Election of ADS."

A Further Discussion of Accelerated and Units of Service Depreciation Computations

9-A

© LFor/Shutterstock

ACCELERATED BOOK DEPRECIATION METHODS

As the name would imply, accelerated book depreciation methods write off more depreciation in the first part of the asset's useful life. Thus, they "accelerate" recognizing depreciation expense. The computations of three accelerated depreciation methods are described in this appendix as follows.

Sum-of-the-Year's Digits (SYD) Method

The Sum-of-the-Year's Digits (SYD) accelerated depreciation method computes depreciation by multiplying the depreciable cost of the asset by a fraction. The fraction is the mechanism by which the acceleration is computed. It is calculated as follows:

- The numerator of the SYD fraction starts with the asset's useful life expressed in years and decreases by one each year thereafter. (Thus, for a five-year useful life, the numerators are 5, 4, 3, 2, and 1 respectively.)
- The denominator of the SYD fraction is the sum of the years' digits of the asset's life. (Thus, for a five -year useful life, the sum of $5 + 4 + 3 + 2 + 1$ equals 15, which is the denominator.)

Table 9-A–1 illustrates the computation for each year. The depreciable cost of $10,000 is divided by 15 to arrive at $666.66. Thus, one-fifteenth or $666.66 is multiplied by 5 for the first year ($3,333 depreciation expense), by 4 for the second year ($2,667 depreciation expense), and so on.

Double-Declining Balance (DDB) Method

The Double-Declining Balance (DDB) accelerated depreciation method computes depreciation by multiplying the asset's net book value at the beginning of each year by a constant percentage, or factor. In the case of DDB, the constant factor is twice the straight-line rate (thus "double-declining").

Table 9-A–2 illustrates the computation for each year of a five-year useful life with no salvage value. The double-declining factor is computed as follows:

- $10,000 cost of the fixed asset divided by the asset's useful life of 5 years equals 20% or a factor of 0.20.
- Multiply the 0.20 by 2 (or double) to arrive at the 0.40 double-declining factor.

Table 9-A-1 Sum-of-the-Years' Digits Depreciation: Five-Year Life with No Salvage Value

		Depreciation Computation			
Cost (to Be Depreciated)	Depreciable Cost (for Computation) ×	Sum-of-the-Years' Digits* Fraction** =	Annual Depreciation Expense	Accumulated Depreciation (Reserve for Depreciation)	Net Remaining Undepreciated Cost (Net Book Value)
$10,000					
Year 1	$10,000	5/15	$3,333	$3,333	$6,667
Year 2	10,000	4/15	2,667	6,000	4,000
Year 3	10,000	3/15	2,000	8,000	2,000
Year 4	10,000	2/15	1,333	9,333	667
Year 5	10,000	1/15	667	10,000	-0-

*Sum-of-the-Years' Digits = 15 = (1 + 2 + 3 + 4 + 5).
**One-fifteenth of $10,000 = $666.66.

Table 9-A–2 Double-Declining Balance Depreciation: Five-Year Life with No Salvage Value

	Cost (to Be Depreciated)	Carry-forward Book Value (for Computation)	×	Double Declining Balance Factor	=	Annual Depreciation Expense	Accumulated Depreciation (Reserve for Depreciation)	Net Remaining Undepreciated Cost (Net Book Value)
	$10,000							
Year 1		$10,000		0.40*		$4,000	$4,000	$6,000
Year 2		6,000		0.40		2,400	6,400	3,600
Year 3		3,600		0.40		1,440	7,840	2,160
Year 4		2,160		S/L**		1,080	8,920	1,080
Year 5		1,296		S/L		1,080	10,000	-0-

*$10,000 divided by 5 years equals 0.20 times 2 (double) equals 0.40 factor.
**Double-Declining Balance changes to straight-line method when straight-line yields a higher depreciation. (See Table 9-A–3.)

The computation continues as follows:

- For Year 1, $10,000 times 0.40 equals $4,000 Year 1 depreciation expense. Accumulated depreciation for Year 1 also equals $4,000. The accumulated depreciation of $4,000 is subtracted from the $10,000 cost to arrive at the net remaining undepreciated cost, or net book value, of $6,000 at the end of Year 1.
- For Year 2, the factor of 0.40 is multiplied times the $6,000 net book value to equal $2,400 Year 2 depreciation expense. The Year 2 depreciation of $2,400 is added to the accumulated depreciation for a total of $6,400 ($4,000 plus $2,400 equals $6,400). The $6,400 is subtracted from the $10,000 cost to arrive at the net remaining undepreciated cost, or net book value, of $3,600 at the end of Year 2.
- For Year 3, the factor of 0.40 is multiplied times the $3,600 net book value to equal $1,440 Year 3 depreciation expense. The Year 3 depreciation of $1,440 is added to the accumulated depreciation for a total of $7,840 ($6,400 plus $1,440 equals $7,840). The $7,840 is subtracted from the $10,000 cost to arrive at the net remaining undepreciated cost, or net book value, of $2,160 at the end of Year 3.

The declining balance method has a peculiarity in that it switches back to the straight-line method at the point where the straight-line computation yields a higher annual depreciation than does the declining balance computation. Thus, as we arrive at Year 4 in this example, we must test the double-declining computation against the straight-line computation.

- To compute Year 4 double declining, the factor of 0.40 is multiplied times the net book value of $2,160 to arrive at a DDB of $864.
- To compute a comparative Year 4 by the straight-line method, the remaining net book value of $2,160 is divided by the remaining years of useful life, which in this case would be 2 years. Thus $2,160 divided by 2 years equals straight-line depreciation per year for Year 4 and for Year 5 of $1,080 per year.
- The Year 4 straight-line method is greater ($1,080) than the Year 4 DDB ($864). Thus the switch to straight line is made for the remaining Year 4 and Year 5, as illustrated in Table 9-A–2.

The point at which the straight-line method overtakes the declining balance method varies, of course, with the method and with the number of years of useful life. **Table 9-A–3** illustrates

Table 9-A–3 Declining Balance Rates by Property Class

Property Class	Method	Declining Balance Rate	Year*
3-year	200% DB	66.667%	3rd
5-year	200% DB	40.000%	4th
7-year	200% DB	28.571%	5th
10-year	200% DB	20.00%	7th
15-year	150% DB	10.0%	7th
20-year	150% DB	7.5%	9th

*Indicates the first year for which the straight-line depreciation method gives an equal or greater deduction.
Reproduced from Internal Revenue Service, Publication 964, "How to Depreciate Property," p. 43.

the first year for which the straight-line depreciation method gives an equal or greater deduction. (Note that the Five-year Property Class [or Useful Life Class] for 200% declining balance [or double-declining balance] shows the fourth year as the point at which the switch to straight line would be made. This is consistent with our example in Table 9-A–2.)

150% Declining Balance Method

The 150% Declining Balance (150% DB) accelerated depreciation method also computes depreciation by multiplying the asset's net book value at the beginning of each year by a constant percentage, or factor. In the case of 150% DB, however, the constant factor is half again or 150% of the straight-line rate.

Table 9-A–4 illustrates the computation for each year of a five-year useful life with no salvage value. The 150% DB factor is computed as follows:

- $10,000 cost of the fixed asset divided by the asset's useful life of 5 years equals 20% or a factor of 0.20.
- Multiply the 0.20 by 150% (or half again) to arrive at the 0.30 150% DB factor.

The 150% DB computation follows the same pattern as the double-declining example just described, with two exceptions:

- The factor applied is 0.30 per year, as just explained.
- The 150% DB switches to straight line in Year 3 instead of Year 4 as in the previous example.

Units of Service or Units of Production (UOP) Depreciation Method

The Units of Service or Units of Production (UOP) method computes depreciation by assigning a fixed amount of depreciation to each unit of service or output that is produced by equipment. The "Units of Production" is a manufacturer's term for manufacturing, or producing, a product. "Units of Service" more properly describes the medical equipment providing services in healthcare organizations.

Instead of a useful life in years, equipment depreciated by the UOP method is assigned a fixed total amount of units of service. This fixed amount is the overall total for the life of the equipment. Then the number of units of service actually provided each year is depreciated.

Table 9-A–5 illustrates the UOP method. The depreciation per unit of service is computed as follows:

- The total depreciable units of service over 5 years are determined to be 5,000 units. The equipment cost to be depreciated of $10,000 is divided by 5,000 units to arrive at depreciation of $2.00 per unit.
- Units of Service in Year 1 total 1,000. Thus 1,000 units times $2.00 per unit equals $2,000 Year 1 depreciation.
- Units of Service in Year 2 total 900. Thus 900 units times $2.00 per unit equals $1,800 Year 2 depreciation.

The computation continues in this manner until the total 5,000 units of service are exhausted. The equipment is then fully depreciated.

Table 9-A–4 150% Declining Balance Depreciation: Five-Year Life with No Salvage Value

	Cost (to Be Depreciated)	Depreciation Computation					Accumulated Depreciation (Reserve for Depreciation)	Net Remaining Undepreciated Cost (Net Book Value)
		Carry-Forward Book Value (for Computation)	×	150% Declining Balance Factor	=	Annual Depreciation Expense		
	$10,000							
Year 1		$10,000		0.30*		$3,000	$3,000	$7,000
Year 2		7,000		0.30		2,100	5,100	4,900
Year 3		4,900		S/L**		1,663	6,733	3,267
Year 4		3,267		S/L		1,633	8,366	1,634
Year 5		1,634		S/L		1,634	10,000	-0-

*$10,000 divided by 5 years equals 0.20 times half again (150%) equals 0.30 factor.
**150% Declining Balance changes to straight-line method when straight-line yields a higher depreciation.

Table 9-A-5 Units of Service (Units of Production) Depreciation: Five-Years of Service with No Salvage Value

Depreciation Computation

	Cost (to Be Depreciated)	Units of Service per Year	×	Depreciation per Unit	=	Annual Depreciation Expense	Accumulated Depreciation (Reserve for Depreciation)	Net Remaining Undepreciated Cost (Net Book Value)
	$10,000							
Year 1		$1,000		$2.00*		$2,000	$2,000	$8,000
Year 2		900		2.00		1,800	3,800	6,200
Year 3		800		2.00		1,600	5,400	4,600
Year 4		1,100		2.00		2,200	7,600	2,400
Year 5		1,200		2.00		2,400	10,000	-0-
Total Units		5,000						

*$10,000 divided by total units (5,000) equals depreciation per unit of $2.00.

Staffing: Methods, Operations, and Regulations

STAFFING REQUIREMENTS

In most businesses, a position is filled if the employee works five days a week, generally Monday through Friday. But in health care, many positions must be filled, or covered, all seven days of the week. Furthermore, in most businesses, a position is filled for that day if the employee works an eight-hour day—from 9:00 AM to 5:00 PM, for example. But in health care, many positions must also be filled, or covered, 24 hours a day. The patients need care on Saturday and Sunday, as well as Monday through Friday, and patients need care around the clock, 24 hours a day.

Thus, healthcare employees work in shifts. The shifts are often 8-hour shifts, because three such shifts times 8 hours apiece equals 24-hour coverage. Some facilities have gone to 12-hour shifts. In their case, two 12-hour shifts equal 24-hour coverage. The manager is responsible for seeing that an employee is present and working for each position and for every shift required for that position. Therefore, it is necessary to understand and use the staffing measurement known as the full-time equivalent (FTE). Two different approaches are used to compute FTEs: the annualizing method and the scheduled-position method. Full-time equivalent is a measure to express the equivalent of an employee (annualized) or a position (staffed) for the full time required. We examine both methods in this chapter.

FTEs FOR ANNUALIZING POSITIONS

Why Annualize?

Annualizing is necessary because each employee that is eligible for benefits (such as vacation days) will not be on duty for the full number of hours paid for by the organization.

Progress Notes

After completing this chapter, you should be able to

1. Understand the difference between productive time and nonproductive time.
2. Understand computing full-time equivalents to annualize staff positions.
3. Understand computing full-time equivalents to fill a scheduled position.
4. Tie cost to staffing.
5. Describe regulatory requirements that affect staffing.

Annualizing thus allows the full cost of the position to be computed through a burden approach. In the burden approach, the net hours desired are inflated, or burdened, in order to arrive at the gross number of paid hours that will be needed to obtain the desired number of net hours on duty from the employee.

Productive Versus Nonproductive Time

Productive time actually equates to the employee's net hours on duty when performing the functions in his or her job description. Nonproductive time is paid-for time when the employee is not on duty: that is, not producing and therefore "nonproductive." Paid-for vacation days, holidays, personal leave days, and/or sick days are all nonproductive time.[1]

Exhibit 10–1 illustrates productive time (net days when on duty) versus nonproductive time (additional days paid for but not worked). In Exhibit 10–1, Bob, the security guard, is paid for 260 days per year (total paid days) but works for only 235 days per year. The 235 days are productive time, and the remaining 25 days of holidays, sick days, vacation days, and education days are nonproductive time.

Exhibit 10–1 Metropolis Clinic Security Guard Staffing

The Metropolis laboratory area has its own security guard from 8:30 AM to 4:30 PM seven days per week. Bob, the security guard for the clinic area, is a full-time Metropolis employee.

He works as follows:

1. The area assigned to Bob is covered seven days per week for every week of the year. Therefore,

Total days in business year	364

2. Bob doesn't work on weekends   (104)

(2 days per week × 52 weeks = 104 days)

Bob's paid days total per year amount to   260

(5 days per week × 52 weeks = 260 days)

3. During the year Bob gets paid for:

Holidays	9
Sick days	7
Vacation days	7
Education days	2
	(25)

4. Net paid days Bob actually works   235

Jim, a police officer, works part time as a security guard for the Metropolis laboratory area. Jim works on the days when Bob is off, as follows:

Weekends	104
Bob's holidays	9
Bob's sick days	7
Bob's vacation days	7
Bob's education days	2
	129

5. Paid days Jim works   129

6. Total days lab area security guard position is covered   364

FTE for Annualizing Positions Defined

For purposes of annualizing positions, the definition of FTE is as follows: the equivalent of one full-time employee paid for one year, including both productive and nonproductive (vacation, sick, holiday, education, etc.) time. Two employees each working half-time for one year would be the same as one FTE.

Staffing Calculations to Annualize Positions

Exhibit 10–2 contains a two-step process to perform the staffing calculation by the annualizing method. The first step computes the net paid days worked. In this step, the number of paid days per year is first arrived at; then paid days not worked are deducted to arrive at net paid days worked. The second step of the staffing calculation converts the net paid days worked to a factor. In the example in Exhibit 10–2, the factor averages out to about 1.6.

This calculation is for a 24-hour around-the-clock staffing schedule. Thus, the 364 in the step 2 formula equates to a 24-hour staffing expectation. **Exhibit 10–3** illustrates such a master staffing plan.

Exhibit 10–2 Basic Calculation for Annualizing Master Staffing Plan

Step 1: How Many Net Paid Days Are Worked?
- (a) A *business year* has 364 days.
- (b) In this example the employee works five days per week. The other two days off are not paid for. Thus two days off per week times 52 weeks equals 104 *nonpaid days.*
- (c) Therefore, the number of *paid days per year* equals 364 less 104, or 260 days.
- (d) But not all paid days per year are worked. In this example, each employee (RN, LPN, and Nurse Assistant [NA]) receives 35 *personal leave days.* (The personal leave days are intended to include holidays, sick leave, and vacation days.)
- (e) In addition, these employees are entitled to *continuing professional education (CPE) days.* These are also paid days not worked, as follows: RNs = 5 days; LPNs = 3 days; NAs = 2 days.
- (f) Therefore the *net paid days worked* are as follows:

$$RN = 260 \text{ days } (35) (5) = 220$$
$$LPN = 260 \text{ days } (35) (3) = 222$$
$$NA = 260 \text{ days } (35) (2) = 223$$

Step 2: How Are Net Paid Days Worked Converted to a Factor?
The factor is calculated by dividing total days in the business year (364) by the net paid days worked, as follows:

$$RN = 364/220 = 1.6545$$
$$LPN = 364/222 = 1.6396$$
$$NA = 364/223 = 1.6323$$

Courtesy of J. J. Baker and R. W. Baker, Dallas, Texas.

Exhibit 10–3 Master Staffing Plan for Nursing Unit

8-Hour Shifts	RNs	LPNs	NAs
Day Shift	3	1	6
Evening Shift	2	2	5
Night Shift	1	2	2
24-Hour Total	6	5	13

Courtesy of J.J. Baker and R.W. Baker, Dallas, Texas.

NUMBER OF EMPLOYEES REQUIRED TO FILL A POSITION: ANOTHER WAY TO CALCULATE FTES

Why Calculate by Position?

The calculation of number of FTEs by the scheduled-position method—in other words, to fill a position—is used in controlling, planning, and decision making. **Exhibit 10–4** sets out the schedule and the FTE computation. A summarized explanation of the calculation in Exhibit10–4 is as follows. One full-time employee (as shown) works 40 hours per week. One 8-hour shift per day times 7 days per week equals 56 hours on duty. Therefore, to cover 7 days per week, or 56 hours, requires 1.4 times a 40-hour employee (56 hours divided by 40 hours equals 1.4), or 1.4 FTEs.

Staffing Calculations to Fill Scheduled Positions

The term "staffing," as used here, means the assigning of staff to fill scheduled positions. The staffing measure used to compute coverage is also called the FTE. It measures what proportion of one single full-time employee is required to equate the hours required (i.e., full-time equivalent) for a particular position. For example, the cast room has to be staffed 24 hours a day, 7 days a week because it supports the emergency room, and therefore has to provide service at any time. In this example, the employees are paid for an 8-hour shift. The three shifts required to fill the position for 24 hours are called the day shift (7:00 AM to 3:00 PM), the evening shift (3:00 PM to 11:00 PM), and the night shift (11:00 PM to 7:00 AM).

Exhibit 10–4 Staffing Requirements Example

Emergency Department Scheduling for Eight-Hour Shifts:

24-Hour Scheduling

Position:	Shift 1 Day	Shift 2 Evening	Shift 3 Night	=	Total
Emergency Room Intake	1	1	1	=	3 8-hour shifts
To Cover Position 7 Days per Week Equals FTEs of:	1.4	1.4	1.4	=	4.2 FTEs

One full-time employee works 40 hours per week. One 8-hour shift per day times 7 days per week equals 56 hours on duty. Therefore, to cover 7 days per week or 56 hours requires 1.4 times a 40-hour employee (56 hours divided by 40 hours equals 1.4), or 1.4 FTEs.

One 8-hour shift times 5 days per week equals a 40-hour work week. One 40-hour work week times 52 weeks equals a person-year of 2,080 hours. Therefore, one person-year of 2,080 hours equals a full-time position filled for one full year. This measure is our baseline.

It takes seven days to fill the day shift cast room position from Monday through Sunday, as required. Seven days is 140% of five days (seven divided by five equals 140%), or, expressed another way, is 1.4. The FTE for the day shift cast room position is 1.4. If a seven-day schedule is required, the FTE will be 1.4.

This method of computing FTEs uses a basic 40-hour work week (or a 37-hour work week, or whatever is the case in the particular institution). The method computes a figure that will be necessary to fill the position for the desired length of time, measuring this figure against the standard basic work week. For example, if the standard work week is 40 hours and a receptionist position is to be filled for just 20 hours per week, then the FTE for that position would be 0.5 FTE (20 hours to fill the position divided by a 40-hour standard work week). **Table 10–1** illustrates the difference between a standard work year at 40 hours per week and a standard work year at 37.5 hours per week.

Tying Cost to Staffing

In the case of the annualizing method, the factor of 1.6 already has this organization's vacation, holiday, sick pay, and other nonproductive days accounted for in the formula (review Exhibit 10–2 to check out this fact). Therefore, this factor is multiplied times the base hourly rate (the net rate) paid to compute cost.

In the case of the scheduled-position method, however, the FTE figure of 1.4 will be multiplied times a burdened hourly rate. The burden on the hourly rate reflects the vacation, holiday, sick pay, and other nonproductive days accounted for in the formula (review Exhibit 10–4 to see the difference). The scheduled-position method is often used in the forecasting of new programs and services.

Actual cost is attached to staffing in the books and records through a subsidiary journal and a basic transaction record. **Exhibit 10–5** illustrates a subsidiary journal in which employee hours worked for a one-week period are recorded. Both regular and overtime hours are noted.

Table 10–1 Calculations to Staff the Operating Room

Job Position	No. of FTEs	No. of Annual Hours Paid at 2,080 Hours*	No. of Annual Hours Paid at 1,950 Hours**
Supervisor	2.2	4,576	4,290
Techs	3.0	6,240	5,850
RNs	7.7	16,016	15,015
LPNs	1.2	2,496	2,340
Aides, orderlies	1.0	2,080	1,950
Clerical	1.2	2,496	2,340
Totals	16.3	33,904	31,785

*40 hours per week × 52 weeks = 2,080.

**37.5 hours per week × 52 weeks = 1,950.

Exhibit 10–5 Example of a Payroll Register

Metropolis Health System
Payroll Register

Week Ended   June 10, ___

| Employee No. | Name | Hours Worked | | | Rate | Base Pay | Overtime Premiums | Gross Earnings | Deductions | | | Net Pay |
		Regular	Overtime	Total					Federal Income Tax	Social Security	Medicare Tax	
1071	J.F. Green	40	2	42	14.00	588.00	14.00	602.00	90.30	37.32	8.73	465.65
1084	C.B. Brown	40		40	14.00	560.00		560.00	84.00	34.72	8.62	432.66
1090	K.D. Grey	40		40	10.00	400.00		400.00	60.00	24.80	6.16	309.04
1092	R.N. Black	40	5	45	10.00	450.00	25.00	475.00	71.25	29.45	6.89	367.41

Courtesy of Resource Group, Ltd., Dallas, Texas.

The hourly rate, base pay, and overtime premiums are noted, and gross earnings are computed. Deductions are noted and deducted from gross earnings to compute the net pay for each employee in the final column.

Exhibit 10–6 illustrates a time card for one employee for a week-long period. This type of record, whether it is generated by a time clock or an electronic entry, is the original record upon which the payroll process is based. Thus, it is considered a basic transaction record. In this example, time in and time out are recorded daily. The resulting regular and overtime hours are recorded separately for each day worked. Although the appearance of the time card may vary, and it may be recorded within a computer instead of on a hard copy, the essential transaction is the same: this recording of daily time is where the payroll process begins.

Exhibit 10–7 represents an emergency department staffing report. Actual productive time is shown in columns 1 and 2, with regular time in column 1 and overtime in column 2. Nonproductive time is shown in column 3, and columns 1, 2, and 3 are totaled to arrive at column 4, labeled "Total [actual] Hours." The final actual figure is the FTE figure in column 5.

The report is biweekly and thus is for a 2-week period. The standard work week amounts to 40 hours, so the biweekly standard work period amounts to 80 hours. Note the first line

Exhibit 10–6 Example of a Time Record

Metropolis Health System
Time Card

Employee __J.F. Green__   No. __1071__

Department __3__   Week ending __June 10__

Day	Regular				Overtime		Hours	
	In	Out	In	Out	In	Out	Regular	Overtime
Monday	8:00	12:01	1:02	5:04			8	
Tuesday	7:56	12:00	12:59	5:03	6:00	8:00	8	2
Wednesday	7:57	12:02	12:58	5:00			8	
Thursday	8:00	12:00	1:00	5:01			8	
Friday	7:59	12:01	1:01	5:02			8	
Saturday								
Sunday								
				Total regular hours			40	
				Total overtime				2

Courtesy of Resource Group, Ltd., Dallas, Texas.

Exhibit 10–7 Comparative Hours Staffing Report

PR 2301

Dept. No. 3421
Emergency Room

Biweekly Comparative Hours Report
for the Payroll Period Ending Sept. 20, _____

| | | Actual | | | | | Budget | | | | Variance | | |
	Job Code	Regular Time (1)	Overtime (2)	Non-Productive (3)	Total Hours (4)	FTEs (5)	Productive (6)	Non-Productive (7)	Total Hours (8)	FTEs (9)	Number Hours (10)	Number FTEs (11)	Percent (12)
Mgr Nursing Service	11075	80	0	0	80	1.0	69.8	10.2	80	1	0	0	0
Supv Charge Nurse	11403	383.2	0.1	79	462.3	5.8	456	64	520	6.5	57.7	0.7	11.1%
Medical Assistant	12007	6.2	0		6.2	0.1	0	0	0	0	-6.2	-0.1	100.0%
Staff RN	13401	2010.5	32.8	285.8	2329.1	29.1	2012.8	240.8	2253.6	28.2	-75.5	-0.9	-3.4%
Relief Charge Nurse	13403	81.9	4.3	0	86.2	1.1	0	0	0	0	-86.2	-1.1	100.0%
Orderly/Transporter	15483	203.8	38	20	261.8	3.3	279.8	35.3	315.1	3.9	53.3	0.6	16.9%
ER Tech	22483	244.6	27.5	67.9	340	4.3	336.2	34.5	370.7	4.6	30.7	0.3	8.3%
Secretary	22730	58.1	0	0	58.1	0.7	50.5	5.9	56.4	0.7	-1.7	0.0	-3.0%
Unit Coordinator	22780	555.1	35.6	74.9	665.6	8.3	505.4	53.8	559.2	7	-106.4	-1.3	-19.0%
Preadmission Testing Clerk	22818	0	6.5	0	6.5	0.1	0	0	0	0	-6.5	-0.1	100.0%
Patient Registrar	22873	617.5	78.6	105.7	801.8	10.0	718.2	57.8	776	9.7	-25.8	-0.3	-3.3%
Lead Patient Registrar	22874	0	0	0	0	0.0	73.8	6.2	80	1	80.0	1.0	100.0%
Patient Registrar (weekend)	22876	36.7	0	0	36.7	0.5	0	0	0	0	-36.7	-0.5	100.0%
Overtime	29998	0	0	0	0	0.0	38.5	0	38.5	0.5	38.5	0.5	100.0%
Department Totals		4277.6	223.4	633.3	5134.3	64.3	4541	508.5	5049.5	63.1	-84.8	-1.2	0.0

Courtesy of Resource Group, Ltd., Dallas, Texas.

item, which is for the manager of the emergency department nursing service. The actual hours worked in column 4 amount to 80, and the actual FTE figure in column 5 is 1.0. We can tell from this line item that the second method of computing FTEs—the FTE computation to fill scheduled positions—has been used in this case. Columns 7 through 9 report budgeted time and FTEs, and columns 10 through 12 report the variance in actual from budget. The budget and variance portions of this report structure will be more thoroughly discussed in the chapter about operating budgets.

In summary, hours worked and pay rates are essential ingredients of staffing plans, budgets, and forecasts. Appropriate staffing is the responsibility of the manager.

REGULATORY REQUIREMENTS REGARDING STAFFING

As if staffing a healthcare organization wasn't complex enough because of the typical need to cover 24 hours a day, there are regulatory requirements that impact staffing configurations.

The IMPACT Act Staffing Report Requirements

This complexity is no more apparent than in the new (2016) skilled nursing facility staffing requirements embodied in P.L. 113-185, the Improving Medicare Post-Acute Care Transformation Act of 2014 (the IMPACT Act). In essence, the Centers for Medicare and Medicaid Services (CMS) are now seeking improved reporting on nursing home staffing.

Regulatory Specifics About Staffing Reports

The first set of regulatory specifics is contained in the Final Rule for the FY 2016 Prospective Payment System under the heading "Staffing Data Collection."[2] The regulation had its genesis in the Affordable Care Act, P.L. 111-148. Section 1128I(g) specifies that a facility is required to "electronically submit…direct care staffing information, including information for agency and contract staff, based on payroll and other verifiable and auditable data in a uniform format according to specifications established by the Secretary in consultation with (stakeholders)."[3]

The direct care staffing information submitted to CMS then appears on the Nursing Home Compare website.[4] Note the phrase "verifiable and auditable data." Previously, facilities could self-report such staffing information, but this information did not have to be "verifiable and auditable."

Additional Reporting Requirements

Additional requirements are also spelled out in the statute. Specifications in the CMS regulation state that the following must be included in the report:

- The category of work a certified employee performs (such as whether the employee is a registered nurse, licensed practical nurse, licensed vocational nurse, certified nursing assistant, therapist, or other medical personnel)
- Resident census data
- Information on resident case mix
- Information on employee turnover and tenure
- The hours of care provided by each category of certified employees per resident per day[5]

This information must be reported on a regular basis. Also, information for agency and contract staff must be kept separate from the information submitted for employee staffing.

We draw your attention to the two phrases requiring the following: the category of work a certified employee performs and the hours of care provided by each category of certified employees per resident per day. What can your organization do to ensure compliance with these requirements that is both "verifiable and auditable"?

For example, which documentation within your system should be retained? To what level of detail should it be retained, and for how long? What guidance can be found, either from government sources or from your professional organizations? And if such guidance is made available, how do your own records compare? What adjustments or additions should be made?

We can also expect that these specific requirements will evolve over time. While the first set of regulatory specifics is set out within the FY 2016 PPS final rule, we can expect that refinements to these requirements will be forthcoming over each succeeding year, as experience provides evidence for the needed adjustments.

Funding Provided for Report Improvements

The IMPACT Act provides a one-time allocation of $11 million to implement these improvements to the Nursing Home Compare website.[6] (Additional details about the Nursing Home Compare website and its 5-Star Rating appear in the chapter titled, "Standardizing Measures and Payment in Post-Acute Care: New Requirements".)

From a public domain perspective, Medicare.gov/Nursing Home Compare serves as a useful reference enabling consumers to assess staffing results among Medicare and Medicaid participating nursing homes. Staffing data are submitted by the facility and are adjusted for the needs of nursing home residents.

State Certificate-of-Need (CON) Laws and Regulations

Additional regulatory sources have had an impact on staffing. Central to health planning in the United States are Certificate-of-Need (CON) regulations. To place CON in its proper context, a brief overview of health planning is in order.

Health Planning Background

Shortly after Medicare was enacted into law in 1965, the Comprehensive Health Planning and Services Act (CHP) was passed in 1966. It was noteworthy insofar as it encouraged states to use health planning to remedy geographic disparities in access to care. This was an application of planning that went beyond just allocating funds for hospital construction as in the historically important Hospital Survey and Construction Act of 1946, popularly known as the Hill–Burton Act.[7]

Planning was carried out by state-level CHP-A agencies and local CHP-B agencies. The former was charged with developing a statewide, comprehensive plan for the delivery of health services in each state; the latter were responsible for assessing the health-services needs of populations in their designated areas, determining the availability of resources, and developing a plan that specified what was required to meet those needs.[8]

While it is beyond the scope of this text to analyze in depth why the CHP program didn't deliver as promised, suffice it to say that it had no resource development component. Resources that were necessary to meet a community's needs had to be sought outside the CHP program's parameters. In effect, then, CHP's impact on staffing was immeasurable.

Congress sought to rectify CHP's shortcomings by enacting the National Health Planning and Resources Development Act in 1974. The Act created state-level organizations that were charged with developing and implementing the state health plan. Operationally, though, it was the health systems agencies (HSAs), local organizations, that served a regulatory function. They were charged with developing annual plans to improve health services in their regions.[9]

The Certificate-of-Need (CON) Program

The regulatory leverage that states used to act on proposals for changes in health services was (and is) the Certificate-of-Need (CON) program. The program was originally aimed at hospitals and nursing homes that were permitted to spend funds on services, facilities, and equipment only if a need had been identified in the HSA plan for their region. The basic assumption underlying CON regulation is that excess capacity (in the form of facility overbuilding) directly results in healthcare price inflation.[10] The 1974 law required all 50 states to have a structure in place involving the submitting of proposals and obtaining approval from a state health planning agency.

In 1986, the National Health Planning and Resources Development Act was repealed, along with its federal funding. Despite numerous changes since, 36 states retain some type of CON program, law, or agency according to the National Conference of State Legislatures.[11] These states tend to concentrate activities on outpatient facilities and long-term care. This is largely due to the trend toward free-standing, physician-owned facilities that constitute an increasing segment of the healthcare market.

How Do CON-Related Regulations Affect Staffing?

State CON-related regulations affect staffing across different types of facilities. For example, if a hospital CON is filed seeking approval for a new surgical wing, staffing needs must be included in the application along with facility and equipment requirements. If a nursing home is seeking to expand its bed capacity, new staff such as RNs, LPNs, and possibly even therapists will be required. If a home care agency is seeking to increase its geographic reach and expand its program capacity, new nursing–related and social work staff will be required.

A prime example of state regulatory requirements on minimum staffing levels in nursing homes may be found in Nursing Home Staffing Standards in State Statutes and Regulations.[12] It depicts minimum staffing standards for skilled nursing or nursing facilities. For example, for every state it lists three variables:

1. A Sufficient Staff Statement (i.e., Licensed to meet the needs of individual residents)
2. Staff Requirement (i.e., RN, LPN/LVN per hour/per bed)
3. Direct Care Requirements (i.e., Two people on duty at all times)

This site is a useful planning tool.

SUMMARY

Staffing operations throughout the U.S. are obviously impacted by regulations about staffing and staffing reports. And desired expansion and related operational issues in 36 states are naturally affected by applicable certificate of need requirements.

INFORMATION CHECKPOINT

What is needed?	The original record of time and the subsidiary journal summary.
Where is it found?	The original record can be found at any check-in point; the subsidiary journal summary can be found with a supervisor in charge of staffing for a unit, division, and so on.
How is it used?	It is reviewed as historical evidence of results achieved. It is also reviewed by managers seeking to perform future staffing in an efficient manner.

KEY TERMS

Certificate of Need (CON)
Full-Time Equivalents (FTEs)
Nonproductive Time
Productive Time
Staffing

DISCUSSION QUESTIONS

1. Are you or your immediate supervisor responsible for staffing?
2. If so, do you use a computerized program?
3. Do you believe a computerized program is better? If so, why?
4. Does your organization report time as "productive" and "nonproductive"?
5. If not, do you believe it should? What do you believe the benefits would be?
6. If your state has certificate-of-need (CON) regulations in place, has your organization made a CON request in the recent past? If so, was it successful? Please describe.

NOTES

1. J. J. Baker, *Prospective Payment for Long-Term Care: An Annual Guide* (Gaithersburg, MD: Aspen Publishers, Inc., 1999).
2. 80 FR 46462 (Aug. 4, 2015).
3. Ibid.
4. "What is Nursing Home Compare?", Medicare.gov, http://www.medicare.gov/nursinghomecompare/About/What-Is-NHC.html
5. 80 FR 46462.
6. SSA Sec. 1819(i).
7. R. I. Field, Health Care Regulation in America: Complexity, Confrontation, and Compromise (New York, NY: Oxford University Press, 2007).

8. P. L. Barton, *Understanding the U.S. Health Services System* (4th ed.) (Chicago, IL: Health Administration Press, 2010).

9. Field, *Health Care Regulation.*

10. Ibid.

11. National Conference of State Legislatures, "CON—Certificate of Need State Laws," http://www.ncsl.org/research/health/con-certificate-of-need-state-laws.aspx, accessed June 9, 2016.

12. Charlene Harrington, "Nursing Home Staffing Standards in State Statutes and Regulations," The National Long-Term Care Ombudsman Resource Center, http://ltcombudsman .org/uploads/files/support/Harrington-state-staffing-table-2010_(1).pdf, accessed June 12, 2016.

# PART IV

Report and Measure Financial Results

Reporting as a Tool

UNDERSTANDING THE MAJOR REPORTS

It is not our intention to convert you into an accountant. Therefore, our discussion of the major financial reports will center on the concept of each report and not on the precise accounting entries that are necessary to make the statement balance. The first concept we will discuss is that of cash versus accrual accounting. In cash basis accounting, a transaction does not enter the books until cash is either received or paid out. In accrual accounting, revenue is recorded when it is earned—not when payment is received—and expenses are recorded when they are incurred—not when they are paid.[1] Most healthcare organizations operate on the accrual basis.

There are four basic financial statements. You can think of them as a set. They include the balance sheet, the statement of revenue and expense, the statement of fund balance or net worth, and the statement of cash flows. The four major reports we are about to examine—the financial statements—have been prepared using the accrual method.

BALANCE SHEET

The balance sheet records what an organization owns, what it owes, and basically, what it is worth (although the terminology uses *fund balance* rather than *worth* or *equity* for nonprofit organizations). The balance sheet balances. That is, the total of what the organization owns—its assets—equals the combined total of what the organization owes and what it is worth—its liabilities and its net worth, or its fund balance. This balancing of the elements in the balance sheet can be visualized as

$$\text{Assets} = \text{Liabilities} + \text{Net Worth/Fund Balance}$$

Progress Notes

After completing this chapter, you should be able to

1. Review a balance sheet and understand its components.
2. Review a statement of revenue and expense and understand its components.
3. Understand the basic concept of cash flows.
4. Know what a subsidiary report is.

Another characteristic of the balance sheet is that it is stated at a particular point in time. A common analogy is that a balance sheet is like a snapshot: it freezes the figures and reports them as of a certain date.

Exhibit 11–1 illustrates these concepts. A single date (not a period of time) is at the top of the statement (this is the snapshot). The clinic balance sheet reflects two years in two columns, with the most current date on the left and the prior period on the right. Total assets for the current left-hand column amount to $963,000. Total liabilities and fund balance also amount to $963,000; the balance sheet balances. The total liabilities amount to $545,000 and the total fund balances amount to $418,000. The total of the two, of course, makes up the $963,000 shown at the bottom of the statement.

Three types of assets are shown: current assets; property, plant, and equipment; and other assets. Current assets are supposed to be convertible into cash within one year—thus "current" assets. Property, plant, and equipment, however, represent long-term assets. Other assets represent noncurrent items.

Two types of liabilities are shown: current liabilities and long-term debt. Current liabilities are those expected to be paid within the next year—thus "current" liabilities. Long-term debt is not due within a year. (In fact, most long-term debt is due over a period of many years.) The amount of long-term debt that will be due within the next year ($52,000) has been subtracted from the long-term debt amount and has been moved up into the current liabilities section. This treatment is consistent with the concept of "current."

Once again, because our intent is not to make an accountant of you, we will not be discussing generally accepted accounting principles (GAAP) either. Financial accounting and the resulting reports intended for third-party use must be prepared in accordance with GAAP. However, managerial accounting for internal purposes in the organization does not necessarily have to adhere to GAAP. One of the requirements of GAAP is that unrestricted fund balances be separated from restricted fund balances on the statements, so you see two appropriate line items (restricted and unrestricted) in the fund balance section.

We should also mention that the standards underlying generally accepted accounting principles within the United States are produced by the Financial Accounting Standards Board (FASB). Sometime in the (probable) near future U.S. publicly held companies may be required to adopt certain international accounting standards as produced by the International Accounting Standards Board (IASB). Benefits would include global comparability and consistency in accounting standards and financial reports while barriers to such adoption include funding, maintenance, application, and governance.[2] Any further discussion of these accounting issues is beyond the scope of this text.

STATEMENT OF REVENUE AND EXPENSE

The formula for a very condensed statement of revenue and expense would look like this:

$$\text{Operating Revenue} - \text{Operating Expenses} = \text{Operating Income}$$

A statement of revenue and expense covers a period of time (rather than one single date or point in time). The concept is that revenue, or inflow, less expenses, or outflow, results in an excess of revenue over expenses if the year has been good, or perhaps an excess of expenses over revenue (resulting in a loss) if the year has been bad.

Exhibit 11–1 Westside Clinic Balance Sheet

Assets	December 31, 20×4		December 31, 20×3	
Current Assets				
Cash and cash equivalents		$190,000		$145,000
Accounts receivable (net)		250,000		300,000
Inventories		25,000		20,000
Prepaid Insurance		5,000		3,000
Total Current Assets		$470,000		$468,000
Property, Plant, and Equipment				
Land	$100,000		$100,000	
Buildings (net)	0		0	
Equipment (net)	260,000		300,000	
Net Property, Plant, and Equipment		360,000		400,000
Other Assets				
Investments	$133,000		$32,000	
Total Other Assets		133,000		32,000
Total Assets		$963,000		$900,000
Liabilities and Fund Balance				
Current Liabilities				
Current maturities of long-term debt	$52,000		$48,000	
Accounts payable and accrued expenses	293,000		302,000	
Total Current Liabilities		$345,000		$350,000
Long-Term Debt	$252,000		$300,000	
Less Current Maturities of Long-Term Debt	−52,000		−48,000	
Net Long-Term Debt		200,000		252,000
Total Liabilities		$545,000		$602,000
Fund Balances				
Unrestricted fund balance	$418,000		$298,000	
Restricted fund balance	0		0	
Total Fund Balances		418,000		298,000
Total Liabilities and Fund Balance		$963,000		$900,000

Exhibit 11–2 sets out the result of operations for two years, with the most current period in the left column. If the balance sheet is a snapshot, then the statement of revenue and expenses is a diary, because it is a record of transactions over the period of a year. Operating

Exhibit 11–2 Westside Clinic Statement of Revenue and Expenses

	For the Year Ending	
Revenue	December 31, 20×4	December 31, 20×3
Net Patient Service Revenue	$2,000,000	$1,850,000
Total Operating Revenue	$2,000,000	$1,850,000
Operating Expenses		
Medical/surgical services	$600,000	$575,000
Therapy services	860,000	806,000
Other professional services	80,000	75,000
Support services	220,000	220,000
General services	65,000	60,000
Depreciation	40,000	40,000
Interest	20,000	24,000
Total Operating Expenses	1,885,000	1,800,000
Income from Operations	$115,000	$50,000
Nonoperating Gains (Losses)		
Interest Income	$5,000	$2,000
Net Nonoperating Gains	5,000	2,000
Revenue and Gains in Excess of Expenses and Losses	$120,000	$52,000
Increase in Unrestricted Fund Balance	$120,000	$52,000

revenues and operating expenses are set out first, with the result being income from operations of $115,000 ($2,000,000 less $1,885,000). Then other transactions are reported; in this case, interest income of $5,000 under the heading "Nonoperating Gains (Losses)." The total of $120,000 ($115,000 plus $5,000) is reported as an increase in fund balance. This figure carries forward to the next major report, known as the statement of changes in fund balance.

STATEMENT OF CHANGES IN FUND BALANCE/NET WORTH

Remember that our formula for a basic statement of revenue and expense looked like this:

$$\text{Operating Revenue} - \text{Operating Expenses} = \text{Operating Income}$$

The excess of revenue over expenses flows back into equity or fund balance through the mechanism of the statement of fund balance/net worth. **Exhibit 11–3** shows a balance at the first of the year, then it adds the excess of revenue over expenses (in the amount of $115,000)

Exhibit 11–3 Westside Clinic Statement of Changes in Fund Balance

	For the Year Ending	
Statement of Changes in Fund Balance	December 31, 20X4	December 31, 20X3
Balance First of Year	$298,000	$246,000
Revenue in Excess of Expenses	115,000	50,000
Interest Income	5,000	2,000
Balance End of Year	$418,000	$298,000

plus some interest income (in the amount of $5,000) to arrive at the balance at the end of the year.

If you refer back to the balance sheet, you will see the $418,000 balance at the end of the year appearing on it. So we can think of the balance sheet, the statement of revenue and expenses, and the statement of changes in fund balance/net worth as locked together, with the statement of changes in fund balance being the mechanism that links the other two statements.

But there is one more major report—the statement of cash flows—and we will examine it next.

STATEMENT OF CASH FLOWS

To perceive why a statement of cash flows is necessary, we must first revisit the concept of accrual basis accounting. If cash is not paid or received when revenues and expenses are entered on the books—the usual situation in accrual accounting—what happens? The other side of the entry for revenues is accounts receivable, and the other side of the entry for expenses is accounts payable. These accounts rest on the balance sheet and have not yet been turned into cash. Another characteristic of accrual accounting is the recognition of depreciation. A capital asset—a piece of equipment, for example—is purchased for $20,000. It has a usable life of five years. So depreciation expense is recognized in each of the five years until the $20,000 is used up, or depreciated. (Land is an exception to this rule: it is never depreciated.) Depreciation is recognized within each year as an expense, but it does not represent a cash expense. This is a concept that now enters into the statement of cash flows.

Exhibit 11–4 presents the current period cash flow. In effect, this statement takes the accrual basis statements and converts them to a cash flow for the period through a series of reconciling adjustments that account for the noncash amounts.

Understanding the cash/noncash concept makes sense of this statement. The starting point is the income from operations, the subtotal from the statement of revenue and expense. Depreciation and interest are added back, and changes in asset and liability accounts, both positive and negative, are recognized. These adjustments account for operating activities. Next, capital and related financing activities are addressed, then investing activities are adjusted. The result is a net increase in cash and cash equivalents of $45,000 in our example. This figure is added to the cash balance at the beginning of the year ($145,000) to arrive at the cash balance at the end of the year ($190,000). Now refer back to the balance sheet, and you will find the cash balance is indeed $190,000. So the fourth major report—the statement of cash flows—interlocks with the other three major reports.

Exhibit 11–4 Westside Clinic Statement of Cash Flows

Statement of Cash Flows	For the Year Ending	
	December 31, 20×4	December 31, 20×3
Operating Activities		
Income from Operations	$115,000	$50,000
Adjustments to reconcile income from operations to net cash flows from operating activities		
Depreciation and amortization	40,000	40,000
Interest expense	20,000	24,000
Changes in asset and liability accounts		
Patient accounts receivable	50,000	−250,000
Inventories	−5,000	−5,000
Prepaid expenses and other assets	−2,000	−1,000
Accounts payable and accrued expenses	−9,000	185,000
Net Cash Flow from Operating Activities	$209,000	$43,000
Cash Flows from Noncapital Financing Activities	0	0
Cash Flows from Capital and Related Financing Activities		
Acquisition of equipment	$ 0	$ (300,000)
Proceeds from loan for equipment	0	300,000
Interest paid on long-term obligations	−20,000	0
Repayment of long-term obligations	−48,000	0
Net Cash Flows from Capital and Related Financing Activities	−68,000	0
Cash Flows from Investing Activities		
Interest income received	$5,000	$2,000
Investments purchased (net)	−101,000	0
Net Cash Flows from Investing Activities	−96,000	2,000
Net Increase (Decrease) in Cash and Cash Equivalents	$45,000	$45,000
Cash and Cash Equivalents, Beginning of Year	145,000	100,000
Cash and Cash Equivalents, End of Year	$190,000	$145,000

SUBSIDIARY REPORTS

The subsidiary reports are just that; subsidiary to the major reports. These reports support the major reports by providing more detail. For example, patient service revenue totals on the statement of revenue and expenses are often expanded in more detail on a subsidiary report. The same thing is true of operating expense. These reports are called "schedules" instead of "statements"—a sure sign that they are subsidiary reports.

SUMMARY

The four major reports fit together; each makes its own contribution to the whole. A checklist for balance sheet review (**Exhibit 11–5**) and a checklist for review of the statement of revenue and expense (**Exhibit 11–6**) are provided.

Exhibit 11–5 Checklist for the Balance Sheet Review

> 1. What is the date on the balance sheet?
> 2. Are there large discrepancies in balances between the prior year and the current year?
> 3. Did total assets increase over the prior year?
> 4. Did current assets increase, decrease, or stay about the same?
> 5. Did current liabilities increase, decrease, or stay about the same?
> 6. Did land, plant, and equipment increase or decrease significantly over the prior year?
> 7. Did long-term debt increase or decrease significantly over the prior year?

Exhibit 11–6 Checklist for Review of the Statement of Revenue and Expense

> 1. What is the period reported on the statement of revenue and expense?
> 2. Is it one year or a shorter period? If it is a shorter period, why is that?
> 3. Are there large discrepancies in balances between the prior year operations and the current year operations?
> 4. Did total operating revenue increase over the prior year?
> 5. Did total operating expenses increase, decrease, or stay about the same? Is any particular line item unusually large or small?
> 6. Did income from operations increase, decrease, or stay about the same?
> 7. Are there unusual nonoperating gains or losses?
> 8. Did the current year result in an excess of revenue over expense? Is it as much as the prior year?
> 9. Did long-term debt increase or decrease significantly over the prior year?

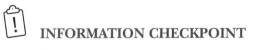 **INFORMATION CHECKPOINT**

What is needed?	A set of financial statements, ideally containing the four major reports plus subsidiary reports for additional detail.
Where is it found?	Possibly in the files of your supervisor or in the finance office or in the office of the administrator.

How is it used?   Study the financial statement to see how they fit together; use the checklists included in this chapter to assist in your review. Understanding how the statements work will give you another valuable managerial tool.

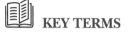

KEY TERMS

Accrual Basis Accounting
Balance Sheet
Cash Basis Accounting
Statement of Cash Flows
Statement of Fund Balance/Net Worth
Statement of Revenue and Expense
Subsidiary Reports

DISCUSSION QUESTIONS

1. Can you give an example of an asset? A liability?
2. Does the concept of revenue less expense equaling an increase in equity or fund balance make sense to you? If not, why not?
3. Are you familiar with the current maturity of long-term debt? What example of it can you give in your own life (either at work or at home)?
4. Do you get a chance to review financial statements at your place of work? Would you like to? Why?

NOTES

1. S. A. Finkler, et al., *Essentials of Cost Accounting for Health Care Organizations*, 3rd ed. (Sudbury MA: Jones & Bartlett Publishers, 2007).
2. K. Tysiac, "Still in Flux: Future of IFRS in U.S. Remains Unclear After SEC report," *Journal of Accountancy* (September 2012), www.journalofaccountancy.com/Issues/2012/Sep/20126059.htm

Financial and Operating Ratios as Performance Measures

12

THE IMPORTANCE OF RATIOS

Ratios are convenient and uniform measures that are widely adopted in healthcare financial management. They are important because they are so widely used, especially because they are used for credit analysis. But a ratio is only a number. It has to be considered within the context of the operation. There is another caveat: ratio analysis should be conducted as a comparative analysis. In other words, one ratio standing alone with nothing to compare it with does not mean very much. When interpreting ratios, the differences between periods must be considered, and the reasons for such differences should be sought. It is a good practice to compare results with equivalent computations from outside the organization—regional figures from similar institutions would be a good example of such outside sources. Caution and good managerial judgment must always be exercised when working with ratios.

Financial ratios basically pull together two elements of the financial statements: one expressed as the numerator and one as the denominator. To calculate a ratio, divide the bottom number (the denominator) into the top number (the numerator). The Case Study that is entitled "Comparative Analysis (Financial Ratios and Benchmarking) Helps Turn Around a Hospital" uses financial ratios as indicators of financial position. We highly recommend that you spend time with this Case Study, as it will add depth and background to the contents of this chapter.

In this chapter we examine liquidity, solvency, and profitability ratios. **Exhibit 12–1** sets out eight basic ratios that are widely used in healthcare organizations: four liquidity types, two solvency types, and two profitability types. All are discussed in this chapter.

Progress Notes

After completing this chapter, you should be able to

1. Understand four types of liquidity ratios.
2. Understand two types of solvency ratios.
3. Understand two types of profitability ratios.
4. Successfully compute ratios.

Exhibit 12–1 Eight Basic Ratios Used in Health Care

Liquidity Ratios

1. Current Ratio

$$\frac{\text{Current Assets}}{\text{Current Liabilities}}$$

2. Quick Ratio

$$\frac{\text{Cash and Cash Equivalents} + \text{Net Receivables}}{\text{Current Liabilities}}$$

3. Days Cash on Hand (DCOH)

$$\frac{\text{Unrestricted Cash and Cash Equivalents}}{\text{Cash Operation Expenses} \div \text{No. of Days in Period (365)}}$$

4. Days Receivables

$$\frac{\text{Net Receivables}}{\text{Net Credit Revenues} \div \text{No. of Days in Period (365)}}$$

Solvency Ratios

5. Debt Service Coverage Ratio (DSCR)

$$\frac{\text{Change in Unrestricted Net Assets (net income)} + \text{Interest, Depreciation, Amortization}}{\text{Maximum Annual Debt Service}}$$

6. Liabilities to Fund Balance

$$\frac{\text{Total Liabilities}}{\text{Unrestricted Fund Balances}}$$

Profitability Ratios

7. Operating Margin (%)

$$\frac{\text{Operating Income (Loss)}}{\text{Total Operating Revenues}}$$

8. Return on Total Assets (%)

$$\frac{\text{EBIT (Earnings Before Interest and Taxes)}}{\text{Total Assets}}$$

Courtesy of Resource Group, Ltd., Dallas, Texas.

LIQUIDITY RATIOS

Liquidity ratios reflect the ability of the organization to meet its current obligations. Liquidity ratios measure short-term sufficiency. As the name implies, they measure the ability of the organization to "be liquid": in other words, to have sufficient cash—or assets that can be converted to cash—on hand.

Current Ratio

The current ratio equals current assets divided by current liabilities. For instance, consider this example:

$$\frac{\text{Current Assets}}{\text{Current Liabilities}} = \frac{\$120,000}{\$60,000} = 2 \text{ to } 1$$

This ratio is considered to be a measure of short-term debt-paying ability. However, it must be carefully interpreted. The standard by which the current ratio is measured is 2 to 1, as computed.

Quick Ratio

The quick ratio equals cash plus short-term investments plus net receivables divided by current liabilities:

$$\frac{\text{Cash and Cash Eqivalents + Net Receivables}}{\text{Current Liabilities}} = \frac{\$65,000}{\$60,000} = 1.08 \text{ to } 1$$

The standard by which the quick ratio is measured is generally 1 to 1. This computation, at 1.08 to 1, is a little better than the standard.

This ratio is considered to be an even more severe test of short-term debt-paying ability (even more than the current ratio). The quick ratio is also known as the acid-test ratio, for obvious reasons.

Days Cash on Hand

The days cash on hand (DCOH) equals unrestricted cash and investments divided by cash operating expenses divided by 365:

$$\frac{\text{Unrestricted Cash and Cash Equivalents}}{\substack{\text{Cash Operating Expenses} \\ \div \text{ No. of Days in Period}}} = \frac{\$330,000}{\$11,000} = 30 \text{ days}$$

There is no concrete standard for this computation.

This ratio indicates cash on hand in relation to the amount of daily operating expense. This example indicates the organization has 30 days worth of operating expenses represented in the amount of (unrestricted) cash on hand.

Days Receivables

The days receivables computation is represented as net receivables divided by net credit revenues divided by 365:

$$\frac{\text{Net Receivables}}{\text{Net Credit Revenue/No. of Days in Period}} = \frac{\$720,000}{\$12,000} = 60 \text{ days}$$

This computation represents the number of days in receivables. The older a receivable is, the more difficult it becomes to collect. Therefore, this computation is a measure of worth as well as performance.

There is no hard and fast rule for this computation because much depends on the mix of payers in your organization. This example indicates that the organization has 60 days worth of credit revenue tied up in net receivables. This computation is a common measure of billing and collection performance. There are many "days receivables" regional and national figures to compare with your own organization's computation.

Figure 12–1 shows how the information for the numerator and the denominator of each calculation is obtained. It takes the Westside Clinic balance sheet and the statement of revenue and expense that were discussed in the preceding chapter and illustrates the source of each figure in the four ratios just discussed. The multiple computations for days cash on hand and for days receivables are further broken down into a three-step process. If you study Figure 12–1 and work with the Case Study entitled "Comparative Analysis (Financial Ratios and Benchmarking) Helps Turn Around a Hospital", you will soon master this process.

SOLVENCY RATIOS

Solvency ratios reflect the ability of the organization to pay the annual interest and principal obligations on its long-term debt. As the name implies, they measure the ability of the organization to "be solvent": in other words, to have sufficient resources to meet its long-term obligations.

Debt Service Coverage Ratio

The debt service coverage ratio (DSCR) is represented as change in unrestricted net assets (net income) plus interest, depreciation, and amortization divided by maximum annual debt service:

$$\frac{\substack{\text{Change in Unrestricted Net Assets (Net Income)} \\ + \text{ Interest, Depreciation, and Amortization}}}{\text{Maximum Annual Debt Service}} = \frac{\$250,000}{\$100,000} = 2.5$$

This ratio is universally used in credit analysis and figures prominently in the Mini-Case Study.

Each lending institution has its particular criteria for the DSCR. Lending agreements often have a provision that requires the DSCR to be maintained at or above a certain figure.

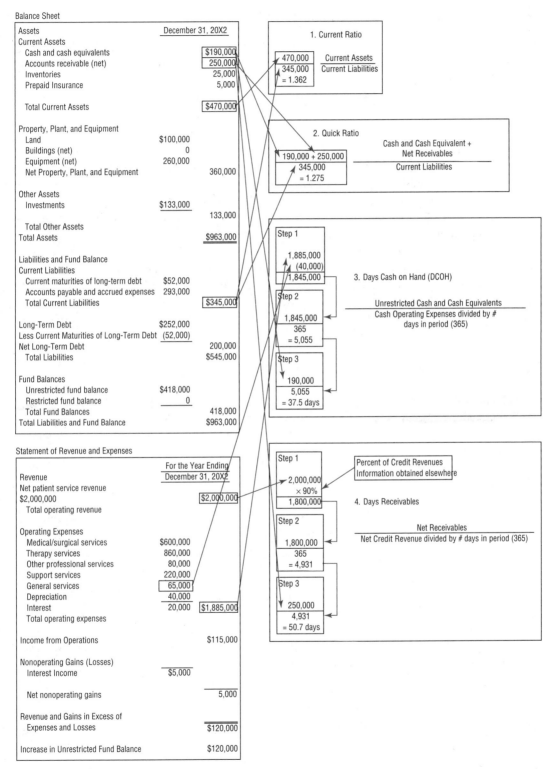

Figure 12–1 Examples of Liquidity Ratio Calculations.
Courtesy of Resource Group, Ltd, Dallas, Texas.

Liabilities to Fund Balance (or Debt to Net Worth)

The liabilities to fund balance or net worth computation is represented as total liabilities divided by unrestricted net assets (i.e., fund balances or net worth) or total debt divided by tangible net worth:

$$\frac{\text{Total Liabilities}}{\text{Unrestricted Fund Balances}} = \frac{\$2,000,000}{\$2,250,000} = 0.80$$

This figure is a quick indicator of debt load.

Another indicator that is more severe is long-term debt to net worth (fund balance), which is computed as long-term debt divided by fund balance. This computation is somewhat equivalent to the quick ratio discussed previously in its restrictiveness to net worth computation.

A mirror image of total liabilities to fund balance is total assets to fund balance, which is computed as total assets divided by fund balance.

Figure 12–2 shows how the information for the numerator and the denominator of each calculation is obtained. This figure again takes the Westside Clinic balance sheet and statement of revenue and expense that were discussed in the preceding chapter and illustrates the source of each figure in the two solvency ratios just discussed, along with each figure in the two profitability ratios still to be discussed. When multiple computations are necessary, they are further broken down into a two-step process.

PROFITABILITY RATIOS

Profitability ratios reflect the ability of the organization to operate with an excess of operating revenue over operating expense. Nonprofit organizations may not call this result a profit, but the measurement ratios are still generally called profitability ratios, whether they are applied to for-profit or nonprofit organizations.

Operating Margin

The operating margin, which is generally expressed as a percentage, is represented as operating income (loss) divided by total operating revenues:

$$\frac{\text{Operating Income (Loss)}}{\text{Total Operating Revenues}} = \frac{\$250,000}{\$5,000,000} = 5.0\%$$

This ratio is used for a number of managerial purposes and also sometimes enters into credit analysis. It is therefore a multipurpose measure. It is so universal that many outside sources are available for comparative purposes. The result of the computation must still be carefully considered because of variables in each period being compared.

Return on Total Assets

The return on total assets is represented as earnings before interest and taxes (EBIT) divided by total assets:

$$\frac{\text{EBIT}}{\text{Total Assets}} = \frac{\$400,000}{\$4,000,000} = 10\%$$

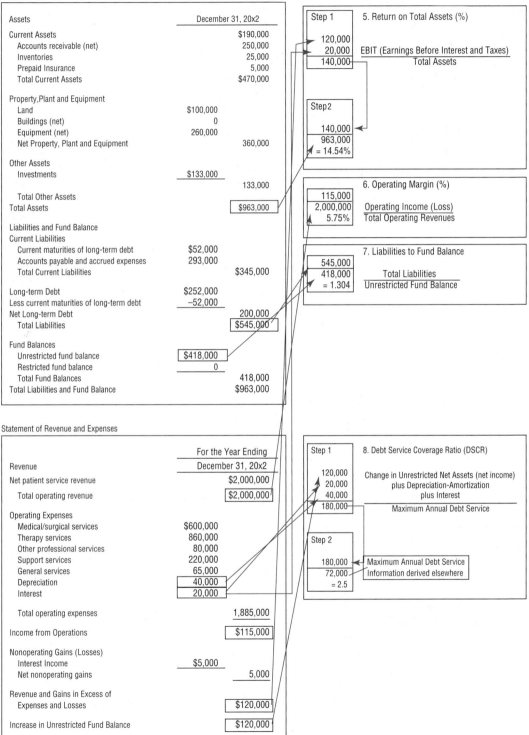

Figure 12–2 Examples of Solvency and Profitability Ratio Calculations.
Courtesy of Resource Group, Ltd, Dallas, Texas.

This is a broad measure in common use. Note the acronym EBIT, as its use is widespread in credit analysis circles. (Some analysts use an alternative computation for Return on Total Assets. They compute this ratio as Net Income divided by Total Assets.)

This concludes the description of solvency and profitability ratios. Again, if you study Figure 12–2 and work with the Case Study entitled "Comparative Analysis (Financial Ratios and Benchmarking) Helps Turn Around a Hospital", you will master this process too.

INFORMATION CHECKPOINT

What is needed?	Reports that use ratios as measures.
Where is it found?	Possibly in your supervisor's file; in the administrator's office; in the chief executive officer's office.
How is it used?	Use as a measure against outside benchmarks (as discussed in this chapter); also use as internal benchmarks for departments/divisions/units; also use as benchmarks at various points over time.

KEY TERMS

Current Ratio
Days Cash on Hand (DCOH)
Days Receivables
Debt Service Coverage Ratio (DSCR)
Liabilities to Fund Balance
Liquidity Ratios
Operating Margin
Profitability Ratios
Quick Ratio
Return on Total Assets
Solvency Ratios

DISCUSSION QUESTIONS

1. Are there ratios in the reports you receive at your workplace?
2. If so, do you use them? How?
3. If not, do you believe ratios should be on the reports? Which reports?
4. Can you think of good outside sources that could be used to obtain ratios for comparative purposes? If the outside information was available, what ratios would you choose to use? Why?

The Time Value of Money

PURPOSE

The purpose of these computations is to evaluate the use of money. The manager has many options as to where resources of the organization should be spent.[1] These calculations provide guides to assist in evaluating the alternatives.

UNADJUSTED RATE OF RETURN

The unadjusted rate of return is a relatively unsophisticated return-on-investment method, and the answer is only an estimate, containing no precision. The computation of the unadjusted rate of return is as follows:

$$\frac{\text{Average Annual Net Income}}{\text{Original Investment Amount}} = \text{Rate of Return}$$

OR

$$\frac{\text{Average Annual Net Income}}{\text{Average Investment Amount}} = \text{Rate of Return}$$

The original investment amount is a matter of record. The average investment amount is arrived at by taking the total unrecovered asset cost at the beginning of estimated useful life plus the unrecovered asset cost at the end of estimated useful life and dividing by two. This method has the advantage of accommodating whatever depreciation method has been chosen by the organization. This method is sometimes called the accountant's method because information necessary for the computation is obtained from the financial statements.

Progress Notes

After completing this chapter, you should be able to

1. Compute an unadjusted rate of return.
2. Understand how to use a present-value table.
3. Compute an internal rate of return.
4. Understand the payback period theory.

PRESENT-VALUE ANALYSIS

The concept of present-value analysis is based on the time value of money. Inherent in this concept is the fact that the value of a dollar today is more than the value of a dollar in the future: thus the "present value" terminology. Furthermore, the further in the future the receipt of your dollar occurs, the less it is worth. Think of a dollar bill dwindling in size more and more as its receipt stretches further and further into the future. This is the concept of present-value analysis.

We learned about compound interest in math class. We learned that

$500 invested at the beginning of year 1
.05   earns interest (assumed) at a rate of 5% for one year,
$525 and we have a compound amount at the end of year 1 amounting to $525,
.05   which earns interest (assumed) at the rate of 5% for another year,
$551 and we have a compound amount at the end of year 2 amounting to $551 (rounded), and so on.

Using this concept, it is possible to restate the present values of $1 to be paid out or received at the end of each of these years. It is possible to use equations, but that is not necessary because we have present-value tables (also called "look-up tables," because one can "look-up" the answer). A present-value table is included at the end of this chapter in Appendix 13-A. All of the figures on the present-value table represent the value of a dollar. The interest rate available on this version of the table is on the horizontal columns and ranges from 1% to 20%. The number of years in the period is on the vertical; in this version of the table, the number of years ranges from 1 to 30. To look up a present value, find the column for the proper interest. Then find the line for the proper number of years. Then trace down the interest column and across the number-of-years line item. The point where the two lines meet is the number (or factor) that represents the value of $1 according to your assumptions. For example, find the year 10 by reading down the left-hand column labeled "Year." Then read across that line until you find the column labeled "10%." The point where the two lines meet is found to be 0.3855. The present value of $1 under these assumptions (10 year/10%) is about 38.5 cents (shown as 0.3855 on the table).

Besides using the look-up table, you can also compute this factor on a business analyst calculator. A reference to business analyst calculators is contained in the Appendix entitled "Web-Based and Software Learning Tools." This can be found at the end of this text. Besides using either the look-up table or the business calculator, you can use a function on your computer spreadsheet to produce the factor. The important point is this: no matter which method you use, you should get the same answer.

Now that you have the present value of $1, by whichever method, it is simple to find the present value of any other number. You merely multiply the other number by the factor you found on the table—or in the calculator or the computer. Say, for example, you want to find the present value of $8,000 under the assumption used above (10 years/10%). You simply multiply $8,000 by the factor of 0.3855 you found in the table. The present value of $8,000 is $3,084 (or $8,000 times 0.3855).

A compound interest table is also included at the end of this chapter in Appendix 13-B, along with a table showing the present value of an annuity of $1.00 in Appendix 13-C, so that you have the tools for computation at your disposal.

INTERNAL RATE OF RETURN

The internal rate of return (IRR) is another return on investment method. It uses a discounted cash flow technique. The internal rate of return is the rate of interest that discounts future net inflows (from the proposed investment) down to the amount invested. The return for a particular investment can therefore be known. The IRR recognizes the elements contained in the previous two methods discussed, but it goes further. It also recognizes the time pattern in which the earnings occur. This means more precision in the computation because IRR calculates from period to period, whereas the other two methods rely on an average investment.

The IRR computation is not very complicated. The computation requires two assumptions and three steps to compute. Assumption 1: Find the initial cost of the investment. Assumption 2: Find the estimated annual net cash inflow the investment will generate. Assumption 3: Find the useful life of the asset (generally expressed in number of years, known as periods for this computation). Step 1: Divide the initial cost of the investment (Assumption 1) by the estimated annual net cash inflow it will generate (Assumption 2). The answer is a ratio. Step 2: Now use the look-up table. Find the number of periods (Assumption 3). Step 3: Look across the line for the number of periods and find the column that approximates the ratio computed in Step 1. That column contains the interest rate representing the rate of return.

How is IRR used? It can take the rate of return obtained and restate it. The restated figure represents the maximum rate of interest that can be paid for capital over the entire span of the investment without incurring a loss. (You can think of that restated figure as a kind of break-even point for investment purposes.) The fact that a rate of return can be computed is the benefit of using an IRR method.

PAYBACK PERIOD

The payback period is the length of time required for the cash coming in from an investment to equal the amount of cash originally spent when the investment was acquired. In other words, if we invested $1,000, under a particular set of assumptions, how long would it take to get our $1,000 back? The payback period concept is used extensively in evaluating whether to invest in a plant and/or equipment. In that case, the question can be restated as follows: If we invested $1,200,000 in a magnetic resonance imaging machine, under a particular set of assumptions, how long would it take to get the hospital's $1,200,000 back?

The assumptions are key to the computation of the payback period. In the case of equipment, volume of usage is a critical assumption and is sometimes very difficult to predict. Therefore, it is prudent to run more than one payback period computation based on different circumstances. Generally a "best case" and a "worst case" run are made.

The computation itself is simple, although it has multiple steps. The trick is to break it into segments.

For example, Doctor Green is considering the purchase of a machine for his office laboratory. It will cost $300,000. He wants to find the payback period for this piece of equipment. To begin, Dr. Green needs to make the following assumptions. Assumption 1: Purchase price of the equipment. Assumption 2: Useful life of the equipment. Assumption 3: Revenue the machine will generate per year. Assumption 4: Direct operating costs associated with earning the revenue. Assumption 5: Depreciation expense per year (computed as purchase price per Assumption 1 divided by useful life per Assumption 2).

Dr. Green's five assumptions are as follows:

1. Purchase price of equipment = $300,000
2. Useful life of the equipment = 10 years
3. Revenue the machine will generate per year = $10,000 after taxes
4. Direct operating costs associated with earning the revenue = $150,000
5. Depreciation expense per year = $30,000

Now that the assumptions are in place, the payback period computation can be made. It is in three steps, as follows:

Step 1: Find the machine's expected net income after taxes.

Revenue (Assumption #3)		$200,000
Less		
Direct operating costs		
(Assumption 4)	$150,000	
Depreciation		
(Assumption 5)	30,000	
		180,000
Net income before taxes		$20,000
Less income taxes of 50%		10,000
Net income after taxes		$10,000

Step 2: Find the net annual cash inflow after taxes the machine is expected to generate (in other words, convert the net income to a cash basis).

Net income after taxes	$10,000
Add back depreciation (a noncash expenditure)	30,000
Annual net cash inflow after taxes	$40,000

Step 3: Compute the payback period.

$$\frac{\text{Investment}}{\text{Net Annual Cash Flow after Taxes}} = \frac{\$300,000 \text{ Machine Cost*}}{\$40,000**} = 7.5 \text{ year Payback Period}$$

*Assumption 1 above
**per Step 2 above

The machine will pay back its investment under these assumptions in 7.5 years.

Payback period computations are very common when equipment purchases are being evaluated. The evaluation process itself is the final subject we consider in this chapter.

EVALUATIONS

Evaluating the use of resources in healthcare organizations is an important task. There are never enough resources to go around, and it is important to use an objective process to evaluate which investments will be made by the organization. A uniform use of a chosen method of evaluating return on investment and/or payback period makes the evaluation process more manageable.

It is important to choose a method that is understood by the managers who will be using it. It is equally important to choose a method that can be readily calculated. If a multiple-page worksheet has to be constructed to set up the assumptions for a modestly priced piece of equipment, the evaluation method is probably too complex. This comment actually touches on the cost-benefit of performing the evaluation.

Sometimes a computer program is chosen that performs a uniform computation of investment returns and payback periods. Such a program is a suitable choice if the managers who use it understand the printouts it produces. Understanding both input and output is key for the managers. In summary, evaluations should be objective, the process should not be too cumbersome, and the responsible managers should understand how the computation was achieved.

RESOURCES

Three look-up tables are presented as appendices to this chapter. They include the following:

A. Present-Value Table (the present value of $1.00)
B. Compound Interest Table (the future value of $1.00)
C. Present Value of an Annuity of $1.00

These tables provide an ongoing resource for you.

INFORMATION CHECKPOINT

What is needed?	Information sufficient to perform these calculations.
Where is it found?	In the files of your supervisor; also in the office of the financial analyst; probably also in the strategic planning office.
How is it used?	To measure the time value of money.

KEY TERMS

Internal Rate of Return
Payback Period
Present-Value Analysis
Time Value of Money
Unadjusted Rate of Return

DISCUSSION QUESTIONS

1. Can you compute an unadjusted rate of return now? Would you use it? Why?
2. Are you able to use the present-value look-up table now? Would you prefer a computer to compute it?

3. Have you seen the payback period concept used in your workplace? If not, do you think it ought to be used? What are your reasons?
4. Have you had a chance to participate in an evaluation of an equipment purchase at your workplace? If so, would you have done it differently if you had supervised the evaluation? Why?

NOTE

1. S. Williamson et al., *Fundamentals of Strategic Planning for Healthcare Organizations* (New York: The Haworth Press, 1997).

APPENDIX 13-A

Present-Value Table
(The Present Value of $1.00)

Year	1%	2%	3%	4%	5%	6%	7%	8%	9%	10%
1	0.9901	0.9804	0.9709	0.9615	0.9524	0.9434	0.9346	0.9259	0.9174	0.9091
2	0.9803	0.9613	0.9426	0.9246	0.9070	0.8900	0.8734	0.8573	0.8417	0.8264
3	0.9706	0.9423	0.9151	0.8890	0.8638	0.8396	0.8163	0.7938	0.7722	0.7513
4	0.9610	0.9238	0.8885	0.8548	0.8227	0.7921	0.7629	0.7350	0.7084	0.6830
5	0.9515	0.9057	0.8626	0.8219	0.7835	0.7473	0.7130	0.6806	0.6499	0.6209
6	0.9420	0.8880	0.8375	0.7903	0.7462	0.7050	0.6663	0.6302	0.5963	0.5645
7	0.9327	0.8706	0.8131	0.7599	0.7107	0.6651	0.6227	0.5835	0.5470	0.5132
8	0.9235	0.8535	0.7894	0.7307	0.6768	0.6274	0.5820	0.5403	0.5019	0.4665
9	0.9143	0.8368	0.7664	0.7026	0.6446	0.5919	0.5439	0.5002	0.4604	0.4241
10	0.9053	0.8203	0.7441	0.6756	0.6139	0.5584	0.5083	0.4632	0.4224	0.3855
11	0.8963	0.8043	0.7224	0.6496	0.5847	0.5268	0.4751	0.4289	0.3875	0.3505
12	0.8874	0.7885	0.7014	0.6246	0.5568	0.4970	0.4440	0.3971	0.3555	0.3186
13	0.8787	0.7730	0.6810	0.6006	0.5303	0.4688	0.4150	0.3677	0.3262	0.2987
14	0.8700	0.7579	0.6611	0.5775	0.5051	0.4423	0.3878	0.3405	0.2992	0.2633
15	0.8613	0.7430	0.6419	0.5553	0.4810	0.4173	0.3624	0.3152	0.2745	0.2394
16	0.8528	0.7284	0.6232	0.5339	0.4581	0.3936	0.3387	0.2919	0.2519	0.2176
17	0.8444	0.7142	0.6050	0.5134	0.4363	0.3714	0.3166	0.2703	0.2311	0.1978
18	0.8360	0.7002	0.5874	0.4936	0.4155	0.3503	0.2959	0.2502	0.2120	0.1799
19	0.8277	0.6864	0.5703	0.4746	0.3957	0.3305	0.2765	0.2317	0.1945	0.1635
20	0.8195	0.6730	0.5537	0.4564	0.3769	0.3118	0.2584	0.2145	0.1784	0.1486
21	0.8114	0.6598	0.5375	0.4388	0.3589	0.2942	0.2415	0.1987	0.1637	0.1351
22	0.8034	0.6468	0.5219	0.4220	0.3418	0.2775	0.2257	0.1839	0.1502	0.1228
23	0.7954	0.6342	0.5067	0.4057	0.3256	0.2618	0.2109	0.1703	0.1378	0.1117
24	0.7876	0.6217	0.4919	0.3901	0.3101	0.2470	0.1971	0.1577	0.1264	0.1015
25	0.7798	0.6095	0.4776	0.3751	0.2953	0.2330	0.1842	0.1460	0.1160	0.0923
26	0.7720	0.5976	0.4637	0.3607	0.2812	0.2198	0.1722	0.1352	0.1064	0.0839
27	0.7644	0.5859	0.4502	0.3468	0.2678	0.2074	0.1609	0.1252	0.0976	0.0763
28	0.7568	0.5744	0.4371	0.3335	0.2552	0.1956	0.1504	0.1159	0.0895	0.0693
29	0.7493	0.5631	0.4243	0.3207	0.2429	0.1846	0.1406	0.1073	0.0822	0.0630
30	0.7419	0.5521	0.4120	0.3083	0.2314	0.1741	0.1314	0.0994	0.0754	0.0573

Year	11%	12%	13%	14%	15%	16%	17%	18%	19%	20%
1	0.9009	0.8929	0.8850	0.8772	0.8696	0.8621	0.8547	0.8475	0.8403	0.8333
2	0.8116	0.7972	0.7831	0.7695	0.7561	0.7432	0.7305	0.7182	0.7062	0.6944
3	0.7312	0.7118	0.6913	0.6750	0.6575	0.6407	0.6244	0.6086	0.5934	0.5787
4	0.6587	0.6355	0.6133	0.5921	0.5718	0.5523	0.5337	0.5158	0.4987	0.4823
5	0.5935	0.5674	0.5428	0.5194	0.4972	0.4761	0.4561	0.4371	0.4190	0.4019
6	0.5346	0.5066	0.4803	0.4556	0.4323	0.4104	0.3898	0.3704	0.3521	0.3349
7	0.4817	0.4523	0.4251	0.3996	0.3759	0.3538	0.3332	0.3139	0.2959	0.2791
8	0.4339	0.4039	0.3762	0.3506	0.3269	0.3050	0.2848	0.2660	0.2487	0.2326
9	0.3909	0.3606	0.3329	0.3075	0.2843	0.2630	0.2434	0.2255	0.2090	0.1938
10	0.3522	0.3220	0.2946	0.2697	0.2472	0.2267	0.2080	0.1911	0.1756	0.1615
11	0.3173	0.2875	0.2607	0.2366	0.2149	0.1954	0.1778	0.1619	0.1476	0.1346
12	0.2858	0.2567	0.2307	0.2076	0.1869	0.1685	0.1520	0.1372	0.1240	0.1122
13	0.2575	0.2292	0.2042	0.1821	0.1625	0.1452	0.1299	0.1163	0.1042	0.0935
14	0.2320	0.2046	0.1807	0.1597	0.1413	0.1252	0.1110	0.0985	0.0876	0.0779
15	0.2090	0.1827	0.1599	0.1401	0.1229	0.1079	0.0949	0.0835	0.0736	0.0649
16	0.1883	0.1631	0.1415	0.1229	0.1069	0.0930	0.0811	0.0708	0.0618	0.0541
17	0.1696	0.1456	0.1252	0.1078	0.0929	0.0802	0.0693	0.0600	0.0520	0.0451
18	0.1528	0.1300	0.1108	0.0946	0.0808	0.0691	0.0592	0.0508	0.0437	0.0376
19	0.1377	0.1161	0.0981	0.0829	0.0703	0.0596	0.0506	0.0431	0.0367	0.0313
20	0.1240	0.1037	0.0868	0.0728	0.0611	0.0514	0.0433	0.0365	0.0308	0.0261
21	0.1117	0.0926	0.0768	0.0638	0.0531	0.0443	0.0370	0.0309	0.0259	0.0217
22	0.1007	0.0826	0.0680	0.0560	0.0462	0.0382	0.0316	0.0262	0.0218	0.0181
23	0.0907	0.0738	0.0601	0.0491	0.0402	0.0329	0.0270	0.0222	0.0183	0.0151
24	0.0817	0.0659	0.0532	0.0431	0.0349	0.0284	0.0231	0.0188	0.0154	0.0126
25	0.0736	0.0588	0.0471	0.0378	0.0304	0.0245	0.0197	0.0160	0.0129	0.0105
26	0.0663	0.0525	0.0417	0.0331	0.0264	0.0211	0.0169	0.0135	0.0109	0.0087
27	0.0597	0.0469	0.0369	0.0291	0.0230	0.0182	0.0144	0.0115	0.0091	0.0073
28	0.0538	0.0419	0.0326	0.0255	0.0200	0.0157	0.0123	0.0097	0.0077	0.0061
29	0.0485	0.0374	0.0289	0.0224	0.0174	0.0135	0.0105	0.0082	0.0064	0.0051
30	0.0437	0.0334	0.0256	0.0196	0.0151	0.0116	0.0090	0.0070	0.0054	0.0042

Compound Interest Table 13-B

Compound Interest of $1.00
(The Future Amount of $1.00)

Year	1%	2%	3%	4%	5%	6%	7%	8%	9%	10%
1	1.010	1.020	1.030	1.040	1.050	1.060	1.070	1.080	1.090	1.100
2	1.020	1.040	1.061	1.082	1.102	1.124	1.145	1.166	1.188	1.210
3	1.030	1.061	1.093	1.125	1.156	1.191	1.225	1.260	1.295	1.331
4	1.041	1.082	1.126	1.170	1.216	1.262	1.311	1.360	1.412	1.464
5	1.051	1.104	1.159	1.217	1.276	1.338	1.403	1.469	1.539	1.611
6	1.062	1.120	1.194	1.265	1.340	1.419	1.501	1.587	1.677	1.772
7	1.072	1.149	1.230	1.316	1.407	1.504	1.606	1.714	1.828	1.949
8	1.083	1.172	1.267	1.369	1.477	1.594	1.718	1.851	1.993	2.144
9	1.094	1.195	1.305	1.423	1.551	1.689	1.838	1.999	2.172	2.358
10	1.105	1.219	1.344	1.480	1.629	1.791	1.967	2.159	2.367	2.594
11	1.116	1.243	1.384	1.539	1.710	1.898	2.105	2.332	2.580	2.853
12	1.127	1.268	1.426	1.601	1.796	2.012	2.252	2.518	2.813	3.138
13	1.138	1.294	1.469	1.665	1.886	2.133	2.410	2.720	3.066	3.452
14	1.149	1.319	1.513	1.732	1.980	2.261	2.579	2.937	3.342	3.797
15	1.161	1.346	1.558	1.801	2.079	2.397	2.759	3.172	3.642	4.177
16	1.173	1.373	1.605	1.873	2.183	2.540	2.952	3.426	3.970	4.595
17	1.184	1.400	1.653	1.948	2.292	2.693	3.159	3.700	4.328	5.054
18	1.196	1.428	1.702	2.026	2.407	2.854	3.380	3.996	4.717	5.560
19	1.208	1.457	1.754	2.107	2.527	3.026	3.617	4.316	5.142	6.116
20	1.220	1.486	1.806	2.191	2.653	3.207	3.870	4.661	5.604	6.728
25	1.282	1.641	2.094	2.666	3.386	4.292	5.427	6.848	8.632	10.835
30	1.348	1.811	2.427	3.243	4.322	5.743	7.612	10.063	13.268	17.449

Year	12%	14%	16%	18%	20%	24%	28%	32%	40%	50%
1	1.120	1.140	1.160	1.180	1.200	1.240	1.280	1.320	1.400	1.500
2	1.254	1.300	1.346	1.392	1.440	1.538	1.638	1.742	1.960	2.250
3	1.405	1.482	1.561	1.643	1.728	1.907	2.067	2.300	2.744	3.375
4	1.574	1.689	1.811	1.939	2.074	2.364	2.684	3.036	3.842	5.062
5	1.762	1.925	2.100	2.288	2.488	2.932	3.436	4.007	5.378	7.594
6	1.974	2.195	2.436	2.700	2.986	3.635	4.398	5.290	7.530	11.391
7	2.211	2.502	2.826	3.185	3.583	4.508	5.629	6.983	10.541	17.086
8	2.476	2.853	3.278	3.759	4.300	5.590	7.206	9.217	14.758	25.629
9	2.773	3.252	3.803	4.435	5.160	6.931	9.223	12.166	20.661	38.443
10	3.106	3.707	4.411	5.234	6.192	8.594	11.806	16.060	28.925	57.665
11	3.479	4.226	5.117	6.176	7.430	10.657	15.112	21.199	40.496	86.498
12	3.896	4.818	5.936	7.288	8.916	13.215	19.343	27.983	56.694	129.746
13	4.363	5.492	6.886	8.599	10.699	16.386	24.759	36.937	79.372	194.619
14	4.887	6.261	7.988	10.147	12.839	20.319	31.691	48.757	111.120	291.929
15	5.474	7.138	9.266	11.074	15.407	25.196	40.565	64.350	155.568	437.894
16	6.130	8.137	10.748	14.129	18.488	31.243	51.923	84.954	217.795	656.840
17	6.866	9.276	12.468	16.672	22.186	38.741	66.461	112.140	304.914	985.260
18	7.690	10.575	14.463	19.673	26.623	48.039	85.071	148.020	426.879	1477.900
19	8.613	12.056	16.777	23.214	31.948	59.568	108.890	195.390	597.630	2216.800
20	9.646	13.743	19.461	27.393	38.338	73.864	139.380	257.920	836.683	3325.300
25	17.000	26.462	40.874	62.669	95.396	216.542	478.900	1033.600	4499.880	25251.000
30	29.960	50.950	85.850	143.371	237.376	634.820	1645.500	4142.100	24201.432	191750.000

Present Value of an Annuity of $1.00

13-C

© LFor/Shutterstock

Periods	2%	4%	6%	8%	10%	12%	14%	16%	18%	20%	Periods
1	0.980	0.962	0.943	0.926	0.909	0.893	0.877	0.862	0.848	0.833	1
2	1.942	1.886	1.833	1.783	1.736	1.690	1.647	1.605	1.566	1.528	2
3	2.884	2.775	2.673	2.577	2.487	2.402	2.322	2.246	2.174	2.107	3
4	3.808	3.630	3.465	3.312	3.170	3.037	2.914	2.798	2.690	2.589	4
5	4.713	4.452	4.212	3.993	3.791	3.605	3.433	3.274	3.127	2.991	5
6	5.601	5.242	4.917	4.623	4.355	4.111	3.889	3.685	3.498	3.326	6
7	6.472	6.002	5.582	5.206	4.868	4.564	4.288	4.039	3.812	3.605	7
8	7.325	6.733	6.210	5.747	5.335	4.968	4.639	4.344	4.078	3.837	8
9	8.162	7.435	6.802	6.247	5.759	5.328	4.946	4.607	4.303	4.031	9
10	8.983	8.111	7.360	6.710	6.145	5.650	5.216	4.833	4.494	4.193	10
15	12.849	11.118	9.712	8.560	7.606	6.811	6.142	5.576	5.092	4.676	15
20	16.351	13.590	11.470	9.818	8.514	7.469	6.623	5.929	5.353	4.870	20
25	19.523	15.622	12.783	10.675	9.077	7.843	6.873	6.097	5.467	4.948	25

PART

V

Tools to Review and Manage Comparative Data

Trend Analysis, Common Sizing, and Forecasted Data

COMMON SIZING

The process of common sizing puts information on the same relative basis. Generally, common sizing involves converting dollar amounts to percentages. If, for example, total revenue of $200,000 equals 100%, then radiology revenue of $20,000 will equal 10% of that total. Converting dollars to percentages allows comparative analysis. In other words, comparing the percentages allows a common basis of comparison. Common sizing is sometimes called "vertical analysis" (because the computation of the percentages is vertical).

Although such comparisons on the basis of percentages can, and should, be performed on your own organization's data, comparisons can also be made between or among various organizations. For example, **Table 14–1** shows how common sizing allows a comparison of liabilities for three different hospitals. In each case, the total liabilities equal 100%. Then the current liabilities of hospital 1, for example, are divided by total liabilities to find the proportionate percentage attributable to that line item (100,000 divided by 500,000 equals 20%; 400,000 divided by 500,000 equals 80%). When all the percentages have been computed, add them to make sure they add to 100%. If you use a computer, computation of these percentages is available as a spreadsheet function.

Another example of comparative analysis is contained in **Table 14-2**. In this case, general services expenses for three hospitals are compared. Once again, the total expense for each hospital becomes 100%, and the relative percentage for each of the four line items is computed ($320,000 divided by $800,000 equals 40% and so on). The advantage of comparative analysis is illustrated by the "laundry" line item, where the dollar amounts are $80,000, $300,000, and $90,000 respectively. Yet each of these amounts is 10% of the total expense for the particular hospital.

Progress Notes

After completing this chapter, you should be able to

1. Understand and use common sizing.
2. Understand and use trend analysis.
3. Understand five types of forecast assumptions.
4. Understand capacity level issues in forecasts.

149

Table 14–1 Common Sizing Liability Information

	Same Year for All Three Hospitals					
	Hospital 1		Hospital 2		Hospital 3	
Current liabilities	$100,000	20%	$500,000	25%	$400,000	80%
Long-term debt	400,000	80%	1,500,000	75%	100,000	20%
Total liabilities	$500,000	100%	$2,000,000	100%	$500,000	100%

Table 14–2 Common Sizing Expense Information

	Same Year for All Three Hospitals					
	Hospital 1		Hospital 2		Hospital 3	
General services expense						
Dietary	$320,000	40%	$1,260,000	42%	$450,000	50%
Maintenance	280,000	35%	990,000	33%	135,000	15%
Laundry	80,000	10%	300,000	10%	90,000	10%
Housekeeping	120,000	15%	450,000	15%	225,000	25%
Total GS expense	$800,000	100%	$3,000,000	100%	$900,000	100%

TREND ANALYSIS

The process of trend analysis compares figures over several time periods. Once again, dollar amounts are converted to percentages to obtain a relative basis for purposes of comparison, but now the comparison is across time. If, for example, radiology revenue was $20,000 this period but was only $15,000 for the previous period, the difference between the two is $5,000. The difference of $5,000 equates to a 33.3% difference because trend analysis is computed on the earlier of the two years: that is, the base year (thus, 5,000 divided by 15,000 equals 33.3%). Trend analysis is sometimes called "horizontal analysis" (because the computation of the percentage of difference is horizontal).

An example of horizontal analysis is contained in **Table 14–3**. In this case, the liabilities of hospital 1 for year 1 are compared with the liabilities of hospital 1's year 2. Current liabilities, for example, were $100,000 in year 1 and are $150,000 in year 2, a difference of $50,000. To arrive at a percentage of difference for comparative purposes, the $50,000 difference is divided by the year 1 base figure of $100,000 to compute the relative differential (thus, 50,000 divided by 100,000 is 50%).

Table 14–3 Trend Analysis for Liabilities

	Hospital 1					
	Year 1		Year 2		Difference	
Current liabilities	$100,000	20%	$150,000	25%	$50,000	50%
Long-term debt	400,000	80%	450,000	75%	50,000	12.5%
Total liabilities	$500,000	100%	$600,000	100%	$100,000	–

Another example of comparative analysis is contained in **Table 14–4**. In this case, general services expenses for two years in hospital 1 are compared. The difference between year 1 and year 2 for each line item is computed in dollars; then the dollar difference figure is divided by the year 1 base figure to obtain a percentage difference for purposes of comparison. Thus, housekeeping expense in year 1 was $120,000, and in year 2 was $180,000, resulting in a difference of $60,000. The difference amounts to 50% ($60,000 difference divided by $120,000 year 1 equals 50%). In Table 14–4, two of the four line items have negative differences: that is, year 2 was less than year 1, resulting in a negative figure. Also, the dollar figure difference is $100,000 when added down (subtract the negative figures from the positive figures; thus, $85,000 plus $60,000 minus $10,000 minus $35,000 equals $100,000). The dollar figure difference is also $100,000 when added across ($900,000 minus $800,000 equals $100,000).

ANALYZING OPERATING DATA

Comparative analysis is an important tool for managers, and it is worth investing the time to become familiar with both horizontal and vertical analysis. Managers will generally analyze their own organization's data most of the time (rather than performing comparisons against other organizations). With that fact in mind, we examine operating room operating data (no pun intended) that incorporate both common sizing and trend analysis.

Table 14–5 sets out 32 expense items. The expense amount in dollars for each line item is set out for the current year in the left column (beginning with $60,517). The expense amount in dollars for each line item is set out for the prior year in the third column of the analysis (beginning with $68,177). The difference in dollars, labeled "Annual Increase (Decrease)," appears in the sixth column of the analysis (beginning with [$7,660]). Vertical analysis has been performed for the current year, and the percentage results appear in the second column (beginning with 4.97%). Vertical analysis has also been performed for the prior year, and those percentage results appear in the fourth column (beginning with 5.70%). Horizontal analysis has been performed on each line item, and those percentage items appear in the far right column (beginning with 12.66%). This table is a good example of the type of operating data reports that managers receive for planning and control purposes.

Comparative analysis is especially important to managers because it creates a common ground to make judgments for planning, control, and decision-making purposes. Using comparative data is the subject of the following chapter.

Table 14–4 Trend Analysis for Expenses

	Hospital 1					
	Year 1		Year 2		Difference	
General services expense						
Dietary	$320,000	40%	$405,000	45%	$85,000	26.5%
Maintenance	280,000	35%	270,000	30%	(10,000)	(3.5)%
Laundry	80,000	10%	45,000	5%	(35,000)	(43.5)%
Housekeeping	120,000	15%	180,000	20%	60,000	50.0%
Total GS expense	$800,000	100%	$900,000	100%	$100,000	–

Table 14–5 Vertical and Horizontal Analysis for the Operating Room

Comparative Expenses

Account	12-Month Current Year	%	12-Month Prior Year	%	Annual Increase (Decrease)	% of Change
Social Security	60,517	4.97	68,177	5.70	(7,660)	−12.66
Pension	20,675	1.70	23,473	1.96	(2,798)	−13.53
Health Insurance	8,422	0.69	18,507	1.55	(10,085)	−119.75
Child Care	4,564	0.37	4,334	0.36	230	5.04
Patient Accounting	155,356	12.76	123,254	10.30	32,102	20.66
Admitting	110,254	9.05	101,040	8.45	9,214	8.36
Medical Records	91,718	7.53	94,304	7.88	(2,586)	−2.82
Dietary	27,526	2.26	35,646	2.98	(8,120)	−29.50
Medical Waste	2,377	0.20	3,187	0.27	(810)	−34.08
Sterile Procedures	78,720	6.46	70,725	5.91	7,995	10.16
Laundry	40,693	3.34	40,463	3.38	230	0.57
Depreciation—Equipment	87,378	7.18	61,144	5.11	26,234	30.02
Depreciation—Building	41,377	3.40	45,450	3.80	(4,073)	−9.84
Amortization—Interest	(5,819)	−0.48	1,767	0.15	(7,586)	130.37
Insurance	4,216	0.35	7,836	0.65	(3,620)	−85.86
Administration	57,966	4.76	56,309	4.71	1,657	2.86
Medical Staff	1,722	0.14	5,130	0.43	(3,408)	−197.91
Community Relations	49,813	4.09	40,618	3.39	9,195	18.46
Materials Management	64,573	5.30	72,305	6.04	(7,732)	−11.97
Human Resources	31,066	2.55	13,276	1.11	17,790	57.27
Nursing Administration	82,471	6.77	92,666	7.75	(10,195)	−12.36
Data Processing	17,815	1.46	16,119	1.35	1,696	9.52
Fiscal	17,700	1.45	16,748	1.40	952	5.38
Telephone	2,839	0.23	2,569	0.21	270	9.51
Utilities	26,406	2.17	38,689	3.23	(12,283)	−46.52
Plant	77,597	6.37	84,128	7.03	(6,531)	−8.42
Environmental Services	32,874	2.70	37,354	3.12	(4,480)	−13.63
Safety	2,016	0.17	2,179	0.18	(163)	−8.09
Quality Management	10,016	0.82	8,146	0.68	1,870	18.67
Medical Staff	9,444	0.78	9,391	0.78	53	0.56
Continuous Quality Improvement	4,895	0.40	0	0.00	4,895	100.00
EE Health	569	0.05	1,513	0.13	(944)	−165.91
Total Allocated	1,217,756	100.00	1,196,447	100.00	21,309	1.75
All Other Expenses	1,211,608	—	—	—	—	—
Total Expense	2,429,364	—	—	—	—	—

IMPORTANCE OF FORECASTS

The dictionary defines "to forecast" as "to calculate or predict some future event or condition, usually as a result of study and analysis of available pertinent data."[1]

From the manager's viewpoint, forecasted data are information used for purposes of planning for the future. Forecasting, to some degree or another, is often required when producing budgets. (Budgets are the subject of two of the following chapters.) It is pretty simple today to create "what if" scenarios on the computer. But the important thing for managers to remember is that assumptions directly affect the results of forecasts.

Forecasts Versus Projections

Forecasts are different than projections, although both are considered to be "prospective" and thus "future" financial statements. Forecasts are based on assumptions that are expected to exist, and that reflect actions that are expected to occur. Projections, on the other hand, are views further into the future. Because they are further into the future, we "project" future events, projects, or operations using a set of presumed, or hypothetical, assumptions.

We are discussing forecasts in this chapter rather than projections. Therefore, these forecasts are relatively short term and can be based on realistic assumptions that we expect to exist, along with actions that we can reasonably expect to occur.

Forecasting Approaches

The approach to producing a forecast usually involves three different sources of information and forecast assumptions:

- The first level derives from the personnel who are directly involved in the department or unit. They know the operation and can provide important ground-level detail.
- The second level comes from electronic and statistical information, including trend analysis. Electronic reports can provide a thicket of information, and there is a skill to selecting relevant information for forecasting purposes.
- The third level represents executive-level judgment that is typically applied to a preliminary rough draft of the forecast. For example, adjusting volume upward or downward due to the anticipated future impact of local competition would most likely be an executive-level judgment.

The amount and type of electronic information that is readily available greatly affects the forecast difficulty. Electronic templates and standardized worksheets may also greatly influence the final forecast results.

Common Types of Forecasts in Healthcare Organizations

The three most common types of forecasts found in most healthcare organizations include revenue forecasts, staffing forecasts, and operating expense forecasts. (The operating expense forecast, which is not as common, would generally cover those operating expenses other than labor.) This section will discuss revenue and staffing forecasts, as they are what most managers will need to deal with.

OPERATING REVENUE FORECASTS

Operating revenue forecasts are inputs into the operating budget. Forecast types and their assumptions are discussed in this section.

Types of Revenue Forecasts

Forecasts of revenue will cover varying time periods. Longer-range multi-year forecasts are useful for executive decision making regarding the future of the organization. **Figure 14–1** illustrates a multi-year forecast.

A single-year forecast is generally for the coming year and is thus a short-range forecast. Reliable forecasts of revenue are a vital part of the organization's planning process and are an input into the operating budget. **Figure 14–2** illustrates a short-range forecast. Note that the graph in Figure 14–2 could be by month instead of by quarter as shown.

Building Revenue Forecast Assumptions

Five important issues regarding revenue forecast assumptions are discussed here.

Utilization Assumptions

In health care, significant changes in utilization patterns can be occurring that need to be taken into account in the manager's forecast assumptions. The inexorable shift to shorter lengths of stay for hospital inpatients over the last decade is an example of a basic shift in utilization patterns.

Patient Mix Assumptions

It is important to specify anticipated patient mix as well as his or her anticipated utilization or volume. By "patient mix" we mean whether the individual is a Medicare patient, a Medicaid patient, a patient covered by private insurance, or a private pay patient. When payers are thus identified, this information allows the appropriate payments to be associated with the service utilization assumptions.

Contractual Allowance Assumptions

The forecasted utilization of a service (or its volume) assumption is multiplied by the appropriate rate, or charges, in order to arrive at forecasted revenue stated in dollars. A word of

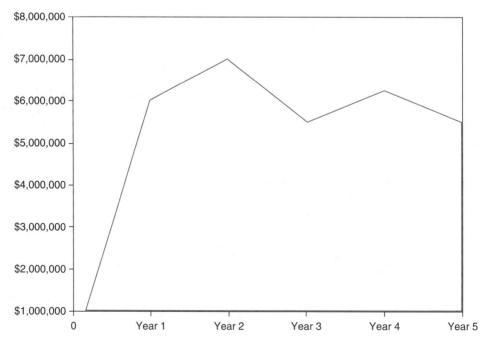

Figure 14–1 Five-Year Operating Revenue Forecast.

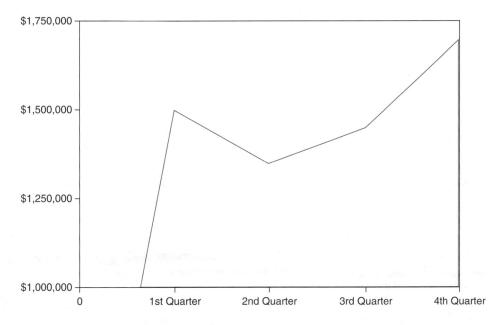

Figure 14–2 One-Year Operating Revenue Forecast.

warning, however: revenue forecasted at "gross charges" is not a valid figure. Instead, revenue stated at "allowed charges" is the proper figure to use. Virtually all payers, including Medicare, Medicaid, and private insurers, will pay a stipulated amount for a particular service. But the amounts these different payers have agreed to pay for the same service will vary. How to handle the issue? Through a contractual allowance, as defined here:

- Gross Charge: Amount for a service as shown on the claim form; a uniform charge generally greater than most expected payments received for the service.
- Allowed Charge: Net amount that the particular payer's contract or participation agreement will recognize, or "allow," for a certain service.
- Contractual Allowance: Difference (between the gross charge and the allowed charge) that is recorded as a reduction of the gross charge within the accounting cycle.

(It should also be noted that part of the payer's allowed charge is generally due from the patient, and the remaining portion of the allowed charge is actually due from the payer.)

Trend Analysis Assumptions

One of the basic purposes of performing trend analysis is to compare data between or among years and to see the trends. If such trends are found, then it makes sense to take them into account in your forecast. A word of warning, however: the manager must determine whether the data used for comparison in the trend analysis are comparable data.

Payer Change Assumptions

Trend analysis is retrospective; that is, it is using historical data from a past period. Forecasting is prospective; that is, it is projecting into the future. If changes, say, in regulatory requirements for payment are made this year, then that fact has to be taken into account.

STAFFING FORECASTS

Staffing forecasts are also inputs into the operating budget. We have addressed staffing computations, costs, and reports in a previous chapter. This section builds upon that information in order to produce a staffing forecast. Thus forecast considerations, components, and assumptions are addressed in this section.

Staffing Forecast Considerations

Staffing forecasts are a very common type of forecast required of managers. Three important considerations when preparing staffing forecasts are discussed here.

Controllable Versus Noncontrollable Expenses

The concept of responsibility centers and controllable versus noncontrollable expenses has been discussed earlier in this book. Essentially, controllable costs are subject to a manager's own decision making, whereas noncontrollable costs are outside that manager's power. It is extremely difficult to make staffing forecasts with any degree of accuracy if noncontrollable expenses are included in the manager's forecast. The organization's structure must be recognized and taken into account when setting up assumptions for staffing forecasts. Shared services across lines of authority are workable in theory, but often do not work in actuality. **Figure 14–3** gives an example of the essential "business units" under the supervision of a director of nurses. Note the responsibility centers and the support centers on this organization chart.

Required Minimum Staff Levels

Regulatory healthcare standards may set minimum staff levels for providing service in a particular unit. These minimum levels cannot be ignored in the forecast process.

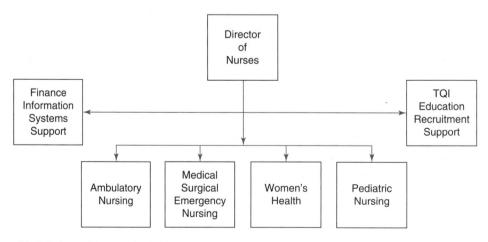

Figure 14–3 Primary Nursing Staff Classification by Line of Authority.
Courtesy of Resource Group, Ltd., Dallas, Texas.

Labor Market Issues in Staffing Forecasts

We most often hear about a chronic lack of adequate staff, and certain parts of the country do have a continual shortage of certain qualified professional healthcare staff. Yet other parts of the country can have an overabundance during that same period. The status of the local labor market has a direct impact on staffing forecasts. The impact is in dollars: when there are plenty of staff available, the hourly rate to attract staff may go down, but when there is a shortage of available qualified staff, the hourly rate has to go up. As strange as it may seem, this elemental economic fact is sometimes not taken into account in forecasting assumptions.

Staffing Forecast Components

In many cases a staffing plan is first created, and the staffing forecast follows after the plan is reviewed and refined. Four components are typically required, as follows. **Figure 14–4** illustrates the sequence.

Scheduling Requirements

Scheduling requirements should encompass all hours and days required to cover each position. For example, see the exhibit in the discussion about staffing (Chapter 10) that illustrates a single security guard position and the number of units required.

Master Staffing Plan

The master staffing plan should include all units and all hours and days required to cover all positions within the units. For example, see the exhibit in the discussion about staffing that illustrates entire units by shift, covering 24 hours per day times 7 days a week.

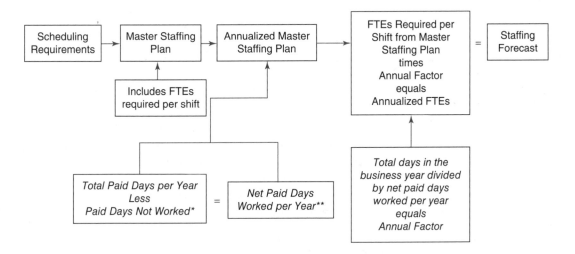

*Paid Days Not Worked = Nonproductive Days
**Net Paid Days Worked = Productive Days

Figure 14–4 Components of the Staffing Forecast.

Computation Sequence to Annualize the Master Staffing Plan

The annualizing sequence is as follows. (This sequence is illustrated visually in Figure 14–4. An example in worksheet form appears in the chapter about staffing.)

- Compute Productive and Nonproductive Days and Net Paid Days
  The proportion of productive days (net paid days) versus nonproductive days (paid days not worked) will be based on the organization's policy as to paying for days not worked. For example, see Step 1 in the Staffing chapter's exhibit for such a computation, including "Net Paid Days." (Holidays, sick days, vacation days, and education days composed the "Paid Days Not Worked" in the worksheet example within the Staffing chapter's exhibit.)
- Convert Net Paid Days Worked to an Annual Factor
  The total days in the business year divided by net paid days worked equals a factor. Step 2 in the Staffing chapter's exhibit illustrates this computation.
- Calculate the Annual FTEs Using the Factors
  Finally, use the factor to calculate the FTEs required to fully cover the position's shifts all year long. For example, in the Staffing chapter's exhibit, the RN FTE would be 1.6 (1.6106195).

The resulting staffing forecast reflects 24 hour per day 7 days per week annual FTEs to cover all shifts.

CAPACITY LEVEL ISSUES IN FORECASTING

In the manufacturing industry, capacity levels relate to the production of, say, widgets. In the world of health care, capacity relates to services; that is, the ability to produce or provide specific healthcare services.

Space and Equipment Availability

The ability to provide services is automatically limited by the availability of both space and the proper equipment to provide certain specific services. Forecasts need to take a realistic view of these capacity levels.

Staffing Availability

Capacity is a tricky assumption to make in staffing forecasts. In some programs, particularly those in a startup phase, overcapacity (too much staff available for the amount of work required) is a problem. In some other organizations, under capacity (a chronic lack of adequate staff) is the problem. Forecasting assumptions, in the best of all worlds, take these difficulties into account. See the Mini-Case Study that demonstrates this problem of staffing in the context of the Women, Infants, and Children (WIC) federal program.[2]

Example of Forecasting Maximum Service Capacity

Exhibit 14–1 illustrates the array of elements that should be taken into account when computing maximum capacity levels. This computation is important because your forecast should take maximum capacity into account. (Alternative assumptions can also be made, of course. See the sensitivity analysis discussion in a following chapter.)

Exhibit 14–1 Capacity Level Checkpoints for an Outpatient Infusion Center

Outpatient Infusion Center Capacity Level Checkpoints

\# infusion chairs .... 3 chairs

\# staff.. 1 RN

\# weekly operating hours...................... 40 hours

\# of hours per patient infusion............. average 2 hours (for purposes of this example)

Work Flow Description

For each infusion the nurse must perform the following steps (generalized for this purpose; actual protocol is more specific):

1. Obtain and review the patient's chart
2. Obtain and prepare the appropriate drug for infusion
3. Interview the patient
4. Prepare the patient and commence the infusion
5. Monitor and record progress throughout the ongoing infusion
6. Observe the patient upon completion of the infusion
7. Complete charting

Work Flow Comments

It is impossible for one nurse to start patients' infusions in all three chairs simultaneously. Thus the theoretical treatment sequence might be as follows:

- Assume one half-hour for patient number one's Steps 1 through 4.
- Once patient number one is at Step 5, the nurse can begin the protocol for patient number two.
- Assume another one half-hour for patient number two's Steps 1 through 4.
- Once patient number two is at Step 5, theoretically the nurse can begin the protocol for patient number three.

This sequence should work, assuming all factors work smoothly; that is, the appropriate drugs in the proper amounts are at hand, the patients show up on time, and no one patient demands an unusual amount of the nurse's attention. (For example, a new patient will require more attention.)

Daily Infusion Center Capacity Level Assumption

Patient scheduling is never entirely smooth, and patient reactions during infusions are never predictable. Therefore, we realistically assume the following: Chair #1 = 3 patients per day, Chair #2 = 2 patients per day, and Chair #3 = 2 patients per day, for a daily total of 7 patients infused.

SUMMARY

In summary, the ultimate accuracy of a forecast rests on the strength of its assumptions.

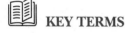 **INFORMATION CHECKPOINT**

What is needed?	An example of a staffing forecast created in your organization.
Where is it found?	In the files of the supervisor who is responsible for staffing.
How is it used?	Use the example to learn the nature of the assumptions that were used and the setup of the forecast itself.

KEY TERMS

Common Sizing
Controllable Expenses
Forecasts
Noncontrollable Expenses
Patient Mix
Trend Analysis
Vertical Analysis

DISCUSSION QUESTIONS

1. Do any of the reports you receive in the course of your work use trend analysis? Why do you think so?
2. Do any of the reports you receive in the course of your work use common sizing? Why do you think so?
3. Are you or your immediate supervisor involved with staffing decisions? If so, are you aware of how staffing forecasts are prepared in your organization? Describe an example.
4. Have you, in the course of your work, become involved in problems with capacity level issues such as space and equipment availability? If so, would forecasting have assisted in solving such problems? Describe why.

NOTES

1. *Merriam Webster's Collegiate Dictionary*, 10th ed., s.v. "Forecast."
2. B. A. Brotman, M. Bumgarner, and P. Prime, "Client Flow through the Women, Infants, and Children Public Health Program," *Journal of Health Care Finance*, 25, no. 1 (1998): 72–77.

Using Comparative Data

© LFor/Shutterstock

OVERVIEW

Comparative data can become an important tool for the manager. It is important, however, to fully understand the requirements and the uses of such data.

COMPARABILITY REQUIREMENTS

True comparability needs to meet three criteria: consistency, verification, and unit measurement. Each is discussed in this section.

Consistency

Three equally important elements of consistency should be considered as follows.

Time Periods

Time periods should be consistent. For example, a 10-month period should not be compared to a 12-month period. Instead, the 10-month period should be annualized, as described within this chapter.

Consistent Methodology

The same methods should be used across time periods. For example, the chapter about inventory discusses the use of two inventory methods: first-in, first-out (FIFO) versus last-in, first-out (LIFO). The same inventory method—one or the other—should always be used consistently for both the beginning of the year and the end of the year.

Progress Notes

After completing this chapter, you should be able to

1. Understand the three criteria for true comparability.
2. Understand the four uses of comparative data.
3. Annualize partial-year expenses.
4. Apply inflation factors.
5. Understand basic currency measures.

Inflation Factors

Finally, if multiple years are being compared, should inflation be taken into account? The proper application of an inflation factor is also described within this chapter.

Verification

Basically, can these data be verified? Is it reasonable? If an objective, qualified person reviewed the data, would he or she arrive at the same conclusion and/or results? You may have to do a few tests to determine if the data can in fact be verified. If so, you should retain your back-up data, because it is the evidence that supports your conclusions about verification.

Monetary Unit Measurement

With regard to comparative data, we should ask: "Is all the information being prepared or under review measured by the same monetary unit?" In the United States, we would expect all the data to be expressed in dollars and not in some other currency such as euros (used in much of Europe) or pounds (used in Britain and the United Kingdom). Most of the manager's data will automatically meet this requirement. However, currency conversions are an important part of reporting financial results for companies that have global operations, and consistency in applying such conversions can be a significant factor in expressing financial results.

A MANAGER'S VIEW OF COMPARATIVE DATA

It is important for the manager to always be aware of whether the data he or she is receiving (or preparing) are appropriate for comparison. It is equally important for the manager to perform a comprehensive review, as described here.

The Manager's Responsibility

Whether you as a manager must either review or prepare required data, your responsibility is to recall and apply the elements of consistency. Why? Because such data will typically be used for decision making. If such data are not comparable, then relying upon them can result in poor decisions, with financial consequences in the future. The actual mechanics of making a comparative review are equally important. The deconstruction of a comparative budget review follows.

Comparative Budget Review

The manager needs to know how to effectively review comparative data. To do so, the manager needs to understand, for example, how a budget report format is constructed. In general, the usual operating expense budget that is under review will have a column for actual expenditures, a column for budgeted expenditures, and a column for the difference between the two. Usually, the actual expense column and the budget column will both have a vertical analysis of percentages (as discussed in the preceding chapter). Each different line item will have a horizontal analysis (also discussed in the preceding chapter) that measures the amount of the difference against the budget.

Table 15–1 illustrates the operating expense budget configuration just described. Notice that the "Difference" column has both positive and negative numbers in it (the negative numbers being set off with parentheses). Thus, the positive numbers indicate budget overage, such as the dietary line, which had an actual expense of $405,000 against a budget figure of $400,000, resulting in a $5,000 difference. The next line is maintenance. This department did not exceed its budget, so the difference is in parentheses; the maintenance budget amounted to $290,000, and actual expenses were only $270,000, so the $20,000 difference is in parentheses. In this case, parentheses are good (under budget) and no parentheses is bad (over budget).

USES OF COMPARATIVE DATA

Four common uses of comparisons that the manager will find helpful are discussed in this section.

Compare Current Expenses to Current Budget

Managers are most likely to be responsible for comparing the current expenses of their department, division, unit, or program to their current budget. Of the four types of comparisons discussed in this section, this is the one most commonly in use.

Table 15–1 illustrates a comparison of actual expenses versus budgeted expenses. This format reflects both dollars and percentages, as is most common. Table 15–1 shows the grand totals for each department (Dietary, Maintenance, etc.) contained in General Services expense for this hospital. There is, of course, a detailed budget for each of these departments that adds up to the totals shown on Table 15–1. Thus, for example, all the detailed expenses of the Laundry department (labor, supplies, etc.) are contained in a supporting detailed budget whose total actual expenses amount to $45,000 and whose total budgeted expenses amount to $50,000.

The department manager will be responsible for analyzing and managing the detailed budgets of his or her own department. A manager at a higher level in the organization—the chief financial officer (CFO), perhaps—will be responsible for making a comparative analysis of the overall operations of the organization. This comparative analysis at a higher level will condense each department's details into a departmental grand total, as shown in Table 15–1, for convenience and clarity in review.

Table 15–1 Comparative Analysis of Budget Versus Actual

	Hospital 1					
	Year 2 Actual		Year 2 Budget		Difference	
	$$	%	$$	%	$$	%
General Services Expense						
Dietary	$405,000	45	$400,000	46	$5,000	12.5
Maintenance	270,000	30	290,000	33	(20,000)	(6.9)
Laundry	45,000	5	50,000	6	(5,000)	(10.0)
Housekeeping	180,000	20	130,000	15	50,000	38.5
Total GS Expense	$900,000	100	$870,000	100	$30,000	3.5

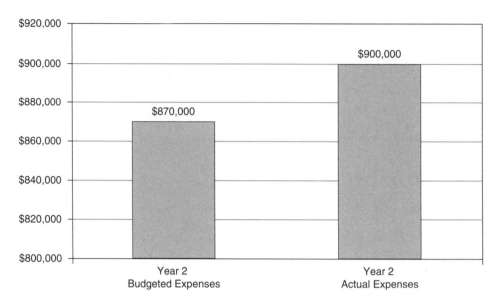

Figure 15–1 A Comparison of Hospital One's Budgeted and Actual Expenses.

The CFO may also convert this comparative data into charts or graphs in order to "tell the story" in a more visual manner. For example, the total General Service expense in Table 15–1 can be readily converted into a graph. **Figure 15–1** illustrates such a graph.

Compare Current Actual Expenses to Prior Periods in Own Organization

Trend analysis, as explained in the preceding chapter, allows comparison of current actual expenses to expenses incurred in prior periods of the same organization. For example, consider total general services expenses of $800,000 for year 1 and $900,000 for year 2. The CFO could easily convert this information into a graph, as shown in **Figure 15–2**. This information might be even more valuable for decision-making input if the CFO used five years instead of the two years that are shown here.

Compare to Other Organizations

Common sizing, as explained in the preceding chapter, allows comparison of your organization to other similar organizations. To illustrate, refer to the table in a preceding chapter (Table 14–1) entitled "Common Sizing Liability Information." Here we see the liabilities of three hospitals that are the same size expressed in both dollars and in percentages. Therefore, our CFO can convert the percentages into an informative graph, as shown in **Figure 15–3**.

Be warned that the basis for some comparisons will be neither useful nor valid. For example, see **Figure 15–4**. Here we have a graph of the grand totals from the table in a preceding chapter (Table 14–2) entitled "Common Sizing Expense Information." The percentages shown are for the General Services departments of each hospital and have been common sized to percentages, as is

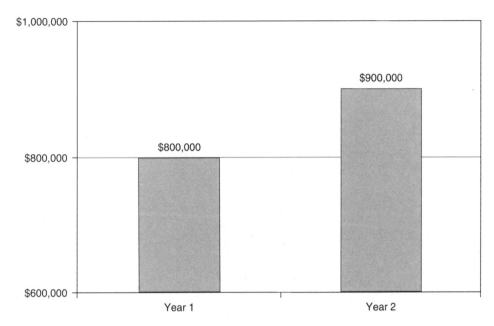

Figure 15–2 A Comparison of Hospital One's Expenses Over Time.

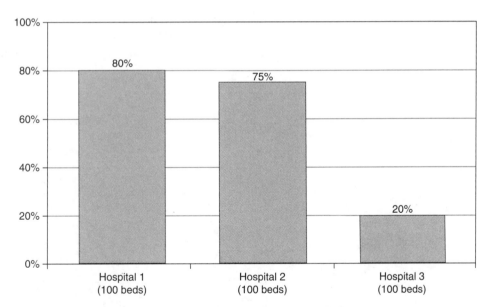

Figure 15–3 A Comparison of Three 100-Bed Hospitals' Long-Term Debt.

perfectly correct. However, Figure 15–4 attempts to compare the total General Services expense (the total of all four general services departments) in dollars. As we can see here, hospital 1 and hospital 3 are both 100 beds, while hospital 2 is 400 beds. Obviously a 400-bed hospital will incur much more expense than a 100-bed hospital, so this graph cannot possibly show a valid comparison among the three organizations.

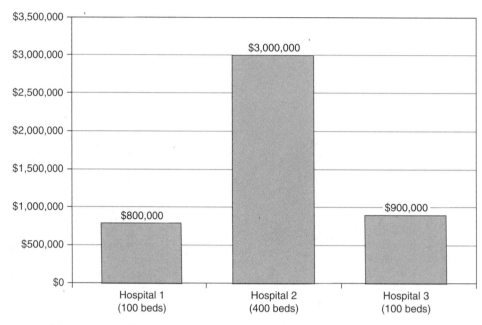

Figure 15–4 A Comparison of Three Hospitals' Total Expenses.

Instead, the CFO should find a standard measure that can be used as a valid basis for comparison. In this case, he or she can choose size (number of beds) for this purpose. The resulting graph is shown in **Figure 15–5**. As you can see, hospital 1's cost per bed is $8,000, computed as follows.

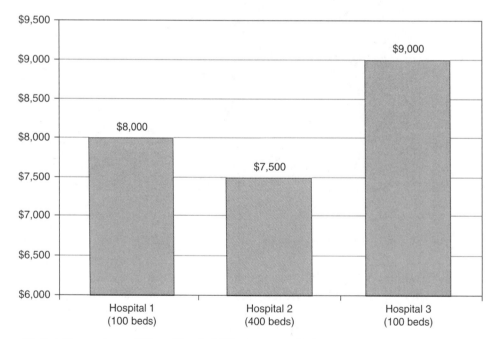

Figure 15–5 A Comparison of Three Hospitals' Expenses per Bed.

The total expense of $800,000 for hospital 1 is divided by 100 beds (its size) to arrive at the $8,000 expense per bed shown on the graph in Figure 15–5. Hospital 2 ($3,000,000 total expense divided by 400 beds to equal $7,500 per bed) and hospital 3 ($900,000 total expense divided by 100 beds to equal $9,000 per bed) have the same computations performed on their equivalent figures.

In actual fact, another step in this computation should be performed in order to make the comparisons completely valid. A per-bed computation implies inpatient expenses incurred, because beds are occupied by admitted inpatients. (Outpatients, on the other hand, use a different mix of services.) Therefore, a more accurate comparison would adjust the overall total expense using one subtotal for inpatients and another subtotal for outpatients. Let us assume, for purposes of illustration, that the CFO of hospital 1 has determined that 70% of General Services expense can be attributed to inpatients and that the remaining 30% can be attributed to outpatients. Let us further assume that hospital 1's General Services expense of $800,000 as shown, is indeed a hospital-wide expense. The CFO would then multiply $800,000 by 70% to arrive at $420,000, representing the inpatient portion of General Services expense.

Compare to Industry Standards

In the example just given in the paragraph above, the CFO has computed his or her own hospital's percentage of inpatient versus outpatient utilization of General Services expense. But this CFO may not have any way to know these equivalent percentages for hospitals 2 and 3. If this is the case, computing the per-bed expense using overall expense, as shown in Figure 15–5, may be the only way to show a three-hospital comparison.

The CFO, however, can use the 70% inpatient and 30% outpatient expense breakdown for another type of comparison. It should be possible to find industry standards that break

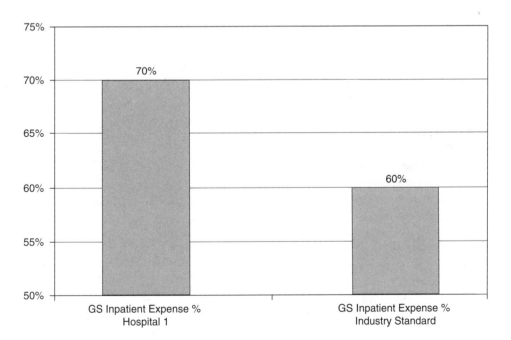

Figure 15–6 A Comparison of Hospital One's GS Inpatient Expenses with Industry Standards.

out inpatient versus outpatient expense percentages. The use of industry standards is of particular use for decision making because it positions the particular organization within a large grouping of facilities that provide a similar set of services.

Healthcare organizations are particularly well suited to use industry standards because both the federal and state governments release a wealth of public information and statistics regarding the provision of health care. **Figure 15–6** illustrates the CFO's graph using such a standard. (The figures shown are for illustration only and do not reflect an actual standard.)

MAKING DATA COMPARABLE

This section discusses annualizing partial-year expenses, along with using inflation factors, standardized measures, and currency measures. The manager needs to know how to make data comparable as a basis for properly preparing and/or reviewing budgets and reports.

Annualizing

Because comparability requires consistency, the manager needs to know how to annualize partial-year expenses. **Table 15–2** sets out the actual 10-month expenses for the operating room. But these expenses are going to be compared against a 12-month budget. What to do? The actual 10-month expenses are converted, or annualized, to a 12-month basis, as shown in the second column of Table 15–2.

These computations were performed on a computer spreadsheet; however, the calculation is as follows. Using the first line as an example, $50,431 is 10-months worth of expenses; therefore, 1 month's expense is one-tenth of $50,431, or $5,043. To annualize for 12-months worth of expenses, the 10-month total of $50,431 is increased by 2 more months at $5,043 apiece ($50,431 plus $5,043 for month 11, plus another $5,043 for month 12, equals $60,517, the annualized 12-month figure for the year).

Table 15–2 Annualizing Operating Room Partial-Year Expenses

	Expenses	
	Actual	Annualized
Account	10 Month	12 Month
Social Security	50,431	60,517
Pension	17,229	20,675
Health Insurance	7,018	8,422
Child Care	3,803	4,564
Patient Accounting	129,463	155,356
Admitting	91,878	110,254
Medical Records	76,432	91,718
Dietary	22,938	27,526
Medical Waste	1,981	2,377
Sterile Procedures	65,600	78,720
Laundry	33,911	40,693
Depreciation— Equipment	72,815	87,378
Depreciation— Building	34,481	41,377
Amortization— Interest	(4,849)	(5,819)
Insurance	3,513	4,216
Administration	48,305	57,966
Medical Staff	1,435	1,722
Community Relations	41,511	49,813
Materials Management	53,811	64,573
Human Resources	25,888	31,066
Nursing Administration	68,726	82,471
Data Processing	14,846	17,815
Fiscal	14,750	17,700
Telephone	2,366	2,839
Utilities	22,005	26,406
Plant	64,664	77,597
Environmental Services	27,395	32,874
Safety	1,680	2,016
Quality Management	8,347	10,016
Medical Staff	7,870	9,444
Continuous Quality Improvement	4,079	4,895
EE Health	474	569
Total Allocated	1,014,796	1,217,756
All Other Expenses	1,009,673	1,211,608
Total Expense	2,024,469	2,429,364

Inflation Factors

Inflation means "an increase in the volume of money and credit relative to available goods and services resulting in a continuing rise in the general price level."[1] An inflation factor is used to compute the effect of inflation.

Let's assume that hospital 1's General Services expenses for year 1 were $800,000, versus $900,000 for year 2. We can assume that these amounts reflect actual dollars expended in each year. But let us also now assume that inflation caused these expenses to rise by 5% in year 2. If the Chief Financial Officer (CFO) decides to take such inflation into account, a government source will be available to provide the appropriate inflation rate. (The 5% in our example is for illustration only and does not reflect an actual rate.)

The inflation factor for this example is expressed as a factor of 1.05 (1.00 plus 5% [expressed as .05] equals 1.05). The CFO might apply the inflation factor to year 1 in order to give it a spending power basis equivalent to that of year 2. (Applying an inflation factor for a two-year comparison is not usually the case, but let us assume the CFO has a good reason for doing so in this case.) The computation would thus be $800,000 year 1 expense times the 1.05 inflation factor equals an inflation-adjusted year 1 expense figure of $840,000.

However, if the CFO wants to apply an inflation factor to a whole series of years, he or she must account for the cumulative effect over time. An example appears in **Table 15–3**. We assume a base of $500,000 and an annual inflation rate of 10%. The inflation factor for the first year is 10%, converted to 1.10, just as in the previous example, and $500,000 multiplied by 1.10 equals $550,000 in nominal dollars.

Beyond the first year, however, we must determine the cumulative inflation factor. For this purpose we turn to the Compound Interest Table. It shows "The Future Amount of $1.00," and appears in Appendix B of the chapter about time value of money. "The Future Amount of $1.00" table has years down the left side (vertical) and percentages across the top (horizontal). We find the 10% column and read down it for years one, two, three, and so on.

As shown in **Table 15–3.2**, the factor for year 2 is 1.210, for year 3 is 1.331, and so on. We carry those factors to column C of **Table 15–3.1**. Now we multiply the $500,000 in column B times the factor for each year to arrive at the cumulative inflated amount in column D. Thus $500,000 times the year 2 factor of 1.210 equals $605,000, and so on.

Currency Measures

Monetary unit measurement, and the related currency measures and currency conversions, are typically beyond most manager's responsibilities. Nevertheless, it is important for the manager to understand that consistency in applying such measures and conversions will be a significant factor in expressing financial results of companies that have global operations.

Therefore, for comparative purposes we must determine if all the information being prepared or under review is measured by the same monetary unit. A few foreign currency examples are illustrated in **Exhibit 15–1**. Currencies are typically converted for financial reporting purposes using the U.S.-dollar foreign exchange rates as of a certain date.

Exchange rates may be expressed in two ways: "in U.S. dollars" or "per U.S. dollars." For example, assume the euro is trading at 1.3333 in U.S. dollars and at 0.7500 per U.S. dollars. That means if you were spending your U.S. dollar in, say, France (part of the "euro area"), it would take a third as much (1.33) in your dollars to buy products priced in euros. If your French friend, on the other hand, was spending euros for products priced in U.S. dollars, he or she

Table 15–3 Applying a Cumulative Inflation Factor

Table 15–3.1

SOURCE OF FACTOR IN COLUMN C BELOW:
From the Compound Interest Look-Up Table
"The Future Amount of $1.00" (Appendix 13-B)

Year	Factors as shown at 10%
1	1.100
2	1.210
3	1.331
4	1.464

Table 15–3.2

(A)	(B)	(C)	(D)
Year	Real Dollars	Cumulative Inflation Factor*	Nominal Dollars**
1	$500,000	$(1.10)^1 = 1.100$	$550,000
2	500,000	$(1.10)^2 = 1.210$	605,000
3	500,000	$(1.10)^3 = 1.331$	665,500
4	500,000	$(1.10)^4 = 1.464$	732,050

*Assume an annual inflation rate of 10%. Thus 1.00 + 0.10 = the 1.10 factor in Column C.
**Column D "Nominal Dollars" equals Column B times Column C.

Exhibit 15–1 Foreign Currency Examples

Country (or Area)	Currency
Canada	Canadian dollar
China	Yuan
Euro Area	Euro
Japan	Yen
Mexico	Peso
United Kingdom	Pound

could buy one-quarter more for his or her money (because the U.S. dollar would be worth only three quarters [0.7500] of the euro at that particular exchange rate).

Standardized Measures

A final word about standardized measures. Standardized measures aid comparability. They especially assist in performance measurement. Types of standardized measures include the typical hospital per-bed measure along with work load measures.

There is, of course, a whole array of uses for standardized measures. Managed care plans, for example, may use a standard set of measures that are applied to every physician who contracts with the plan. Each physician then receives a report from the plan that illustrates his or her performance.

Finally, electronic medical records (as further discussed in following chapters) depend upon standardized input. The input into various fields is standardized (and thus made comparable) by the very nature of the electronic system design.

CONSTRUCTING CHARTS TO SHOW THE DATA

Managers use charts to explain their projects and to report their results. Thus constructing accurate and effective charts is a valuable skill.

Types of Charts

There are four basic chart styles as follows:

- Column chart
- Pie chart
- Bar chart
- Line chart

The column chart's data is presented in vertical columns. The pie chart is typically circular (like a pie, thus its name). The bar chart presents data in horizontal bars. The line chart generally uses multiple lines that track along a grid. **Figures 15-7, 15-8,** and **15-9** illustrate examples of the pie chart, bar chart, and line chart respectively.

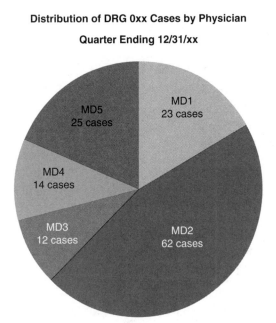

Distribution of DRG 0xx Cases by Physician

Quarter Ending 12/31/xx

Figure 15–7 Distribution of DRG 0xx Cases by Physician.
Modified from R. Hankins & J.J. Baker, *Management Accounting for Health Care Organizations* (Sudbury, MA: Jones & Bartlett 2004). p. 375.

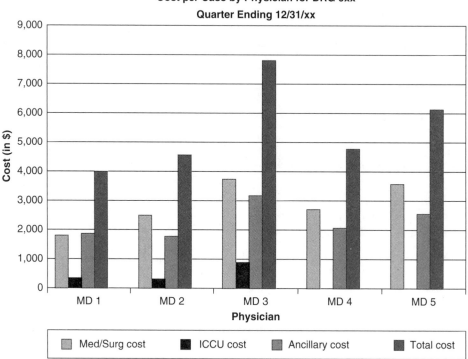

Figure 15–8　Cost per Case by Physician for DRG 0xx.
Modified from R. Hankins & J.J. Baker, *Management Accounting for Health Care Organizations* (Sudbury, MA: Jones & Bartlett 2004). p. 376.

Chart Content and Format

Constructing the chart means answering a series of questions about content and format, as follows:

- What is the subject of the chart?
- What are the specific elements to be included?
- What type of chart will best serve my purpose?
- Is the information accurate and consistent?
- If applicable, is the information comparable?
- What are the dimensions of the chart?
- If applicable, what is the span between high and low?

Chart Templates

A variety of chart templates are now available online. They are generally found within office suite programs. Each template typically offers a drop-down menu for specifics of the format and a second drop-down menu for the chart's data input. Electronic templates also provide quick and easy color choices for your chart presentation. You can experiment with various colors to reach the best combination for your project.

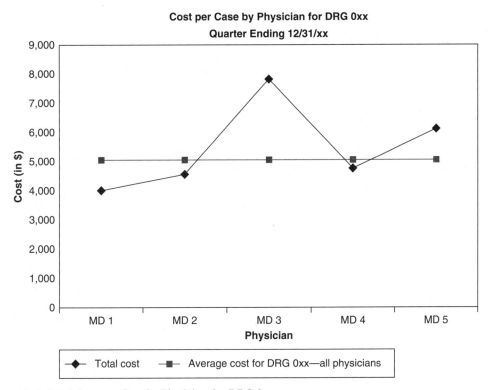

Figure 15–9 Total Cost per Case by Physician for DRG 0xx.
Modified from R. Hankins & J.J. Baker, *Management Accounting for Health Care Organizations* (Sudbury, MA: Jones & Bartlett 2004). p. 377.

To summarize, the chart you construct can be simple or elaborate. It can be black and white or it can be multi-colored. But whatever its style, your chart must contain accurate and comparable data.

INFORMATION CHECKPOINT

What is needed?	Example of a detailed comparative budget review (comparing budget to actual).
Where is it found?	With the supervisor responsible for the budget.
How is it used?	To find whether data are stated in comparable terms between actual amounts and budget amounts.

KEY TERMS

Annualize
Inflation Factor
Monetary Unit

DISCUSSION QUESTIONS

1. Do you believe your organization uses a flexible or static budget? Why do you think so?
2. If you reviewed a budget at your workplace, do you think the major increases and decreases could be explained? If so, why? If not, why not?
3. Have you ever in the course of your work reviewed a report that had been annualized? If so, did you agree with how it appeared to be annualized?
4. Were you also able to see the assumptions used to annualize? If so, were you able to recalculate the results using the same assumptions?
5. Have you ever in the course of your work reviewed a financial report that applied inflation factors? If so, were you able to see the assumptions used to apply the factors? If not, why not? Please describe.

NOTE

1. *Merriam Webster's Collegiate Dictionary*, 10th ed., s.v. "Inflation."

# PART VI

Construct and Evaluate Budgets

Operating Budgets

OVERVIEW

A budget is an organization-wide instrument. The organization's objectives define the specific activities to be performed, how they will be assembled, and the particular levels of operation, whereas the organization's performance standards or norms set out the anticipated levels of individual performance. The budget is the instrument through which activities are quantified in financial terms.

Objectives for the Budgeting Process

A healthcare standard view of budgeting is illustrated by the American Hospital Association's (AHA's) objectives for the budgeting process:

1. To provide a written expression, in quantitative terms, of a hospital's policies and plans.
2. To provide a basis for the evaluation of financial performance in accordance with a hospital's policies and plans.
3. To provide a useful tool for the control of costs.
4. To create cost awareness throughout the organization.[1]

Operating Budgets Versus Capital Expenditure Budgets

Operating budgets generally deal with actual short-term revenues and expenses necessary to operate the facility. The usual period covered is the next year (a 12-month period). Capital expenditure budgets, on the other hand, may cover the next year as well, but are linked into a more futuristic view. Thus, capital expenditure budgets may cover a 5- or even a 10-year period.

Progress Notes

After completing this chapter, you should be able to

1. Understand the difference between operating budgets and capital expenditure budgets.
2. Understand what budget expenses will most likely be identifiable versus allocated expenses.
3. Understand how to build an operating budget.
4. Understand the difference between static and flexible budgets.

BUDGET VIEWPOINTS

Responsibility Centers

In a responsibility center the manager is responsible for a particular set of activities. (We have discussed responsibility centers in a previous chapter.) In the context of operating budgets there are two common types of responsibility centers: cost centers and profit centers. As shown in **Figure 16–1**, in cost centers the manager is responsible for controlling costs. In profit centers the manager is responsible for both costs and revenues. Thus, we expect that a cost center operating budget will show costs only, while a profit center budget should show both revenues and costs.

Transactions Outside the Operating Budget

Certain transactions are outside the operating budget, as shown in **Figure 16–2**. For example, many grants received by healthcare organizations are restricted funds. The monies in a restricted fund are not to be commingled with general operations monies. Also, a restricted fund generally requires altogether separate accounting and reporting.

Foundation transactions are also outside the operating budget. Foundations are legally separate organizations that require separate accounting and reporting of their funds. Therefore, we would not expect any of their costs to be included in operations.

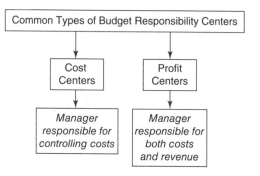

Figure 16–1 Two Common Budget Responsibility Centers.

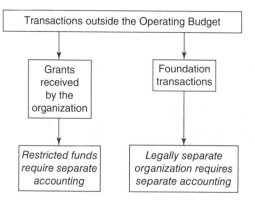

Figure 16–2 Transactions Outside the Operating Budget.

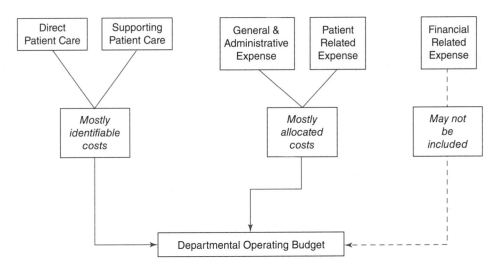

Figure 16–3 Identified Versus Allocated Costs.

BUDGET BASICS: A REVIEW

A brief review of budget basics is advisable as we move into constructing an operating budget.

Identifiable Versus Allocated Budget Costs

Within a departmental budget, certain costs will be specifically identifiable while others will be allocated instead, as shown in **Figure 16–3**:

- Direct patient care and supporting patient care should be mostly identifiable.
- General and administrative expense and patient-related expense will probably be mostly allocated costs.
- Financial-related expense, such as interest expense, may not be included at all in the manager's budget.

Fixed Versus Variable Costs

You will recall that fixed costs do not change in total, even though volume rises or falls (within a wide range). Variable costs, however, rise or fall in proportion to a change (a rise or fall) in volume. You will further recall that volume, in the case of healthcare organizations, generally means number of procedures (outpatient services) or number of patient days (inpatient services) or perhaps, prescriptions filled (pharmacy services). **Figure 16–4** illustrates this principle, while **Exhibit 16–1** provides examples of fixed and variable cost categories that would typically be found within an operating budget.

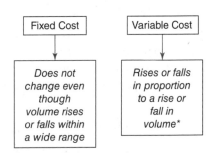

*Examples of volume: Number of procedures or patient days

Figure 16–4 Fixed Versus Variable Costs.

Exhibit 16–1 Fixed and Variable Cost Examples

Operating Expenses	Fixed	Variable
Labor		
Gross Salaries	X	
Employers' Payroll Taxes	X	
Other Employee Benefits	X	
Part-Time Temporary Contract Labor		X
Other Expenses		
Drugs and Medical Supplies		X
Rent	X	
Insurance	X	
Five-Year Equipment Lease	X	

BUILDING AN OPERATING BUDGET: PREPARATION

Appropriate preparation is an important stage in building an operating budget. It is often difficult for the manager to allow adequate time for budget preparation, because this effort is above and beyond his or her daily responsibilities. Understanding the usual stages, or sequence, of budget construction as listed here assists in predicting how much time will be required.

Construction Stages

Operating budget construction stages include the following:

- Plan
- Gather information
- Prepare input
- Construct and submit draft version of budget
- Make required revisions to draft
- Present preliminary budget
- Make required revisions to preliminary budget
- Submit final budget

Input includes both assumptions and calculations; required revisions to the draft version would occur after upper-level management has reviewed the draft. Additional revisions will typically be required after the preliminary budget has been presented. (The preliminary budget almost never becomes the final version without some degree of revision.)

Construction Elements

What will your budget look like? Will it follow guidelines from last year, or will it take on a new form? What will be expected of you, the manager? Understanding the budget construction elements will help you create a budget that is a useful tool.

As part of the preparation process, you should determine the following:

- Format to be used
- Budget scope
- Available resources
- Levels of review
- Time frame

As to format, will templates be available for use? And if so, will they be required? As to budget scope, will your budget become a segment only, to be combined and consolidated in a later stage? If this is so, you may lose some of your line items as you lose control of the final product. Necessary resources made available to you could include, for example, special data processing runs or extra staff assistance to locate required information. The levels of review, along with how many versions of the budget will be required, depend upon the structure and expectations of the particular healthcare organization. And the time frame should be adequate.

BUILDING AN OPERATING BUDGET: CONSTRUCTION

Budget information sources, assumptions, and computations are all vital to proper operating budget construction.

Budget Information Sources

Three primary sources of operating budget information are illustrated in **Figure 16–5**. They include the Operating Revenue Forecast and the Staffing Plan or Forecast, along with a plan or forecast of other operating expenses. As Figure 16–1 illustrated earlier in this chapter, the manager who is responsible for both costs and revenues would require the revenue forecast. If, however, the manager is responsible only for costs (and not for revenues), the revenue forecast would not become part of his or her responsibility.

When the preliminary operating budget is under construction, the capacity-level checkpoints (discussed in a previous chapter) should also be taken into consideration. (This step may be undertaken at a different level and thus may not be your own responsibility.)

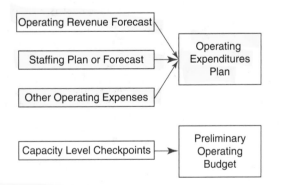

Figure 16–5 Operating Budget Inputs.

Budget Assumptions and Computations

Budget assumptions and computations are somewhat intertwined.

Table 16–1 Nursing Hours Report

Unit		Nursing Hours	
No.	Description	Regular	Overtime
620	S-MED-SURG DIV 5	72,509	6,042
630	N-MED-SURG DIV B	40,248	3,354
640	N-MED SURG DIV D	42,182	3,515
645	N-INTENSIVE CARE UNIT	55,952	4,663
655	S-INTENSIVE CARE UNIT	52,000	4,333
660	S-SURG ICU	21,840	1,820
665	S-STEPDOWN	52,208	4,351

Assumptions

Building a budget means making a series of assumptions. The budget process should begin with a review of strategy and objectives.

Forecasting workload is a critical part of building a budget. The workload should tie into expected volume for the new budget period. Good information is necessary to forecast workload. For example, **Table 16–1** presents total nursing hours by unit. But there is not enough detail in this report to use because it does not indicate, among other things, hours by type of staff and/or staff level. Sufficient information at the proper level of detail is essential in creating a budget.

Another critical assumption in building a budget is whether special projects are going to use resources during the new budget period. Still another factor to consider is whether operations are going to be placed under some type of unusual or inconvenient circumstances during the new budget period. A good example would be renovation of the work area.

Computations

Computations should be supported by their assumptions and should be replicable; that is, another individual should be able to reproduce your computations when using the same assumptions. Computations must also be comparable; that is, the same type of computation must be used by each unit or each department. Thus, when the departmental budgets are combined, they will all be stated on the same basis.

An example of computations that must be comparable is contained in **Figure 16–6**. Recall information about preparation of the Staffing Forecast (an input to the operating budget), which has been described in the preceding chapter about staffing. Now costs must be attached to the forecast for budget purposes. As shown in Figure 16–6, the forecast should first contain annual FTEs and Total Paid Days Required. When cost is attached to the cost of Annual Paid Days Required, that cost should include Gross Salaries and Employee Benefit Costs. If

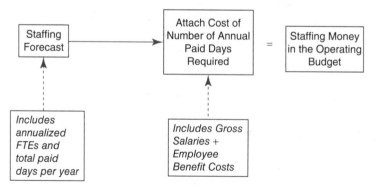

Figure 16–6 Staffing Money in the Operating Budget.

one department defines total employee benefit cost one way and another department defines it more broadly, then the resulting combined budget's staffing dollars will not have been computed on a comparable basis. That budget will be flawed.

Finalize and Implement the Budget

The final budget is approved for use after multiple reviews and adjustments of the preliminary budget drafts. The final step is then to implement the new budget. It is important to explain the contents to all involved personnel. It may also be necessary to provide training for new report formats or similar issues.

WORKING WITH STATIC BUDGETS AND FLEXIBLE BUDGETS

Both static budgets and flexible budgets can be useful tools if wielded by a manager who understands both their strengths and their weaknesses.

Definitions and Uses

Definitions and uses of the static budget and the flexible budget are included in this section.

Static Budget

A static budget is essentially based on a single level of operations. After a static budget has been approved and finalized, that single level of operations (volume) is never adjusted. Budgets are measured by how they differ from actual results. Thus, a variance is the difference between an actual result and a budgeted amount when the budgeted amount is a financial variable reported by the accounting system. The variance may or may not be a standard amount, and it may or may not be a benchmark amount.[2]

The computation of a static budget variance only requires one calculation, as follows:

$$\text{Actual Results} - \text{Static Budget Amount} = \text{Static Budget Variance}$$

The basic thing to understand is that static budgeted expense amounts never change, when volume actually changes during the year. In the case of health care, we can use patient days as an example of level of volume, or output. Assume that the budget anticipated 400,000 patient days this year (patient days equating to output of service delivery; thus, 400,000 output units). Further assume that the revenue was budgeted for the expected 400,000 patient days and that the expenses were also budgeted at an appropriate level for the expected 400,000 patient days. Now assume that only 360,000, or 90%, of the patient days are going to actually be achieved for the year. The budgeted revenues and expenses still reflect the original expectation of 400,000 patient days. This example is a static budget; it is geared toward only one level of activity, and the original level of activity remains constant or static.

Static budgets may be used to plan. When utilized in this way, these budget figures represent a goal for the budget period. **Table 16–2** illustrates this concept. The table shows a goal of 100

Table 16–2 Static Budget: Can Be Used to Plan (a Goal)

	Static Budget Assumptions per Procedure	Static Budget Totals
# Procedures Performed		100
Net Revenue ($200 @)	$200 per procedure =	$20,000
Expenses	[various]	15,000
Operating Income		$5,000

Note: Dollar amounts shown for illustration only.

procedures to be performed during the budget period, along with the revenues and expenses that support that goal.

Flexible Budget

A flexible budget is one that is created using budgeted revenue and/or budgeted cost amounts. A flexible budget is adjusted, or flexed, to the actual level of output achieved (or perhaps expected to be achieved) during the budget period.[3] A flexible budget thus looks toward a range of activity or volume (versus only one level in the static budget).

Flexible budgets became important to health care when diagnosis-related groups (DRGs) were established in hospitals in the 1980s. The development of a flexible budget requires more time and effort than does the development of a static budget. If the organization is budgeting with workload standards, for example, the static budget projects expenses at a single normative level of workload activity, whereas the flexible budget projects expenses at various levels of workload activity.[4]

The concept of the flexible budget addresses workloads, control, and planning. The budget checklists contained in Appendix 16–A are especially applicable to the flexible budget approach.

To build a flexible budget that looks toward a range of volume, or activity, instead of a single static amount, one must first determine the relevant range of volume, or activity:

- Thus, the outer limits of fluctuations are determined by defining the relevant range.
- Next, one must analyze the patterns of the costs expected to occur during the budget period.
- Third, one must separate the costs by behavior (fixed or variable).

Finally, one can prepare the flexible budget—a budget capable of projecting what costs will be incurred at different levels of volume, or activity.

Flexible budgets can readily be used to review the prior performance of the unit, the department, or the organization. When utilized for this purpose, these budget figures will typically include the volume range (for example, a range of number of procedures or number of patient days) discussed above. **Table 16–3** illustrates this concept. The table shows a volume range of 50, 100, and 150 procedures to be performed during the budget period, along with the per-procedure assumptions for revenues and variable expense plus the total fixed expenses that would accompany these procedures.

Table 16–3   Flexible Budget—Used to Review Prior Performance

	(1)	(2)	(3)	(4)
	Flexible Budget Assumptions per Procedure	*Range of #s of Procedures (Volume Range)*		
# Procedures Performed		50	100	150
Net Revenue	$200 per procedure =	$10,000	$20,000	$30,000
Variable Expense	$150 per procedure =	7,500	15,000	22,500
Fixed Expense	[fixed total amount]	1,500	1,500	1,500
Total Expense		$9,000	$17,500	$24,000
Operating Income		$1,000	$3,500	$6,000

Note: Dollar amounts shown for illustration only.

Examples

Examples of both static budgets and flexible budgets appear in this section.

Static Budget Example

A static budget example for an open imaging center appears in **Table 16–4**. The net revenue is computed using a dollar amount per procedure ($400) multiplied by the budgeted total number of procedures performed (1,000 procedures). The total expenses are derived from a variety of sources.

Flexible Budget Example

A flexible budget example for an infusion center located within a physician practice appears in **Table 16–5**. The table shows a volume range of 64, 80, and 96 procedures to be performed

Table 16–4 Static Budget Example for an Open Imaging Center

	Static Budget Assumptions per Procedure	*Static Budget Totals*
# Procedures Performed		1,000
Net Revenue	$400 per procedure =	$400,000
Expenses		
Salaries & Employee Benefits	[various]	$150,000
Supplies	[various]	25,000
Insurance—General	[various]	5,000
Insurance—Malpractice	[various]	10,000
Depreciation—Building	[various]	50,000
Depreciation—Equipment	[various]	100,000
Total Expenses		$340,000
Operating Income		$60,000

Note: Dollar amounts shown for illustration only.

Table 16–5 Flexible Budget Example for Infusion Center Within a Physician Practice

		(1)	(2)	(3)	(4)
		Flexible Budget Assumptions per Procedure	Range of #s of Infusions (Volume Range)		
# Procedures Performed			64	80	96
Net Revenue		$2,250 per infusion =	$144,000	$180,000	$216,000
Variable Expense		$1,500 per infusion =	96,000	120,000	144,000
Fixed Expense		[fixed total amount]	40,000	40,000	40,000
Total Expense			$136,000	$160,000	$184,000
Operating Income			$8,000	$20,000	$32,000

Note: Dollar amounts shown for illustration only.

during the budget period, along with the per-procedure assumptions for revenues and variable expense, plus the total fixed expenses that would accompany these procedures.

BUDGET CONSTRUCTION SUMMARY

There is no one right way to prepare an operating budget. The budget construction depends on factors such as the organizational structure, the reporting system, the manager's scope of responsibility and controllable costs, and so on. **Exhibit 16–2** sets out a series of questions and steps to undertake when commencing to build a budget.

It is also important to note that the budget for operations is usually part of an overall, or comprehensive, financial budget. Responsibility for the comprehensive financial budget always rests with upper-level financial officers of the organization and is beyond the scope of this chapter.

BUDGET REVIEW

The questions discussed in constructing a budget also serve to evaluate an existing budget. Issues of valid and replicable assumptions and comparability are especially essential. Comparative

Exhibit 16–2 Checklist for Building a Budget

1. What is the proposed volume for the new budget period?
2. What is the appropriate inflow (revenues) and outflow (cost of services delivered) relationship?
3. What will the appropriate dollar cost be?
   (Note: this question requires a series of assumptions about the nature of the operation for the new budget period.)
3a. Forecast service-related workload.
3b. Forecast non-service-related workload.
3c. Forecast special project workload if applicable.
3d. Coordinate assumptions for proportionate share of interdepartmental projects.
4. Will additional resources be available?
5. Will this budget accomplish the appropriate managerial objectives for the organization?

analysis, as examined in the preceding chapter, is an important skill to acquire. **Exhibit 16–3** sets out a series of questions and steps to undertake when commencing to review and evaluate a budget.

Exhibit 16–3 Checklist for Reviewing a Budget

1. Is this budget static (not adjusted for volume) or flexible (adjusted for volume during the year)?
2. Are the figures designated as fixed or variable?
3. Is the budget for a defined unit of authority?
4. Are the line items within the budget all expenses (and revenues, if applicable) that are controllable by the manager?
5. Is the format of the budget comparable with that of previous periods so that several reports over time can be compared if so desired?
6. Are actual and budget for the same period?
7. Are the figures annualized?
8. Test one line-item calculation. Is the math for the dollar difference computed correctly? Is the percentage properly computed based on a percentage of the budget figure?

INFORMATION CHECKPOINT

What is needed?	Example of variance analysis performed on a budget.
Where is it found?	Probably with the supervisor who is responsible for the budget.
How is it used?	To see what type of budget it is and to see how it is constructed.

KEY TERMS

Capital Expenditures Budget
Flexible Budget
Operating Budget
Responsibility Center
Static Budget

DISCUSSION QUESTIONS

1. Do you believe your organization uses one or more operating budgets? Why do you think so?
2. Do you believe your organization uses a flexible or a static budget? Why do you think so?

3. If you reviewed a budget at your workplace, do you think the major increases and decreases could be explained?
4. If so, why? If not, why not?

NOTES

1. W. O. Cleverly, *Essentials of Health Care Finance*, 4th ed. (Gaithersburg, MD: Aspen Publishers, Inc., 1997).
2. C. Horngren et al., *Cost Accounting: A Managerial Emphasis*, 9th ed. (Englewood Cliffs, NJ: Prentice Hall, 1998), 227.
3. Ibid., 228.
4. J. R. Pearson et al., "The Flexible Budget Process—A Tool for Cost Containment," *A. J. C. P.*, 84, no. 2 (1985): 202–208.

Creating a DRG Budget for Respiratory Care: The Resource Consumption Approach

16-A

BACKGROUND

This section provides background on how the budget uses diagnosis-related groups (DRGs) and relative value units (RVUs).

Diagnosis-Related Groups

Diagnosis-related groups (DRGs) were developed in the early 1970s by Yale University to describe all types of patient care provided in an acute care hospital.[1] They form a patient classification system that can be used for several purposes, including planning and budgeting. This system is an efficient way to measure case mix and it facilitates comparisons with other hospitals.

Specifically, price-per-case or episodes-of-care reimbursement is intended to represent the resource intensity of hospital care utilized by patients who are classified in the specific DRG. Thus, the case-mix methodology utilized to assign inpatients to DRGs assumes that the resources used during their hospital stay will vary directly with length of stay.[2] As a reimbursement system, the DRG assignment ultimately determines the payment level that the hospital will receive. Yet DRG reimbursement adds to the complexity of preparing an annual budget because the volume and mix of patients to be treated during the rate year is not always clear.

Relative Value Units

Relative Value Units (RVUs) are central to creating the DRG budget for respiratory care. They are used to measure resource consumption as a method of budgeting or the resources consumed by each product. RVUs are mistakenly thought to measure productivity. Every physician within a practice consumes resources, and RVUs therefore measure their resource consumption. RVUs may also be thought of as a measurement of time and effort put in by a physician. Therefore, the value of RVUs is in costing or accurately measuring consumption of resources.

How This Budget Uses DRGs and RVUs

The patient classification system of DRGs is used in this case to classify patients as to their overall diagnosis grouping (thus DRG 190-192 for COPD, as below). Treatments are administered in the hospital's outpatient Respiratory Care Department. Therefore, ICD-10-CM codes (International Classification of Diseases, 10th Revision, Clinical Modifications) are used to identify their actual diagnosis for treatment within the department (thus ICD-10-CM J44.1 = chronic bronchitis and J44.2 = emphysema as below).

In computing projected expenses, RVUs provide the number of minutes-per-treatment and the computation method required in order to measure resource consumption. (Thus, volume for each treatment is converted into RVUs by using minutes-per-treatment.) Departmental expense totals can then be converted to expense per RVU for three categories: labor, supplies, and overhead. (Gross revenues for this budget are computed using established charges as below. Gross revenues are then adjusted by a percentage ["rate"] for each type of payer.)

A DRG BUDGET FOR RESPIRATORY CARE

The hospital's outpatient Respiratory Care Department has been reorganized in response to the increased incidence of DRG 190-192: Chronic Obstructive Pulmonary Disease (COPD). COPD is a progressive disease without a cure, so that the staff's main function will be to manage symptoms. COPD ICD-10 codes include J44.1 for chronic bronchitis and J44.2 for emphysema. This year there were 620 admissions to the department. Treatments ranged from medication administration (65%), which takes 10 minutes; oxygen therapy (24%), which takes 30 minutes; and bronchodilator administration (11%), which takes 15 minutes per treatment. The charges established by the Controller in consultation with the Chief Financial Officer are $61 per medication administration, $310 per oxygen therapy treatment, and $85 per bronchodilator application.

Step 1: Project Volumes

(a) Calculate the current volume for each treatment.

Treatment	Admissions	Volume
Medication Administration	620 × .65	403
Oxygen Therapy	620 × .24	149
Bronchodilators	620 × .11	68
Total		620

(b) Convert the current volumes to RVUs.

Treatment	Minutes	Minutes/GCD*	RVUs/Procedure	Volume	Total RVUs
Medication Administration	10	10/5	2	403	806
Oxygen Therapy	30	30/5	6	149	894
Bronchodilators	15	15/5	3	68	204
Total				620	1,904

*GCD = Greatest Common Denominator (equals 5)

(c) Calculate the projected volume for each treatment

With the expectation of a 6.2% increase in DRG 190-192 for the following year (620 × .062), the department can anticipate an increase of 38 admissions, or 658 total.

Treatment	Admissions	Volume
Medication Administration	658 × .65	428
Oxygen Therapy	658 × .24	158
Bronchodilators	658 × .11	72
Total		658

(d) Convert the projected volumes to RVUs

Treatment	Minutes	Minutes/GCD	RVUs/Procedure	Volume	Total RVUs
Medication Administration	10	10/5	2	428	856
Oxygen Therapy	30	30/5	6	158	948
Bronchodilators	15	15/5	3	72	216
Total				658	2,020

Step 2: Convert Projected Volumes into Projected Revenues

Calculate the projected gross and net revenues by payer; in this example, COPD generally has been an affliction of the elderly, so we are very interested in the projected and gross revenues by Medicare, which covers 82% of our patients. (Note: Medicaid covers 13% of patients, and self-pay patients equal 5%.)

Medicare

Treatment	Projected Charge	Projected Volume	%	Gross Revenue	Rate*	Net Revenue
Medication Admin.	61	428	.82	21,409	.80	17,127
Oxygen Therapy	310	158	.82	40,164	.80	32,131
Bronchodilators	85	72	.82	5,018	.80	4,014
Total		658		66,591		53,272

Note that Projected Charge, Gross Revenue, and Net Revenue are expressed in dollars.
*The DRG rate is 80% of charges.

Medicaid

Treatment	Projected Charge	Projected Volume	%	Gross Revenue	Rate*	Net Revenue
Medication Admin.	61	428	.13	3,394	.83	2,817
Oxygen Therapy	310	158	.13	6,367	.83	5,285
Bronchodilators	85	72	.13	796	.83	661
Total		658		10,557		8,763

Note that Projected Charge, Gross Revenue, and Net Revenue are expressed in dollars.
*The DRG rate is 83% of charges.

Self Pay

Treatment	Projected Charge	Projected Volume %		Gross Revenue Rate*		Net Revenue
Medication Admin.	61	428	.05	1,305	.93	1,214
Oxygen Therapy	310	158	.05	2,449	.93	2,278
Bronchodilators	85	72	.05	306	.93	285
Total		658		4,060		3,777

Note that Projected Charge, Gross Revenue, and Net Revenue are expressed in dollars.
*The Self-Pay rate is 93% because 7% don't pay their bills.

Projected total revenue = $65,812 (53,272 + 8,763 + 3,777 = 65,812)

Step 3: Convert Projected Volumes into Projected Expenses

(a) Calculate current expenses per RVU

DRG 190-192 accounts for 35% of labor, supply, and overhead departmental expenses. The OPD Respiratory Care Department's labor expenses are $179,385, supply expenses are $135,670, and overhead expenses are $286,770.

$179,383 × .35 = 62,784/1,904* = $32.97 labor expense/RVU

$135,670 × .35 = 47,485/1,904 = $24.94 supply expense/RVU

$286,770 × .35 = 100,370/1,904 = $52.72 overhead expense/RVU

(*1904 = Total RVUs)

(b) Calculate projected expenses per RVU for next year

Labor expenses are projected to increase 3%	= 32.97 + .99 =	33.96
Supply expenses are projected to increase 5%	= 24.94 + 1.25 =	26.19
Overhead expenses are not expected to increase = 52.72 + 0	=	52.72
Total		$112.87

(c) Calculate projected expenses per treatment

Treatment	Projected RVUs	Projected Expense/RVU	Total Projected Expense
Medication Admin.	856	$112.87	$96,617
Oxygen Therapy	948	112.87	107,001
Bronchodilators	216	112.87	24,380
Total	2020		$227,998

Step 4: Determine Profit/Loss

Net Revenues	$65,812
Projected Expenses	227,998
Loss	$162,186

Next Steps

In the context of the hospital's overall financial well being, the projected loss is untenable. What strategies can help to mitigate the impact? Can expenses be reduced? Can revenue collection strategies be enhanced by adding more profitable treatments? Is the staffing level optimal? Can we continue the service at a loss by having other profitable services subsidizing Respiratory Care?

NOTES

1. J. A. Bielby, "Evolution of DRGs (2010 update)," *Journal of the American Health Information Management Association*, April 2010, http://library.ahima.org/doc?oid=106590#.V7txWq46HE8
2. P. L. Grimaldi and J. A. Richardson, *Diagnosis Related Groups: A Practitioner's Guide* (Chicago: Pluribus Press, 1983).

Reviewing a Comparative Operating Budget Report

THE COMPARATIVE REPORT TO REVIEW

The following report provides figures for the Memorial Hospital's Operating Room and Recovery Room.

Memorial Hospital Operating Budget
For the Fiscal Year October 1, 20xx to September 30, 20xx

Operating Room

Account #	Item	Actual	Budget	Variance	%Variance
1010-020	RN Salaries	470,640	470,640	(10,930)	(2.3)
1010-030	LPN Salaries	44,685	44,685	(3,451)	(7.8)
1010-040	Other Nursing Salaries	68,390	56,937	11,453	20.1
1010-200	OR Supplies-Req.	54,350	57,162	(2,812)	(4.9)
1010-220	Supplies-Direct Purchase	3,833	3,540	293	8.3
1010-221	Instruments	50,727	52,310	(1,583)	(3.0)
1010-245	Uniform Expense	628	410	218	53.2
1010-605	Periodicals & Books	670	750	(80)	(10.7)
1010-610	Employee Education	4,720	4,192	528	12.6
1010-620	Maintenance	6,387	5,940	447	7.6
1010-730	Purchased Maintenance	9,366	8,550	816	9.5
1010-740	Purchased Service	864	864	0	—

Recovery Room

Account #	Item	Actual	Budget	Variance	%Variance
1012-020	RN Salaries	173,527	174,807	(1,280)	(0.7)%
1012-040	Other Nursing Salaries	26,155	21,617	4,538	21.0
1012-200	Recovery Room Supplies-Req.	10,114	12,375	(2,261)	(18.3)
1012-213	Minor Equipment	422	422	0	—
1012-220	Supplies-Direct Purchase	482	295	187	63.4
1012-610	Employee Education	125	63	62	98.4
1012-620	Maintenance	1,037	758	279	36.8
1012-730	Purchased Maintenance	438	310	128	41.3

Note: Actual, Budget, and Variance are reported in dollars. Data in parentheses () represent negative values.

CHECKLIST QUESTIONS AND ANSWERS FOR THE COMPARATIVE BUDGET REVIEW

1. Q. Is this budget static (not adjusted for volume) or flexible (adjusted for volume during the year?
   A. This budget should be flexible insofar as surgical volume is characterized by variation because of elective surgery versus unplanned (emergency) surgery.
2. Q. Are the figures designated as fixed or variable?
   A. The figures should be designated as fixed and variable (see Variance column).
3. Q. Is the budget for a defined unit of authority?
   A. The budgets are for two interrelated units of authority: the operating and recovery rooms, which fall under the aegis of the Department of Surgery.
4. Q. Are the line items within the budget all expenses (and revenues, if applicable) that are controllable by the manager?
   A. The line items are not all controllable by the manager; see Other Nursing Salaries, Supplies, and Maintenance data, for example.
5. Q. Is the format of the budget comparable with that of previous periods so that several reports over time can be compared if so desired?
   A. The format is comparable. For example, one may compare fiscal year 2018 with 2017 and 2016.
6. Q. Are the actual and budget for the same period?
   A. The actual and budget are for the same period.
7. Q. Are the figures annualized?
   A. The figures are annualized.
8. Q. Test one line-item calculation. Is the math for the dollar difference computed correctly? Is the percentage properly computed based on a percentage of the budget figure?
   A. The calculations are properly computed. Note, for example, "Other Nursing Salaries" in the operating room. The comparison of Actual versus Budget produces a variance that is the most obvious and of the greatest magnitude and significance given the importance of that line item. As a manager, you have to ask: What are the possible causes of the variation?

   Higher-than-budgeted Other Nursing Salaries may be comprised of per diems, nurses' aides, and certified nurse anesthetists (CNAs), the negative variance of which may be attributed to a higher-than-normal absentee rate (nurse burnout) and/or excessive demand.
9. Q. How are the "percent variance" figures calculated?
   A. Using Account #1010-020, Operating Room RN Nursing Salaries, the variance of ($10,930) is divided by the budgeted amount of $470,640, resulting in a +2.3% variance expressed as a percent.

   Likewise, for Account #1010-040, Other Nursing Salaries, the variance of $11,453 is divided by the budgeted amount of $56,937, resulting in a −20.1% variance expressed as a percent.

Capital Expenditure Budgets

OVERVIEW

Capital expenditures involve the acquisition of assets that are long lasting, such as equipment, buildings, and land. Therefore, capital expenditure budgets are usually intended to plan, monitor, and control long-term financial issues. Decisions must be made about the future use of funds in order to complete these types of budgets.

Operations budgets, on the other hand, generally deal with actual short-term revenues and expenses necessary to operate the facility. For example, the Great Shores Health System's operations budgets may usually be created to cover the next year only (a 12-month period), while Great Shores[1] capital expenditure budgets may be created to cover a 5-year span (a 60-month period) or even a 10-year span.

It is also important to note that the budget for capital expenditures is usually part of an overall, or comprehensive, financial budget. Responsibility for the comprehensive financial budget always rests with upper-level financial officers of the organization and is beyond the scope of this chapter.

CREATING THE CAPITAL EXPENDITURE BUDGET

The capital expenditure budget, which may sometimes be identified by another name, such as "capital spending plan," usually consists of two parts. The first part of the budget represents spending for capital assets that have already been acquired and are in place. This spending protects an existing asset; you are essentially spending in order to protect that which you already have. The second part of the budget represents spending for new capital assets. In this

Progress Notes

After completing this chapter, you should be able to

1. Recognize the reason that a capital expenditure budget is necessary.
2. Review the cash flow and the startup cost concept.
3. Understand differences between cash flow reporting methods.
4. Recognize types of capital expenditure budget proposals.
5. Understand about evaluating capital expenditure proposals.

case, you will be expending capital funds to acquire new assets such as equipment, buildings, and land.

The "existing asset" part of the budget forces planning questions about whether existing equipment and buildings should be kept in their present condition (which can involve repair and maintenance expenses), renovated, or replaced. Renovating equipment or buildings implies a large expenditure that would be capitalized. (To be capitalized means the expenditure would be placed on the balance sheet as an additional capital cost that is recognized as an asset.)

The "new capital asset" part of the budget forces more planning questions. In this case, the questions are about new assets. The reasons for new asset spending may involve the following:

- Expansion of capacity in a department or program
- Creation of a new facility, department, or program
- New equipment to improve productivity
- New equipment or space to comply with federal or state requirements

It should also be noted that acquiring new assets results in additional capital costs that will be placed on the balance sheet as assets. For more information, refer to the chapter about assets, liabilities, and net worth.

BUDGET CONSTRUCTION TOOLS

How the capital expenditure budget is constructed may be predetermined by requirements of the organization. Your facility or practice may have a template that must be used. This takes the decision out of your hands. Otherwise, you will have to decide which tool will be most effective to build your capital expenditure budget.

One important tool is net cash flow reporting. The concept of cash flow analysis, usually an important part of the capital expenditure budget, is described later. But how will the cash flow be reported? Four methods are discussed in this section.

Cash Flow Concept

As its title implies, a cash flow analysis illustrates how the project's cash is expected to move over a period of time. Many analyses concentrate only on the cash expenditure for the equipment. (This is, after all, a "capital expenditure" budget.) Other analyses, however, will also take revenue earned into account.

In any case, it is always important to report the net cash flow. While most line items will usually be expenditures, called cash outflow, sometimes there will also be cash receipts, called cash inflow. For example, if a new piece of equipment will replace an old one, and the old replaced equipment will be sold for cash, the cash received from the sale will represent a cash receipt.

Cash flow must also be reported as cumulative. This means the accumulated effect of cash inflows and cash outflows must be added and/or subtracted to show the overall net accumulated result. In our example mentioned previously: where the old equipment might be sold, the cumulative cash flow is illustrated in **Table 17–1**. As you can see, the initial expenditure or cash spent (outflow) is decreased by the cash received (inflow) to produce a net cumulative result.

Table 17–1   Illustration of Cumulative Cash Flow

Line Number		Cash Spent (Outflow)	Cash Received (Inflow)	Cumulative Cash Flow
1	Buy new equipment	(50,000)	—	(50,000)
2	Sell old equipment that is being replaced	—	+6,000	(44,000)

Cash Flow Reporting Methods

Cash flow is typically reported using one of four methods. They include the following:

- Payback method
- Accounting rate of return
- Net present value
- Internal rate of return

A previous chapter of this book has explained and illustrated each of the four methods. Their advantages and disadvantages, for purposes of capital expenditure budgeting, are summarized later.

Payback Method

The payback method is based on cash flow. This method recognizes the cash flows that are necessary to recover the initial cash invested. The payback method is advantageous because it is easy to understand and highlights risks. However, it does not take either profitability or the time value of money into account.

Accounting Rate of Return

The accounting rate of return is based on profitability. However, it does not take the time value of money into account.

Net Present Value

Net present value, or NPV, is a discounted cash flow method. It is based on cash flows in that it takes all the cash (incoming and outgoing) into account over the life of the equipment (or, if applicable, over the life of the relevant project). Although the NPV is based on cash flows, it also takes profitability and the time value of money into account.

Internal Rate of Return

Internal rate of return, or IRR, is also a discounted cash flow method that takes all incoming and outgoing cash into account over the life of the equipment (or the project). It also takes profitability and the time value of money into account.

The use of net present value, the internal rate of return, and so forth, is the vocabulary of capital budgeting. It is also an important part of the language of finance. Therefore, it is important to understand the differences between the four methods. Review the chapter about the time value of money for more detail. Appendix 17-A at the end of this chapter presents a step-by-step method for net present value computation that assists in this understanding.

Budget Inputs

Capital expenditure budget inputs may have to be taken into consideration if the operating budget requires additional capital equipment or space renovations. **Figure 17–1** illustrates these potential inputs.

Startup Cost Concept

If the proposal for capital expenditures incorporates operational expenses, the concept of startup costs must also be taken into consideration. In these cases, management believes the cost of starting up a new service line or a new program should be included as part of the original investment. Although such operational costs do not fall into a strict definition of capital expenditure budgeting, the requirement is common enough to warrant discussion.

FUNDING REQUESTS

This section discusses the process of requesting capital expenditure funds and the types of proposals that might be submitted for consideration.

The Process of Requesting Capital Expenditure Funds

Different departments or divisions often have to compete for capital expenditure funding. The hospital's radiology department director may want new equipment, but so does the surgery department director, and so on. The various requests for funding are often collected and subjected to a review process in order to make decisions about where, and to whom, the available capital expenditure funds will go. While the upper levels of management make overall decisions about future use of funds, the departmental funding requests represent the first step in the overall process.

The process involved for capital expenditure funding requests varies according to the organization. Size plays a part. Due to its sheer size, we would expect a giant hospital to have a more

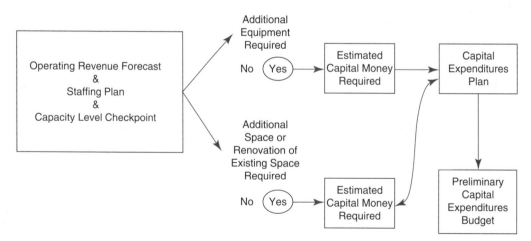

Figure 17–1 Capital Expenditures Budget Inputs.

complex process than, say, a two-physician practice. The corporate culture of the organization plays a part, too. Some organizations are extremely structured, while others are more flexible in their management principles. And in some facilities, politics may also play a part in the process of making and reviewing funding requests.

Types of Capital Expenditure Proposals

The type of proposal affects its size and scope. Proposal types commonly include the following types of requests:

- Acquiring new equipment
- Upgrading existing equipment
- Replacing existing equipment with new equipment
- Funding new programs
- Funding expansion of existing programs
- Acquiring capital assets for future use

Certain of these types may sometimes be paired as either/or choices in capital expenditure proposals. All six types of proposals are discussed in this section.

Acquiring New Equipment

The reason why new equipment is needed must be clearly stated. The acquisition cost must be a reasonable figure that contains all appropriate specifications. The number of years of useful life that can be reasonably expected from the equipment is also an important assumption.

Upgrading Existing Equipment

The reason why an upgrade is necessary must be clearly stated. What is the impact? What will the outcomes be from the upgrade? The upgrade costs must be a reasonable figure that also contains all appropriate specifications. Will the upgrade extend the useful life of the equipment? If so, by how long?

Replacing Existing Equipment with New Equipment

The rationale for replacing existing equipment with new equipment must be clearly stated. Often a comparison may be made between upgrading and replacement in order to make a more compelling argument. The usual arguments in these comparisons revolve around improvements in technology in the new equipment that are more advanced than available upgrades to the old equipment. A favorite argument in favor of the new equipment is increased productivity and/or outcomes.

Funding New Programs

A proposal for new program capital expenditures must take startup costs into account. This type of proposal will generally be more extensive than a straightforward equipment replacement proposal because it involves a new venture without a previous history or proven outcomes.

Funding Expansion of Existing Programs

A proposal for expansion of an existing program is generally easier to prepare than a proposal for a new program. You will have statistics available from the existing program with which to make your arguments. In addition, any startup costs should be negligible for the existing program. The most difficult selling point may be comparison with other departments' funding requests.

Acquiring Capital Assets for Future Use

This type of proposal may be the most difficult to accomplish. Capital expenditures for future long-term use are often postponed by decision makers in cash-strapped organizations who must first fulfill immediate demands for funding. Consider, for example, a metropolitan hospital that is hemmed in on all sides by privately owned property. The hospital will clearly need expansion space in the future. An adjacent privately owned property comes on the market at a price less than its appraised value. Even though the expansion is not scheduled until several years in the future, it would be wise to seriously consider this acquisition of a capital asset for future use.

EVALUATING CAPITAL EXPENDITURE PROPOSALS

Management planning must involve the allocation of available financial resources for projects that promise to reap returns in the future. This applies to both for-profit and not-for-profit organizations.

Hard Choices: Rationing Available Capital

Most businesses, including those providing healthcare services and products, have only a limited amount of capital available for purposes of capital expenditure. It usually becomes necessary, then, to ration the available capital funds. Different organizations approach the rationing process in different ways. However, most organizations will consider the following factors in some fashion or other:

- Necessity for the request
- Cost of capital to the organization
- Return that could be realized on alternative investments

These three factors will probably be considered in a descending sequence of decision making. The overriding question is necessity. Necessity for the request pertains to the criticality of the need. What are the basic reasons for contemplating the capital expenditure? Are these reasons necessary? If so, how necessary?

While necessity is an overarching consideration, the cost of capital to the organization for the proposed capital expenditure is a computation of the sort we have previously discussed in this section. Although the answer to "what is the cost of capital" is provided in the form of a computation, the amount of the answer depends on the method selected to illustrate this cost.

The third element in management's decision-making sequence is what return could be realized on alternative investments of the available capital. This concept is known as "opportunity cost." The term is appropriate. Assume a rationing situation where unlimited funds are not available. Thus, when a choice is made to expend funds on capital project A, an opportunity is lost to expend those same funds on project B or project C. The choice of A thus costs the opportunity to gain benefits from B or C.

To summarize, the decision makers must apply judgment in making all these choices. Thus, the rationing of available capital becomes somewhat of a management art as well as a science.

The Review and Evaluation Process

The degree of attention paid to evaluation and the level of management responsible for making the decisions may be dictated by the overall availability of capital funding and by the amount of funds requested. Evaluation of capital expenditure budget proposals may be objective or subjective. An impartial review process is most desirable.

An objective method usually involves scoring and/or ranking the competing proposals. In scoring, the basic approach generally focuses on a single proposal and evaluates it on a fixed set of criteria. In ranking, the proposal is compared with other proposals and ranked in accordance with a looser set of criteria.

The objective review and evaluation may actually first involve scoring to eliminate the very low-scoring proposals. The remaining higher scoring proposals may then be ranked in accordance with still another set of criteria.

The criteria may, in turn, contain quantitative items such as outcomes and/or productivity and may also contain qualitative items such as whether the proposal is in accordance with the organization's core mission.

Finally, some authorities believe the source of financing the project (whether it is internal or external, for example) should not be relevant to the investment decision. Real-world management, however, has a different view. How the project will be financed may be their first question in the review and evaluation process.

INFORMATION CHECKPOINT

What is needed?	An example of an entire capital expenditure budget or a capital expenditure proposal for a particular project or a specific piece of equipment.
Where is it found?	Probably with your manager or the director of your department or, depending on the dollar amount proposed, perhaps with someone in the finance department.
How is it used?	The use would probably be one time. Can you tell if this is so?

KEY TERMS

Accounting Rate of Return
Capital Budget
Capitalized Asset
Cash Flow Analysis
Cumulative Cash Flow
Internal Rate of Return
Net Present Value

Operations Budget
Opportunity Cost
Payback Method
Unadjusted Rate of Return

DISCUSSION QUESTIONS

1. Have you ever been involved in helping to create any part of a capital expenditure budget?
2. If so, which type of proposal was it? Was the proposal successful?
3. Do you recall whether any of the four cash flow reporting methods were used? If so, which one? Do you now think that was the best choice for the particular proposal?
4. If you were assigned to prepare a capital expenditure budget request, what two people would you most want to have on your team? Why? How would you expect to use them?

NOTE

1. S. A. Finkler, "Flexible Budget Variance Analysis Extended to Patient Acuity and DRGs," *Health Care Management Review*, 10, no. 4 (1985): 21–34.

A Further Discussion of Capital Budgeting Methods

17-A

© LFor/Shutterstock

This appendix presents a further discussion of the four methods of capital budgeting computations presented in this chapter.

ASSUMPTIONS

Item: Assume the purchase of a new piece of laboratory equipment is proposed.

Cost: The laboratory equipment will cost $70,000.

Useful life: It will last five years.

Remaining value (salvage value): The lab equipment will be sold for $10,000 (its salvage value) at the end of the five years.

Cost of capital: The estimated cost of capital for the hospital is 10%.

Cash flow: The addition of this new piece of equipment is expected to generate additional revenue. In fact, the increase of revenue over expenses is expected to amount to $20,000 per year for the five years. The cash flow is therefore expected to be as follows: Year 0 = ($70,000); year 1 = $20,000; year 2 = $20,000; year 3 = $20,000; year 4 = $20,000; year 5 = $20,000. Note that year 0 is a negative figure and years 1 through 5 are positive figures.

PAYBACK METHOD

The payback method calculates how many periods are needed to recover the equipment's initial investment of $70,000. In this case, the periods to be counted are years; thus, there are five years, or five periods as shown in **Table 17-A-1**.

The investment of $70,000 is recovered halfway between year 3 and year 4, when the remaining balance to be recovered equals zero. Therefore, the payback period is three and one-half years, expressed as 3.5 years.

Commentary: The payback method recognizes the cash flows that are necessary to recover the initial cash invested. The payback method is advantageous because it is easy to

Table 17-A-1 Payback Method Input

Year	Cash Flow	Balance
0	(70,000)	(70,000)
1	20,000	(50,000)
2	20,000	(30,000)
3	20,000	(10,000)
4	20,000	10,000
5	20,000	30,000

understand and highlights risks. However, it does not take either profitability or the time value of money into account.

UNADJUSTED RATE OF RETURN (AKA ACCOUNTANT'S RATE OF RETURN)

The unadjusted, or accountant's, rate of return is based on averages. The average accounting income is divided by the average level of investment to arrive at the accounting rate of return. Step 1 computes the average accounting income, Step 2 computes the average level of investment, and Step 3 then calculates the accounting rate of return.

Step 1: In this example, the average accounting income is calculated by deducting depreciation (a non-cash amount) from the annual cash flow.

Step 1.1: First, we must calculate the annual depreciation amount. In this example the depreciation is computed on a straight-line basis, which means the total amount of depreciation will equal the equipment's cost minus its salvage value.

The equipment's cost is $70,000 and its salvage value at the end of its five-year life is estimated to be $10,000. Therefore, the total amount to be depreciated is the difference, or $60,000. To arrive at annual depreciation, the $60,000 is divided by the number of years of useful life, which is five years in this example. Therefore, the annual amount of depreciation is $60,000 divided by five years, or $12,000 per year.

Step 1.2: Next, we must use the depreciation amount to calculate the accounting income per year. In this example, the accounting income represents the cash flow per year of $20,000 as previously computed less the depreciation expense per year of $12,000. The remaining balance net of depreciation is $8,000 as shown in **Table 17-A-2**.

Step 2: In this example, the average level of investment is determined by calculating the average investment represented by the equipment. We determine the average investment by computing its midpoint as follows:

Step 2.1: Determine the total investment by adding the initial investment of $70,000 and the salvage value of $10,000, for a total of $80,000.

Step 2.2: Now divide the total investment of $80,000 by 2. The answer of $40,000 indicates the midpoint of the investment and is considered the average investment over the five-year period of its useful life.

Step 3: The unadjusted or accounting rate of return is now calculated by dividing the average income (Step 1) by the average investment (Step 2). In this example, the unadjusted or accounting rate of return amounts to $80,000 average income divided by $40,000 average investment, or a 20% rate of return.

Table 17-A-2 Accounting Income Input

Year	Cash Flow	Less Depreciation	Balance Net of Depreciation
1	20,000	12,000	8,000
2	20,000	12,000	8,000
3	20,000	12,000	8,000
4	20,000	12,000	8,000
5	20,000	12,000	8,000

Commentary: While the accounting rate of return is based on profitability, it does not take the time value of money into account. That is why it is known as the "unadjusted" rate of return. This method is used by many capital expenditure budget decision makers.

NET PRESENT VALUE

Net present value, or NPV, is a discounted cash flow method. It is based on cash flows in that it takes all the cash (incoming and outgoing) into account over the life of the equipment. **Table 17-A–3** shows the individual steps involved in the computation as follows:

Step 1: Enter the net cash flow on the table. (For this example, the net cash flow has already been calculated; see the middle column of Table 17-A–1. Also enter the salvage value.)

Step 2: Determine the cost of capital (which is 10% in this example). Look up the present value factor for 10% for each period. Also, include the present value factor for the salvage value.

Step 3: Multiply the present value factor for each period times the period's net cash flow.

Step 4: Compute the net present value by first adding the present value answers for each operating period (Years 1 through 5 plus the salvage value) and then by subtracting the initial cash expenditure of $70,000 in Year 0 from the sum of the present value computations. In this example, $70,000 is subtracted from a total of $81,980 to arrive at the net present value of $11,980 as shown in Table 17-A–3.

Commentary: Net present value takes all the cash (incoming and outgoing) into account over the life of the equipment. Even though the net present value is based on cash flow, it also takes profitability and the time value of money into account.

INTERNAL RATE OF RETURN

Internal rate of return, or IRR, computes the actual rate of return that is expected, or assumed, from an investment. The internal rate of return reflects the discount rate at which the investment's net present value equals zero.

The IRR computation will be compared against the cost of capital. In our example the cost of capital is 10%, as set out in our initial assumptions.

The IRR seeks the rate of return that allows the net present value of the project to equal zero. The IRR expresses the rate of return that the organization can expect to earn when investing in the equipment (or the project, as the case may be).

The actual rate of return is determined by trial and error. The authorities say to "guess" and work forward from your initial guess. An easier method to arrive at IRR is to use a business calculator or a computer program and let it perform the computation for you. It is cumbersome, but possible, to arrive at the appropriate IRR by hand. An example follows.

Table 17-A–3 Net Present Value Computations

	Year 0	Year 1	Year 2	Year 3	Year 4	Year 5	Salvage Value
Net Cash Flow	(70,000)	20,000	20,000	20,000	20,000	20,000	10,000
Present value factor (10% cost of capital)	n/a	0.909	0.826	0.751	0.683	0.620	0.620
Present value answers	(70,000)	18,180	16,520	15,020	13,660	12,400	6,200
Net present value = 11,980							

This example solves for an initial investment of $70,000 and a positive cash flow of $20,000 per year for five years. Because the annual amount of $20,000 is the same for each of the five years, we can use the "Present Value of an Annuity of $1" presented in Appendix 13-C for this purpose.

The computation is approached in two steps as follows:

Step 1: Initial investment ($70,000) divided by the annual net cash inflow ($20,000) equals the annuity present value (PV) factor for five periods. We compute 70,000 divided by 20,000 and arrive at a PV factor of 3.5.

Step 2: Now we refer to Appendix 13-C, the "Present Value of an Annuity of $1." We look across the "5" row (because that is the number of periods in our example). We are looking for the column that most closely resembles our PV factor of 3.5. On our table we find 3.605 in the 12% column and 3.433 in the 14% column. Obviously 3.5 will fall somewhere between these amounts. To find what 15% would be, we add the 3.605 to the 3.433 and divide by 2. The answer is 3.519 (3.605 + 3.433 = 7.038; 7.038 divided by 2 = 3.519). Thus we have found, by trial and error, that the rate of return in our example is approximately 15%.

As we have previously stated, an easier method to arrive at IRR is to use a business calculator or a computer program and let it perform the computation for you. The business calculator or computer program will quickly give you a precise answer.

Many capital expenditure budget proposals also compare the rate of return to the organization's cost of capital. In our example, the cost of capital is 10%, so the 15% IRR is clearly greater.

Commentary: Internal rate of return is also a discounted cash flow method that takes all incoming and outgoing cash into account over the life of the equipment (or the project). It, too, takes profitability and the time value of money into account.

# PART VII

Tools to Plan, Monitor, and Control Financial Status

Variance Analysis and Sensitivity Analysis

VARIANCE ANALYSIS OVERVIEW

A variance is, basically, the difference between standard and actual prices and quantities. Variance analysis analyzes these differences. This discussion assumes a flexible budget prepared in accordance with the steps described in the chapters about budgeting.

Flexible budgeting variance analysis was conceived by industry and subsequently discovered by health care. It provides a method to get more information about the composition of departmental expenses.

THREE TYPES OF FLEXIBLE BUDGET VARIANCE

The method subdivides total variance into three types.

Volume Variance

The volume variance is the portion of the overall variance caused by a difference between the expected workload and the actual workload and is calculated as the difference between the total budgeted cost based on a predetermined, expected workload level and the amount that would have been budgeted had the actual workload been known in advance.[1]

Quantity (or Use) Variance

The quantity variance is also known as the use variance or the efficiency variance. It is the portion of the overall variance that is caused by a difference between the budgeted and actual quantity of input needed per unit of output, and

After completing this chapter, you should be able to

1. Understand the three types of flexible budget variance.
2. Perform budget variance.
3. Compute a contribution margin.
4. Perform sensitivity analysis.

is calculated as the difference between the actual quantity of inputs used per unit of output multiplied by the actual output level and the budgeted unit price.

Price (or Spending) Variance

The price variance is also known as the spending or rate variance. This variance is the portion of the overall variance caused by a difference between the actual and expected price of an input and is calculated as the difference between the actual and budgeted unit price, or hourly rate, multiplied by the actual quantity of goods, or labor, consumed per unit of output, and by the actual output level.

TWO-VARIANCE ANALYSIS AND THREE-VARIANCE ANALYSIS COMPARED

Variance analysis can be performed as a two- or a three-variance analysis. (There is also a five-variance analysis that is beyond the scope of this discussion.) The two-variance analysis involves the volume variance as compared with budgeted costs (defined as standard hours for actual production). The three-variance analysis involves the three types of variances defined above. **Figure 18–1** illustrates these elements.

Composition Compared

The makeup of the two-variance analysis is compared with the three-variance analysis in **Figure 18–2**. As is shown, two elements (A and B) remain the same in both methods. The third element (C) is a single amount in the two-variance method but splits into two amounts (C-1 and C-2) in the three-variance method.

Computation Compared

Actual computation is illustrated in **Figure 18–3** for two-variance analysis and **Figure 18–4** for three-variance analysis. The A, B, C, C-1, and C-2 designations are carried forward from Figure 18–2. In Figure 18–3, the two-variance calculation is illustrated, and a proof total computation is supplied at the bottom of the illustration. In Figure 18–4, the three-variance

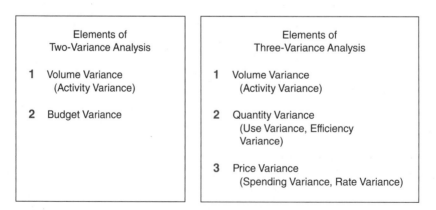

Figure 18–1 Elements of Variance Analysis.

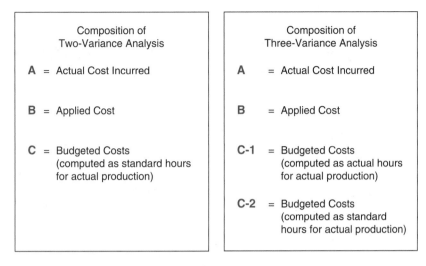

Composition of Two-Variance Analysis	Composition of Three-Variance Analysis
A = Actual Cost Incurred	**A** = Actual Cost Incurred
B = Applied Cost	**B** = Applied Cost
C = Budgeted Costs (computed as standard hours for actual production)	**C-1** = Budgeted Costs (computed as actual hours for actual production) **C-2** = Budgeted Costs (computed as standard hours for actual production)

Figure 18–2 Composition of Two- and Three-Variance Analysis.

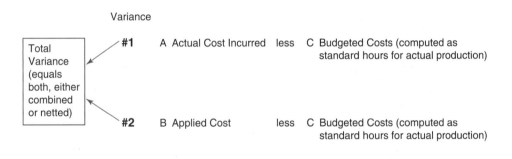

Variance

Total Variance (equals both, either combined or netted)	**#1**	A Actual Cost Incurred	less	C Budgeted Costs (computed as standard hours for actual production)
	#2	B Applied Cost	less	C Budgeted Costs (computed as standard hours for actual production)

Note: To obtain proof total, perform the following calculation:
A, Actual Cost Incurred, less B, Applied Cost = Total Variance

Figure 18–3 A Calculation of Two-Variance Analysis.

calculation is likewise illustrated, and a proof total computation is also supplied at the bottom of the illustration. This set of three illustrations deserves study. If the manager understands the concept presented here, then he or she understands the theory of variance analysis.

Different Names for the Three Variable Cost Elements

Another oddity in variance analysis that contributes to confusion is this: all three variable cost elements—that is, direct materials, direct labor, and variable overhead—can have a price variance and a quantity variance computed. But the variance is not known by the same name in all instances. **Exhibit 18–1** sets out the different names. Even though the names differ, the calculation for all three is the same. Note, too, that variance analysis is primarily a matter of input–output analysis. The inputs represent actual quantities of direct materials, direct labor, and variable overhead used. The outputs represent the services or products delivered (e.g., produced) for

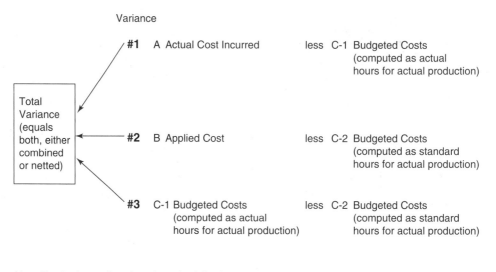

Figure 18–4 Calculation of Three-Variance Analysis.

Exhibit 18–1 Different Names for Materials, Labor, and Overhead Variances

Price or Spending Variance = Materials Price Variance   [for direct materials]
Price or Spending Variance = Labor Rate Variance   [for direct labor]
Price or Spending Variance = Overhead Spending Variance   [for variable overhead]

the applicable time period, expressed in terms of standard quantity (in the case of materials) or of standard hours (in the case of labor). In other words, the standard quantity or standard hours equates to what should have been used (the standard) rather than what was actually used. This is an important point to remember.

THREE EXAMPLES OF VARIANCE ANALYSIS

This section provides three useful examples of variance analysis. The Hospital Rehab Services example is a flexible budget with all the variances expressed in Therapy Minutes (TMs). (Therapy Minutes thus serve as uniform units of measure regarding rehab services.) One of the two examples that follow it is a static budget variance analysis, and the other is a flexible budget example—both are carried forward from examples originating in the chapter about operating budgets.

Example 1: Hospital Rehab Services Variance Analysis

An example of variance analysis in a hospital system is given in **Exhibit 18–2**. It deals with price or spending variance and quantity or use variance. The price variance is expressed in Therapy Minutes (TMs). The quantity variance is broken out into four subtypes—physical, occupation, speech,

Exhibit 18–2 Variance Analysis for Hospital Rehab Services

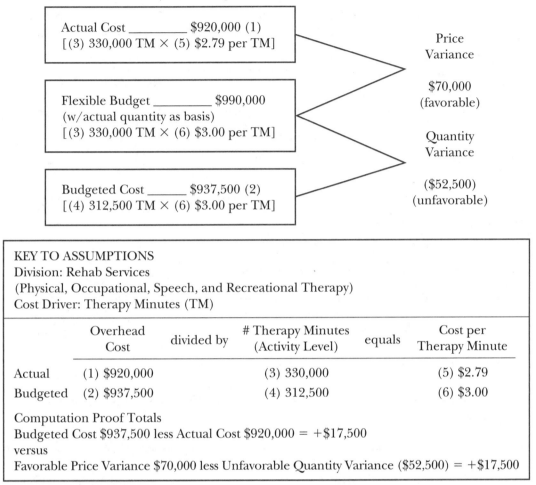

Courtesy of J.J. Baker and R.W. Baker, Dallas, Texas.

and recreational therapy—all of which are expressed in Therapy Minutes. Finally, it is assumed that the budgeted activity level is equal to the standard activity level for purposes of this example.

The flexible budget calculation ($990,000) is based on actual quantity. When the $990,000 is compared with the actual cost of $920,000 for this activity center, a favorable price variance of $70,000 is realized. When the $990,000 is compared with the budgeted cost of $937,500 for this activity center, an unfavorable quantity variance of ($52,500) is realized. Exhibit 18–2 also illustrates the computation of a net proof total amounting to $17,500.

Example 2: Static Budget Variance Analysis for an Open Imaging Center

An example of static budget variance analysis for an open imaging center is given in **Table 18–1**. As shown, the static budget's number of procedures performed totaled 1,000, while the actual number totaled 1,100. The revenue per procedure is $400 for both budget and actual. The net revenue variance is favorable in the amount of $40,000 ($440,000 less $400,000).

Table 18–1 Static Budget Variance Analysis for an Open Imaging Center

	Actual Amounts Incurred	Static Budget Totals	Static Budget Variance
# Procedures Performed	1,100	1,000	—
Net Revenue ($400/procedure)	$440,000	$400,000	$40,000 F
Expenses			
Salaries & Employee Benefits	$170,000	$150,000	$20,000 U
Supplies	40,000	25,000	15,000 U
Insurance—General	5,000	5,000	-0-
Insurance—Malpractice	10,000	10,000	-0-
Depreciation—Building	50,000	50,000	-0-
Depreciation—Equipment	100,000	100,000	-0-
Total Expenses	$375,000	$340,000	$35,000 U
Operating Income	$65,000	$60,000	$5,000 F

Key: "F" = "Favorable" variance, while "U" = "Unfavorable" variance.
Note: Dollar amounts shown for illustration only.

The salaries and employee benefits expense line item exceeded budget by an unfavorable balance of $20,000. Likewise, the supplies expense line item exceeded budget by an unfavorable balance of $15,000. The remaining expenses did not vary; thus the total expense variance is an unfavorable $35,000. The operating income variance equals a favorable $5,000 (the net difference between $40,000 favorable and $35,000 unfavorable).

Example 3: Flexible Budget Variance Analysis for an Infusion Center Within a Physician Practice

An example of flexible budget variance using different terminology is given for an infusion center within a physician practice in **Table 18–2**. Assumptions for revenue, variable expense, and fixed expense are set out below the table itself. An explanation of the computations in Table 18–2 follows.

As to Line 1, Number of Procedures:

Line 1 presents the number of planned procedures (80) and the number of actual procedures (96). Thus the procedures sales volume difference is 16 (96 less 80), and is favorable.

As to Line 2, Net Revenue:

1. Eighty planned budget procedures at $2,250 revenue apiece totals line 2 column E $180,000, while 96 actual procedures at $2,250 apiece totals line 2 column C $216,000.
2. The sales volume difference in column D totals $36,000 ($216,000 less $180,000).
3. To prove this figure, multiply the excess 16 procedures at the top of column D times $2,250 apiece equals the $36,000.

As to Line 3, Variable Expense:

1. The budgeted variable expense for drugs was $1,500 per procedure. Thus, 80 planned budget procedures times $1,500 drug expense apiece totals line 3 column E $120,000.

Table 18–2 Flexible Budget Variance Analysis for Infusion Center Within a Physician Practice

	(A)	(B)	(C)	(D)	(E)
	Actual Amounts at Actual Prices	Flexible Budget Variance	Flexible Budget for Actual Volume	Sales Volume Variance	Static Planning (Master) Budget
# Procedures					
1 Performed	96	—	96	16 F	80
2 Net Revenue	$216,000	—	$216,000	$36,000 F	$180,000
3 Variable Expense	$151,200	$6,000 U	$144,000	$25,200 U	120,000
4 Fixed Expense	44,000	4,000 U	40,000	—	40,000
5 Total Expense	$195,200	$10,000 U	$184,000	$25,200 U	$160,000
6 Operating Income	$20,800	$10,000 U	$32,000	$10,800 F	$20,000

Flexible Budget Variance = $11,200 U   Sales Volume Variance = $12,000 F

Static Budget Variance = $800 F

Assumptions:
Revenue per procedure = $2,250 per static budget and per actual amounts (no increase).
Variable expense (drugs) = $1,500 per static budget; increase to $1,575 actual amounts.
Fixed expense = $40,000 total per static budget; increase in total to $44,000.

Key: "F" = "Favorable" variance, while "U" = "Unfavorable" variance.
Note: Dollar amounts shown for illustration only.

The 96 actual procedures times the planned budget expense of $1,500 apiece totals line 3 column C $144,000. The 96 actual procedures times the actual increased variable drug expense of $1,575 apiece totals line 3 column A $151,200.

2. The total variable expense difference is $31,200 (line 3 column A $151,200 less line 3 column E $120,000).

3. Of this difference, the sales volume difference is line 3 column D $25,200. It is represented by the 16 extra procedures (96 minus 80 equals the 16 extra) times the $1,575 actual variable expense ($1,575 times 16 equals $25,200).

4. The remaining difference is line 3 column B $6,000. It is represented by the rise in expense attributed to the 80 planned budget procedures, or line 3 column B 80 procedures times $75 apiece (the difference between $1,500 and $1,575) equals $6,000. Note that line 3 column B accounts for only the rise in expense for the planned procedures (80), while line 3 column D accounts for the entire variable expense for the increase in sales volume of the extra 16 procedures.

5. Proof total is as follows: the column B $6,000 and the column D $25,200 equals the entire variable expense difference of $31,200 ($151,200 less $120,000 equals $31,200).

As to Line 4, Fixed Expense:

1. The entire $4,000 increase in line 4 fixed expense is attributed to the flexible budget variance, as it does not relate to sales volume.

2. The $4,000 excess expense is an unfavorable variance.

As to Line 5, Total Expense:

Total expenses on line 5 represents, of course, the total of variable and fixed expenses.

As to Line 6, Operating Income:

1. The entire operating income variance amounts to a favorable $800 (line 6 column E static budget of $20,000 minus line 6 column A actual of $20,800 equals $800). The $800 represents the Static Budget Variance.
2. The Flexible Budget Variance equals an unfavorable $11,200 (line 6 column C $32,000 flexible budget for actual volume minus line 6 column A actual $20,800 equals the unfavorable variance of $11,200).
3. The Sales Volume Variance equals a favorable $12,000 (line 6 column C $32,000 less line 6 column E $20,000 equals the favorable variance of $12,000).
4. Proof total is as follows: favorable $12,000 variance less unfavorable variance $11,200 equals the overall static budget variance of $800.

SUMMARY

In closing, when should variances be investigated? Variances will fluctuate within some type of normal range. The trick is to separate normal randomness from those factors requiring correction. The manager would be well advised to calculate the cost–benefit of performing a variance analysis before commencing the analysis.

SENSITIVITY ANALYSIS OVERVIEW

Sensitivity analysis is a "what if" proposition. It answers questions about what may happen if major assumptions change or if certain predicted events do not occur. The "what if" feature allows the manager to plan for a variety of possibilities in different scenarios.

Forecasts almost always should be subjected to sensitivity analysis. As previously defined, a forecast is a view of the organization's future events. Because the future cannot be predicted with absolute precision, forecasts will always contain a degree of uncertainty. Thus "what if" analyses become important to the manager's decision making. For example, "*What* will the radiology department's operating income be *if* the department's revenue is 10% greater than expected?" Or, conversely, "*What* will the radiology department's operating income be *if* the department's revenue is 10% less than expected?"

A common example of sensitivity analysis is computing three levels of forecast revenue: the basic, or most likely level, which is the planned goal; a high (best case) level; and a low (worst case) level. A chart illustrating this three-level concept for revenue appears in **Figure 18–5**.

SENSITIVITY ANALYSIS TOOLS

Manager's tools involving sensitivity analysis that are described in this section include the contribution margin and the contribution income statement; target operating income using the contribution margin method; and finding the break-even point using the contribution margin method.

Contribution Margin and the Contribution Income Statement

The contribution income statement specifically identifies the contribution margin within the income statement format. You will recall that the contribution margin is the difference between revenue and variable costs. The remaining difference is available for fixed costs and operating income.

For example, assume 100 units are sold at $50 each for a total of $5,000 revenue. Further, assume variable costs amount to $30 per unit. One hundred units have been sold, so variable costs amount to $3,000 (100 times $30/unit = $3,000). The contribution margin equals $2,000 ($5,000 revenue less $3,000 variable costs). (For a further discussion of the contribution margin, refer to the chapter about cost behavior and break-even analysis.) Now further assume that fixed costs in this example amount to $1,200. Therefore, the operating income will amount to $800 ($2,000 contribution margin less $1,200 equals $800). The format of a contribution margin income statement will appear as follows:

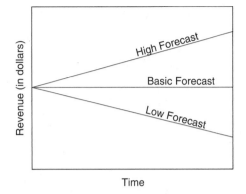

Figure 18–5 Three-Level Revenue Forecast (Sensitivity Analysis).

Revenue	$5,000
Variable costs	3,000
Contribution margin	$2,000
Fixed costs	1,200
Operating income	$800

Target Operating Income Using the Contribution Margin Method

A target operating income computation allows the manager to determine how many units must be sold in order to yield a particular operating income. We will describe the contribution margin method of computing target operating income. This method is particularly useful to the manager because it is easily understood and can be applied in many circumstances. The formula for the contribution margin method of determining target operating income is as follows:

$$N = \frac{\text{Fixed Costs} + \text{Target Operating Income}}{\text{Contribution Margin per Unit}}$$

The necessary inputs for this formula include the following:

- Desired (target) operating income amount
- Unit price for sales
- Variable cost per unit
- Total fixed cost

Let us consider an example:

- Desired (target) operating income amount = $1,600
- Unit price for sales = $100
- Variable cost per unit = $60
- Total fixed cost = $2,000

The contribution margin per unit therefore amounts to $40 ($100 sales price per unit less $60 variable cost per unit), and the formula will appear as follows:

$$N = \frac{\$2,000 + \$1,600}{\$40}$$

$40N = $3,600
  N = $3,600 divided by $40 = 90 units

Therefore: 90 units times $100 unit price for sales = $9,000 required revenue.

We can then create a contribution income statement to prove the formula results, as follows:

Revenue $100/unit × 90 units =	$9,000
Variable costs $60/unit × 90 units =	5,400
Contribution margin	$3,600
Fixed costs	2,000
Desired (target) operating income =	$1,600

In summary, note that this formula is one type of cost-volume-profit (CVP) equation. (For a further discussion of the CVP concept, refer to the chapter about cost behavior and break-even analysis.)

Worksheet Example

Julie Smith is the Metropolis Health System's Director of Community Relations. She has been informed that the Health System will participate in the first area Wellness Gala, to be held at the city convention center. The gala is an annual fundraising event in which a variety of nonprofit organizations each have an opportunity to earn dollars for their cause. Individuals attending the gala will be prepared to, and are expected to, purchase items from the various booths. Julie's boss wants their proceeds to go to the Health System's auxiliary.

It is now Julie's responsibility to make the financial arrangements and to coordinate the Health System's participation in the event. Last year the booth expense was $1,000, and Julie uses this figure as her assumption of fixed cost for the coming year's event. She finds a local vendor who assembles unique gift baskets. Her wholesale cost per basket will be $30 apiece, if she can place the order within 10 days (otherwise, the cost rises after the 10 days expires).

Julie believes the gift baskets will sell at the gala for a sales price of $50 apiece. She prepares a worksheet to determine what dollar amount of sales would be required to earn three ranges of operating income: $5,000, $6,250, and $7,500. **Exhibit 18–3** illustrates Julie's worksheet. Line

Exhibit 18–3 Target Operating Income Worksheet

	Fixed Cost	Variable Cost per Unit	(A)	(B)	(C)
			At $50 Sales Price per Unit, $$ Sales Required to Earn Operating Income of:		
(1)	$1,000	$30	$5,000	$6,250	$7,500
(2)	$1,500	$30	$6,250	$7,500	$8,750

number 1 contains her first set of assumptions: $1,000 fixed cost for the booth rental and $30 variable cost for each basket.

The convention center representative now e-mails Julie with news: due to a recent renovation of the convention center, booth rental fees have increased. It will cost Julie $1,500 for the booth. She then adds line 2 to her worksheet with a second set of assumptions: $1,500 fixed cost for the booth rental and the same $30 variable cost for each basket. She is now prepared to discuss her findings with her boss.

Break-Even Point Using the Contribution Margin Method

You will recall that the break-even point is the point at which operating revenues and costs equal each other and operating income is zero. There is a graph method to illustrate the break-even point (which was previously discussed in the chapter about cost behavior and break-even analysis). In this sensitivity analysis section, we will describe another method to determine the break-even point. It is called the "contribution margin method." The advantage of this method is its transparency. The manager can easily explain his or her results, because the computations can be easily seen and understood.

It is understood that operating income is zero at the break-even point. It follows, then, that the number of units at break-even point can be computed. The formula is as follows:

$$\text{Break-Even Number of Units} = \frac{\text{Fixed Costs}}{\text{Contribution Margin per Unit}}$$

To compute the contribution margin per unit, subtract the variable costs per unit from the sales price per unit. In the Target Operating Income formula inputs as previously described, the sales price per unit was $100 and the variable costs per unit were $60. Thus the contribution margin per unit is $40 ($100 less $60 equals $40).

Using the same inputs, our break-even formula will now appear as follows:

$$\text{Break-Even Number of Units} = \frac{\$2,000}{\$40}$$

Thus the break-even number of units will equal $2,000 divided by $40 = 50 units.

We can create a contribution income statement to prove this formula's results, as follows:

Revenue $100/unit × 50 units =	$5,000
Variable costs $60/unit × 50 units =	3,000
Contribution margin	$2,000
Fixed costs	2,000
Operating income at break even =	$-0-

SUMMARY

Sensitivity analysis, in its various forms, is a useful and flexible tool for planning purposes.

INFORMATION CHECKPOINT

What is needed?	Example of variance analysis performed on a budget.
Where is it found?	Possibly with the supervisor responsible for the budget. More likely, it will be found in the office of the strategic planner or financial analyst charged with actually performing the analysis.
How is it used?	To find where and how variances have occurred during the budget period, in order to manage better in the future.

KEY TERMS

Contribution Income Statement
Contribution Margin
Target Operating Income
Three-Variance Method
Two-Variance Method
Variance Analysis

DISCUSSION QUESTIONS

1. Do you believe variance analysis (or a better variance analysis) would be a good idea at your workplace? If so, why? If not, why not?
2. Are any of the reports you receive in the course of your work ever in a format that includes a contribution margin? If so, what were the circumstances?
3. Have you ever had to compute target operating income? If so, what were the circumstances?

NOTE

1. S. A. Finkler, "Flexible Budget Variance Analysis Extended to Patient Acuity and DRGs," *Health Care Management Review*, 10, no. 4 (1985): 21–34.

Estimates, Benchmarking, and Other Measurement Tools

© LFor/Shutterstock

ESTIMATES OVERVIEW

According to the dictionary, to estimate "… implies a judgment, considered or casual, that precedes or takes the place of actual measuring or counting or testing out."[1]

Such estimates may be of the following:

- amount
- value
- size

The first question should be, "Is it capable of being estimated?" Relying on estimates for input to reports (financial statements, forecasts, budgets, internal monthly statements, etc.) means sacrificing some degree of accuracy.

COMMON USES OF ESTIMATES

Using estimates often involves trade-offs, such as gaining a quick answer that is less accurate. Four common uses of estimates are described here.

Timeliness Considerations

Deadlines may dictate the use of estimates because there is no time allowed to develop more accurate figures. Some managers call these "quick and dirty" results. The quick and dirty estimates may then be followed at a later date by a more detailed report.

Cost/Benefit Considerations

Estimates may be purposely used instead of a more formal forecasting process discussed in a preceding chapter. Situations do arise where an estimate is adequate. The manager

After completing this chapter, you should be able to

1. Understand four common uses of estimates.
2. Estimate ending inventory.
3. Understand the concept of financial benchmarking.
4. Understand the use of the Pareto rule.
5. Compute quartiles for measurement purposes.

223

may decide upon using estimates instead of proceeding with the more formal forecasting process. After assessing the effort and time involved to gather and prepare a forecast, the manager will be making a cost–benefit decision; that is, the cost (of forecasting) equivalent to the benefit (of the more precise information)? Or will estimates adequately serve the purpose? Of course, this manager's decision will depend upon the intended purpose.

Lack of Data

Estimates may also be used out of necessity when there is not enough information available to prepare a full forecast. In this case, there is no choice but to use estimates as an alternative.

Internal Monthly Statements

Estimates may be commonly used in the preparation of short-term financial statements. For example, the monthly statements that managers receive often contain a number of estimated figures that are derived from various ratios and percentages. These estimates will probably have a historical basis because they are typically based on the organization's prior years' operating history. Thus, if bad debts for the last two years averaged 2%, the monthly statements for the current year may estimate bad debts at the same 2%.

EXAMPLE: ESTIMATING THE ENDING PHARMACY INVENTORY

Certain healthcare organizations (or departments) require accounting for inventory. The most common example in health care, of course, is the pharmacy. Internal monthly statements of the pharmacy are not usually expected to reflect the results of an actual physical inventory (unless your organization has an electronic inventory program—and that is another story). So what to do? **Figure 19–1** illustrates the solution.

The computations contained in Figure 19–1 are described as follows:

1. We first add net drug purchases for the period to the beginning drug inventory, thus arriving at the cost of goods (drugs) available for sale. So far, the steps are the same and the

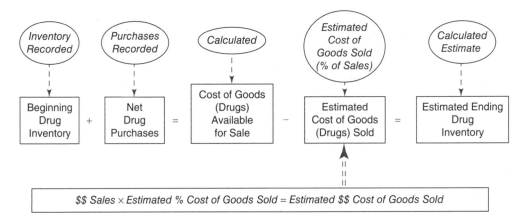

Figure 19–1 Estimating the Ending Pharmacy Inventory.

result would be the same as that in a preceding chapter, where Figure 9–1 illustrated how to record inventory.

2. But now we will compute an estimated cost of goods (drugs) sold. To do this:

First, find the amount of net sales (sales after allowances, discounts, rebates, etc.) for the period.

Then find the percent of net sales that represents cost of goods (drugs) sold in a prior period. This percentage figure is your estimated assumption and it will probably come from the last year's financial report. (For example, $1,000,000 net sales and $800,000 cost of goods [drugs] sold equals 80% cost of goods sold [drugs] for last year. The 80% is your estimated assumption for this calculation.)

Apply this estimated assumption to the net sales for the period. (For example, if the month's drug sales amounted to $70,000, multiply the $70,000 by 80% to arrive at $56,000 for the estimated cost of goods [drugs] sold this month.)

3. Finally, we will compute the estimated ending drug inventory. We subtract the cost of goods (drugs) sold (per Step 2 above) from the cost of goods (drugs) available for sale (per Step 1 above) to arrive at the "Estimated Ending Drug Inventory" for the monthly internal report.

EXAMPLE: ESTIMATED ECONOMIC IMPACT OF A NEW SPECIALTY IN A PHYSICIAN PRACTICE

Estimates can be extremely general, or they can reflect considerable judgment, with line-item detail that has been well thought out. **Figure 19–2** illustrates an example of a general estimate and its subsequent impact.

In this case we have a four-doctor physician practice. The four MDs decide to bring another doctor into the practice. He is a pulmonary specialist. The county is growing rapidly, economically

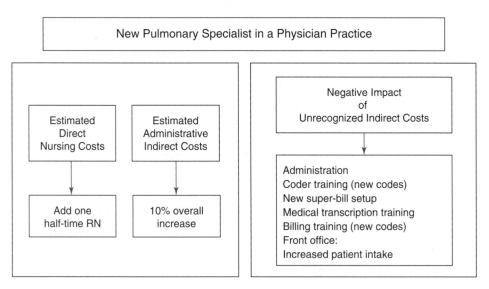

Figure 19–2 Estimated Economic Impact of a New Specialist in a Physician Practice.

speaking, and the local hospital has just expanded. The doctors determine there is a sufficient demand within this growing area to support the services of a pulmonary specialist. They want him to join their practice, even though they have not previously had such a specialty within this practice.

One morning, the senior doctor asks the practice manager to estimate the expense involved in adding the pulmonary specialist to the practice. He wants the report for their four o'clock meeting that afternoon. They must make a decision quickly because the specialist has had another offer.

The practice manager is trying to close the books for the month, but makes some time to produce an estimate. The doctors already know the amount that the specialist wants as a guaranteed salary for the first year, and they have already projected what revenue he should produce for the first year. There is an empty office available that was acquired in the initial lease for purposes of future expansion. Thus, the practice manager needs to estimate the impact on basic practice operational costs. His "quick and dirty" estimate is in two parts.

Part 1: Add one half-time RN for direct support. Assume existing nursing staff can take up any slack.

Part 2: Assume an overall 10% increase in practice administration operating costs. He has no specific basis for the 10% estimate. Instead, he knows that labor is the greatest part of practice administration costs. As a result of his "back of the envelope" calculation he thinks that administrative staff is not overworked at present and can handle tasks imposed by an additional physician. Since he disregards adding any administrative staff, he feels estimating an overall 10% increase for administrative expenses of the practice is adequate.

Three months after the pulmonary specialist has arrived and joined the practice, the senior doctor meets with the practice manager to complain. Operational costs to absorb the new specialist have far exceeded the original estimate. The doctors want an explanation from the practice manager for their meeting the next afternoon.

The practice manager realizes that his estimate did not allow for start-up costs. He composes a memo explaining that the administrative expenses were impacted by start-up costs such as coder training for the new pulmonary codes, the consultants' fees for the new super-bill setup in the office software, training about pulmonary services for the medical records transcriptionist, and training for the office biller regarding the new codes. He also notes the front office problems arising from increased patient intake, which had been underestimated. The original estimates and the negative impact of unrecognized indirect costs are illustrated in Figure 19–2.

OTHER ESTIMATES

Other commonly used computations are actually estimates. The weighted average inventory method is a good example. Weighted average cost is determined by dividing the cost of goods available for sale by the number of units available as described in the preceding chapter about inventory. The resulting average cost of inventory is in fact an estimate.

IMPORTANCE OF A VARIETY OF PERFORMANCE MEASURES

If operations are to be managed most effectively, a variety of performance measures must be in place for the organization. Generally, a broad variety of such measures are available, and different organizations tend to lean toward using one type over another. One healthcare organization, for example, may rely heavily on one type of measure, whereas another organization may rely on a very different measurement profile. Generally speaking, a wider variety of performance measures are evident in organizations that have adopted total quality improvement (TQI).

ADJUSTED PERFORMANCE MEASURES OVER TIME

We have previously discussed how measures over time are very effective when evaluating the use of money. The example given in **Figure 19–3** now combines these measures over time with a two-part case mix adjustment. (*Case mix adjustment* refers to adjusting for the acuity level of the patient. It may also refer to the level of resources required to provide care for the patient with the acuity level.) In this case, the desired measure is cost per discharge. The vertical axis is cost in dollars. The horizontal axis is time, a five-year span in this case. Two lines are plotted: the first is unadjusted for case mix, and the second is case mix adjusted. The unadjusted line rises over the five-year period. However, when the case mix adjustment is taken into account, the plotted line flattens out over time.

BENCHMARKING

Benchmarking is the continuous process of measuring products, services, and activities against the best levels of performance. These best levels may be found inside the organization or outside it. Benchmarks are used to measure performance gaps.

There are three types of benchmarks:

1. A financial variable reported in an accounting system
2. A financial variable not reported in an accounting system
3. A nonfinancial variable

How to Benchmark

The benchmarking method is predicated on the assumption that an exemplary process, similar to the process being examined, can be identified and examined to establish criteria for

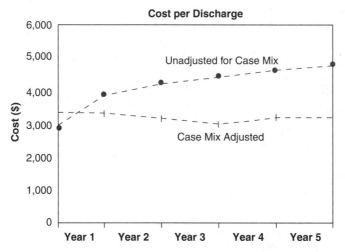

Figure 19–3 Adjusted Performance Measures over Time.

excellence. Benchmarking can be accomplished in one of several ways, including (1) studying the methods and end results of your prime competitors, (2) examining the analogous process of noncompetitors with a world-class reputation, or (3) analyzing processes within your own organization (or health system) that are worthy of being emulated. In any of these three cases, the necessary analysis will rely on one or both of the following methods: parametric analysis or process analysis. In parametric analysis, the characteristics or attributes of similar services or products are examined. In process analysis, the process that serves as a standard for comparison is examined in detail to learn how and why it performs the way it does.

Benchmarking is used for opportunity assessment. Opportunity assessment, used for strategic planning and for process engineering, provides information about the way things should or possibly could be. Benchmarking is a primary information-gathering approach for opportunity assessment when it is used in this way.

Benchmarking in Health Care

Financial benchmarking compares financial measures among benchmarking groups. This is the most common type of "peer group" healthcare benchmarking in use. An example of a healthcare financial benchmarking report is provided in **Table 19–1**. The computation of ratios included in this report has been discussed in preceding chapters. The computation of quartiles is described later in this chapter.

Statistical benchmarking is a related method of benchmarking. In this case, the statistics of utilization and service delivery, on which inflow and outflow are based, are compared with those of certain other hospitals.

Table 19–1 Financial Benchmark Example

Indicator	Total	Upper Quartile	Mid Quartile	Low Quartile
No. of hospitals	500.0	105.0	305.0	90.0
Total margin (%)	4.1	11.0	4.5	−6.0
Occupancy (%)	64.5	65.7	64.0	56.1
Deductions from GPR (%)	29.0	28.5	29.2	31.3
Medicare (%GPR)	53.0	55.1	52.2	50.4
Medicaid (%GPR)	10.0	8.4	9.7	13.7
Self pay (%GPR)	7.0	8.5	7.1	6.4
Managed care plans (%GPR)*	16.0	13.0	17.0	17.5
Other third party (%GPR)	14.0	15.0	14.0	12.0
Outpatient revenue (%GPR)	22.0	25.0	21.8	17.7
No. of days in accounts receivable	75.0	70.0	74.0	80.0
Cash flow as a percentage of total debt	30.0	60.0	27.0	−0.5
Long-term debt as a percentage of total assets	35.0	26.0	36.0	42.0
Change in admissions (2003–2007, %)	−7.0	−3.7	−6.3	−15.8
Change in inpatient days (2003–2007, %)	−6.0	−1.8	−6.5	−11.1

*Note: Managed care plans other than Title XVIII or Title XIX. All amounts are fictitious.
Reproduced with the permission of Wolters Kluwer Law & Business from J.J. Baker, Activity-Based Costing and Activity-Based Management for Health Care, p. 140, © 1998, Aspen Publishers, Inc.

In summary, benchmarking is a comparative method that allows an overview of the individual organization's indicators. Objective measurement criteria are always required for best practices purposes.

ECONOMIC MEASURES

Other performance measures may be made outside the actual confines of the facility. A good example of a widespread performance measure would be the role of community hospitals in the performance of local economies. Nonprofit organizations in particular are concerned about their ability to measure such performance. This case study gives a specific direction for such measurement efforts.

MEASUREMENT TOOLS

Pareto Analysis

Creating benchmarks, especially in an organization committed to continuous quality improvement, ultimately leads managers to explore how to improve some step in a process. Pareto analysis is an analytical tool that employs the Pareto principle and helps in this exploration. Pareto was a 19th-century economist who was a pioneer in applying mathematics to economic theory. His Pareto principle states that 80% of an organization's problems, for example, are caused by 20% of the possible causes: thus the "80/20 Rule."

The usual way to display a Pareto analysis is through the construction of a Pareto diagram. A Pareto diagram displays the important causes of variation, as reflected in data collected on the causes of such variation. **Figure 19–4** presents an example of a Pareto diagram. This example reinforces the idea behind the Pareto analysis: that the majority of problems are due to a small number of identifiable causes.

The chief financial officer of XYZZ Hospital believes that the billing and collection department is inefficient—or, to be more specific, that the process is probably inefficient. An activity analysis is conducted. It shows that billing personnel are spending too much time on unproductive work. This Pareto diagram displays the activities involved in resubmitting denied bills. (Resubmitting denied bills is an inefficient and nonproductive activity, as we have discussed in a preceding chapter.)

Constructing a Pareto diagram is really simple. The first step is to prepare a table that shows the activities recorded, the number of times the activities were observed, and the percentage of the total number of times represented by each count. In Figure 19–4, the total number of times these activities were observed is 43. The number of times that processing denied bills for resubmission (coded as PDB) was observed is 22. Thus, 100 (22/43) = 51%. Similar calculations complete the table. The table of observations is shown in its entirety within the figure.

The Pareto diagram has two vertical axes, the left one corresponding to the "No." column in the table, the right one corresponding to the "%" column in the table. On the horizontal axis, the activities are listed, creating bases of equal length for the rectangles shown in the diagram. The activities are listed in decreasing order of occurrence. Constructing the diagram in this manner means that the most frequently observed activity lies on the left extreme of the diagram and the least frequently observed activity on the right extreme. The heights of the rectangles are drawn to show the frequencies of the activities, and then the sides of the rectangle are drawn.

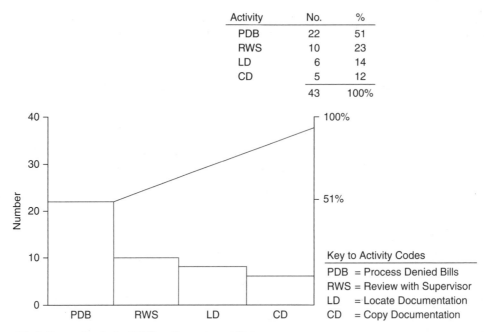

Activity	No.	%
PDB	22	51
RWS	10	23
LD	6	14
CD	5	12
	43	100%

Key to Activity Codes

PDB	= Process Denied Bills
RWS	= Review with Supervisor
LD	= Locate Documentation
CD	= Copy Documentation

Figure 19–4 Pareto Analysis of Billing Department Data.

The next step is to locate the cumulative percentage of the activities, using the right-hand axis. The cumulative percent for the first rectangle, labeled *PDB*, is 51%. (The calculation of the 51% was previously explained.) For the second rectangle from the left, labeled *RWS*, the cumulative percentage is 51 + 23 = 74%. The 74% is plotted over the right-hand side of the rectangle labeled *RWS*. The next cumulative percentage, for the third rectangle from the left, labeled *LD*, is 51 + 23 + 14 = 88%. The 88% is plotted over the right-hand side of the rectangle labeled *LD*. The last cumulative percentage is, of course, 100% (51 + 23 + 14 + 12 = 100%), and it is plotted over the right-hand side of the last rectangle on the right, labeled *CD*.

Now draw straight lines between the plotted cumulative percentages as shown in Figure 19–4. The next step is to label the axes and add a title to the diagram. In Figure 19–4, the tallest rectangle could be lightly shaded to highlight the most frequent activity, suggesting the one that may deserve first priority in problem solving.

In general, the activities requiring priority attention—the "vital few"—will appear on the left of the diagram where the slope of the curve is steepest. Pareto diagrams are often constructed before and after improvement efforts for comparative purposes. When comparing before and after, if the improvement measures are effective, either the order of the bars will change or the curve will be much flatter.

In conclusion, note that many authorities recommend that Pareto analysis take the costs of the activities into account. The concern is that a very frequent problem may nevertheless imply less overall cost than a relatively rare but disastrous problem. Also, before basing a Pareto analysis on frequencies, as this example does, the analyst needs to decide that the seriousness of the problem is roughly proportional to the frequency. If seriousness fails to satisfy this criterion, then activities should be measured in some other way. Figure 19–4 underlines the importance of judging the relevance of the measurements used in a Pareto analysis.

Quartile Computation

Reporting by quartiles is an effective way to show ranges of either financial or statistical results. Quartiles represent a distribution into four classes, each of which contains one-quarter of the whole. Each of the four classes is a quartile. Quartile computation is not very complicated, although several steps are involved. We can use the outpatient revenue line item in Table 19–1 to illustrate the computation of quartile data. (Outpatient revenue, expressed as a percentage of all revenue, is found on the tenth line down from the top in Table 19–1.) We see from the first line that 500 hospitals were in the group used for benchmarking. The median is found for the outpatient revenue of the entire group of hospitals. (Most computer spreadsheet programs offer median computation as an available function.) Then each hospital's revenue is identified as a percentage of this median. These percentages are arrayed. In the case of this report, cutoffs were then made to arrange the arrayed percentages into three groups. The percentages that were between 0 and 25% were designated as the low-quartile group. The percentages that were between 75 and 100% were designated as the upper-quartile group. The percentages that were between 25 and 75% were designated as the mid-quartile group.

The average (also known as the arithmetic mean) of each quartile group is then presented in this report. Thus, the outpatient revenue (expressed as a percentage of gross revenue) for the upper-quartile group in the report is 25.0; for the mid-quartile group, 21.8; and for the low-quartile group, 17.7. (A grand total of the entire 500 hospitals is also computed and presented in the left-hand column; the grand total amounts to 22%.) In summary, quartiles are based on a quantitative method of computation and are an effective way to illustrate a variety of performance measures.

INFORMATION CHECKPOINT

What is needed?	An example of estimates, either used in some way in your work, or published.
Where is it found?	In your own files or from a public source.
How is it used?	Use the example to examine how the estimate was determined, if possible.

KEY TERMS

Benchmarking
Case Mix Adjusted
Estimates
Pareto Analysis
Performance
Performance Measures
Quartiles

DISCUSSION QUESTIONS

1. Have you, in the course of your work, had to estimate items for reports? If so, what type of items? How did you go about estimating?
2. Does your organization use measurements such as the case mix adjustment over time? If not, do you believe they should? Why?
3. Does your organization use financial benchmarking? Would you use it if you had a chance to do so? Why?

NOTE

1. *Merriam Webster's Collegiate Dictionary*, 10th ed., s.v. "Estimate."

Understanding the Impact of Data Analytics and Big Data

INTRODUCTION

This chapter focuses upon the fast-moving field of data analytics and its impact upon the healthcare industry.

DEFINING DATA ANALYTICS

This section defines data analytics and big data.

What Is Data Analytics?

Data analytics represents the process of examining big data to uncover hidden patterns, unknown correlations, and other useful information that can be used to make better decisions.[1]

What Are Healthcare Analytics?

Data analytics applied to the healthcare industry is referred to as healthcare analytics. In addition to helping reveal and understand historical data patterns, healthcare analytics enables new approaches toward strategic forecasting, environmental analyses, competitor assessments, needs assessments, patient-centered care, and improving market knowledge about population health.

What Is Big Data?

Big data refers to large data sets that an organization analyzes for patterns or trends.[2] In other words, big data enhances data analytics by applying more sophisticated analysis techniques, by using new tools, and by sharing expanded data sets that go beyond traditional claims data and are obtained from multiple sources.[3]

Progress Notes

After completing this chapter, you should be able to

1. Define data analytics.
2. Describe healthcare analytics.
3. Define big data and data mining.
4. Recognize the differences among retrospective, predictive, and prospective analytics.
5. Understand the impact of healthcare analytics.

233

Why Is Big Data Different?

Big data typically refers to volumes of data so large that traditional health information technologies and systems can no longer manage or process the information. Also characteristic of big data is the speed at which data is created and must be processed, as well as the array of different data sources and formats.

How Is Data Volume Measured?

The basic unit of data measure is the byte, and larger measures are generally expressed in ascending order, beginning with the byte. Thus, 1024 bytes equal one kilobyte (KB); 1024 kilobytes equal one gigabyte (GB); 1024 gigabytes equals one terabyte (TB); and 1024 terabytes equal one petabyte (PB). The volume measures actually continue upward, as 1024 petabytes equal one exabyte and so on through zettabytes and even yottabytes. **Exhibit 20–1** illustrates these data measure units.

We need to know data volume amounts in order to allow for adequate data storage. While gigabytes used to be adequate, terabytes are fast becoming the standard for data storage. Such storage needs will only continue to grow. Consider, for example, Kaiser Permanente: This health network, with over 9 million members, is believed to have between 26.5 and 44 petabytes of data from electronic health records (EHRs). (And the data include images and annotations along with figures.).[4] To put such volume into perspective, using a byte converter app we find that one terabyte equals 1,099,511,627,776 bytes.[5] Can you imagine how many bytes are in just one petabyte? (And KP has not just one, but 44 petabytes.)

However, health care should focus on the relevance of the data rather than the volume of data collected. Using the data to help reduce costs and improve patient care should be of paramount importance.

What Is Big Data in the Healthcare Industry?

Healthcare industry data are of many types and are derived from many sources. A sampling of these sources includes the following:

- Physicians' written notes and prescriptions
- Medical imaging
- Laboratory data
- Pharmacy data
- Insurance and other administrative data
- Patient data in electronic patient records
- Machine-generated and/or sensor data, such as from monitoring vital signs
- Social media posts (Twitter feeds, blogs, and status updates on Facebook)
- Website pages
- Information that is non-patient specific (emergency care data, news feeds, and medical journal articles)[6]

Exhibit 20–1 Data Volume Measures

Really Big Data, Illustrated		
1024 Bytes	=	One Kilobyte (KB)
1024 Kilobytes	=	One Megabyte (MB)
1024 Megabytes	=	One Gigabyte (GB)
1024 Gigabytes	=	One Terabyte (TB)
1024 Terabytes	=	One Petabyte (PB)
1024 Petabytes	=	One Exabyte (EB)

This totality of data related to patient health care and well being make up big data in the health-care industry. Their appropriate use should lead to better-informed decisions.

TWO BASIC APPROACHES TO DATA ANALYTICS

This section explains two basic approaches to data analytics.

The Retrospective Analytics Approach

Retrospective Analytics identifies trends and problems. It looks at what has already happened (past actions) and draws empirical conclusions. Thus, retrospective analytics, sometimes called descriptive analytics, deals with historical information.

The retrospective-analytics approach can readily remove variations and standardize care. It can be extremely effective in dealing with healthcare tasks such as inventory control or staffing or billing.[7]

The Predictive Analytics Approach

The term often refers to the use of predictive analytics (sometimes used interchangeably with data analytics) or other advanced methods to extract value from data. It does not tell you what will happen in the future. Instead, it analyses the probability of what is likely to happen in the future. We can think of the predictive approach as looking forward, while the retrospective approach looks back. **Figure 20–1** illustrates these approaches.

Working with many sets of data enables views of the organization's operations that are not possible when examining one set of data at a time. Such analysts are seeking relationships that exist in the data. Analyzing data sets or using data analytics helps to find relationships that exist in the data. Finding relationships such as new correlations and business trends, in turn, may lead to opportunities to improve care, reduce costs, and improve operational performance.

Prospective Analytics: A Subset of Predictive Analytics

Prospective analytics is a decision-making tool that can deliver value by providing evidence-based solutions. The following example highlights the differences among retrospective, predictive, and prospective analytics.

Every year on Amateur Rodeo Night, this particular Emergency Department would get many more patients—mostly orthopedic patients. Retrospective analytics allowed the hospital to see

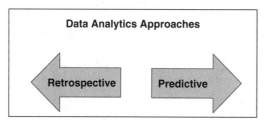

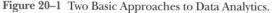

Figure 20–1 Two Basic Approaches to Data Analytics.

how many patients were treated on Rodeo Saturday night compared to the previous 20 or 30 Saturday nights. In other words, retrospective analytics identified the ED's problem.

Predictive analytics told the hospital what the likelihood was that it would need an increase in certain services that would be relevant to these emergency room injuries. (Needing, for example, more X-rays, operating rooms, staff, etc.). In other words, predictive analytics anticipated the problem and allowed future planning.

If, however, prospective analytics had been performed, the hospital could have seen how to specifically adjust resources for the overload. For example, if the X-ray suites were all full, the analytics would suggest which cases could have portable X-rays brought to bedside instead of using the suites. In other words, prospective analytics would have provided possible solutions to the problem that had been identified by retrospective analytics and anticipated by predictive analytics.

DATA ANALYTICS AND HEALTHCARE ANALYTICS SERVE MANY PURPOSES

This section provides examples of how data analytics can be used.

Using Predictive Analytics to Answer a Patient Population Question

From a demographic perspective, predictive analytics can help answer a primary question: Who are the most likely candidates for health services? For example, one hospital learned that their self-pay population was split equally among men and women, with their ages falling mostly between 18 and 26 years old, which led to bad debt problems as well as patients who were less compliant with their care than other age groups. The hospital addressed the issue starting with incentives to reduce bad debt and putting a program in place in which the patients agreed to be compliant with their care if the provider helped them pay the cost of their prescriptions.[7-8]

Using Predictive Analytics in the Human Resources Department

An emerging domain for the application of big data is human resources. The practice of "people analytics" is already transforming how employers hire, fire, and promote.[9] The application of predictive analytics to people's careers is illustrated by the following example. In 2010, Xerox switched to an online evaluation for job applicants that incorporated personality testing, cognitive-skill assessment, and multiple-choice questions about how the applicant would handle specific scenarios that he or she might encounter on the job. An algorithm (a process or set of rules used in calculations) behind the evaluation analyzed the responses, along with factual information gleaned from the candidate's application—as used in conjunction with in-person interviews.

Using a Combination of Retrospective and Prospective Data Analytics

For example, the use of analytics has allowed hospitals to correlate the patient risk of readmission with the actual readmission rate, the total cost of readmission encounters, and the clinical drivers of readmissions. Analytics can also provide a financial model that calculates the overall impact of readmission rate reductions on reimbursement, cost, and value-based purchasing payments.[10]

Using a Sophisticated Analytics Approach to Combat Prescription Drug Fraud

Express Scripts, a national pharmacy benefit management organization, has created the Express Scripts Fraud, Waste, & Abuse Team. The team uses "...industry-leading, proprietary data analytics to uncover patterns of potential fraud or abuse, and scans for behavioral red flags to identify when someone is involved in wrongdoing."[11] The proprietary data analytics are combined with Express Script's Health Decision Science platform (behavioral sciences, clinical specialization, and actionable data) to identify 290 potential indicators of pharmacy fraud.[12]

One case uncovered by the team involved a husband and wife. Over just eight months, the wife obtained over 2,800 tablets from 8 physicians and 5 pharmacies, while the husband obtained almost 4,000 tablets from 9 physicians and 12 pharmacies. The tablets included oxycodone, Endocet, and hydrocodone.[13] The team member goes on to say "...upon contacting several of the physicians we found that in several instances, the couple had signed agreements that prohibited obtaining narcotics from other doctors. However, none of the physicians was aware of the couple's visits to the others."[14]

DATA MINING

This section defines data mining and provides examples of its use.

What Is Data Mining?

The big data "revolution" encompasses yet another semantic variant: Data Mining. This is a process used by organizations to turn raw data into useful information.

How Is Data Mining Used?

By using software to look for patterns in large batches of data, healthcare organizations can learn more about their customers, develop effective marketing strategies, increase utilization, and decrease costs. Data mining depends on effective data collection and working with many sets of data in what is often called a data warehouse.

A Hospital's Clinical Research Example of Data Mining

A noteworthy application of data mining to clinical medicine is occurring at Memorial-Sloan Kettering (MSK) Cancer Center in New York City. MSK scientists leverage the massive amount of data produced by tumor sequencing to learn more about the biology of cancer.[15] They use that leverage to take the genetic discoveries made through analysis and use them to produce more-precise and cost-effective treatments for people with cancer more quickly.

Another Hospital's Patient Safety Research Example of Data Mining

In yet another example, Boston Children's Hospital has teamed with the nonprofit, federally funded MITRE Corporation research center to tackle patient safety issues.[16] In harnessing big data to boost patient safety, they are pulling data together from multiple sources—electronic health records, safety event reports, physiologic monitors, etc.—to gain insights into what may have caused patient harm.

Developing a Protocol Through Data Mining

Using a combination of clinical experience and big data analytics research, The University of Michigan Health System developed a protocol for the administration of blood transfusions.[17]

Associating Clinical Data with Cost Data

In another example illustrating the potential of big data, California-based Kaiser Permanente generated a key data set by associating clinical data with cost data. The result of this important analysis led to the discovery of adverse drug effects from Vioxx, an anti-inflammatory drug, which led to its withdrawal from the market.[18]

IMPACTS OF HEALTHCARE ANALYTICS

The impact of healthcare analytics reaches across the entire industry. Three examples of such impacts follow.

Corporate Acquisition

Noteworthy regarding the growth in the data analytics and cloud computing business is IBM's recent acquisition of Truven Health Analytics for $2.6 billion. The magnitude of the purchase is reflected in the enhanced capabilities of the company's Watson Health Unit, which is a digital repository of health-related information for approximately 300 million patients. Truven's contribution is to add patient-related payment information to a database that already includes data from patients' electronic medical records and medical imaging software.[19] The ultimate goal is to have Watson's artificial intelligence software assist physicians and administrators in improving care and curbing costs.

The Big Data Revolution

Big data creates opportunities and challenges. It's revolutionary insofar that it gives healthcare professionals the ability to use the data to solve problems much more quickly and in new ways to gain greater business insight. It is a disruptive change for healthcare organizations in that it requires new business models.[20]

New tools and statistical techniques are used to extract meaningful information from what was unstructured data. An algorithm, or set of rules or processes, governs the greatly enhanced speed with which problems are solved. The potential benefits in the realm of public health and medicine are being defined in real time.

Collaborative Efforts

By necessity, the generation and utilization of big data in health care involves collaboration between organizations. Optum Labs, a collaborative research and innovation center, has been instrumental in integrating data, generating new knowledge, and translating knowledge into practice. This has necessitated a shift in current patient care practices. Optum's efforts have focused on enabling physicians to utilize big data to improve the care of patients with comorbidities or chronic illnesses.[21] A challenge for Optum amidst their collaborative efforts is to assure an appropriate level of privacy regarding patient information.

Conclusion

Thus, analytics provide the data to reshape healthcare environments in the transition from fee-for-service to value-based reimbursement, and in so doing can help by strategically targeting patients who need preventive care. The upshot is more effective patient-volume forecasting.

Other impacts that result from enhanced data analytics and related data sharing include better coordination of patient care, better use of available resources, better claims and benefit management, and improved prevention of fraud and abuse.

CHALLENGES FOR HEALTHCARE ANALYTICS

The human resources challenge in the use of big data is well illustrated by AT&T's Vision 2020 Plan. The essence of the challenge is to retrain its 280,000 employees to enable them to learn coding skills and make quick business decisions based upon huge volumes of data that are all sorted through software managed in the cloud.[22] In an effort to keep up with competitors such as Google and Amazon, AT&T executives are urging staff to spend 5–10 hours a week in online learning relative to cloud computing. The company is willing to fund a good part of that training. The new systems facilitate collecting more data, quickly analyze information about what people and things are doing, and react.

An ongoing challenge in the use of data analytics is to weigh progress versus privacy: Balancing the promise of big data with consumer privacy and security is an essential consideration. Along with rising digital expectations of practitioners and patients, healthcare IT executives know they face strict requirements related to patient privacy and data protection, leaving them to ponder how to transform their infrastructures and keep data secure.

INFORMATION CHECKPOINT

What is needed?	Find a document or report that shows it has applied data analytics.
Where is it found?	Perhaps in the IT department or in a manager's office.
How is it used?	Its use depends on the item you find. It could be used for planning, for reference, for budgeting, or for training purposes.

KEY TERMS

Big Data
Data Analytics
Data Mining
Healthcare Analytics
Predictive Analytics
Prospective Analytics
Retrospective Analytics

DISCUSSION QUESTIONS

1. Is your organization using big data resources to address clinical and/or administrative issues? If so, for what purposes have they been utilized?
2. Have you or your area of work been involved in using big data and data analytics to uncover and examine patterns or trends? Please describe.
3. Consider your organization and the context in which it operates. What would be your recommendations for using big data?

NOTES

1. SAS, "Big Data Analytics," www.sas.com/en_us/insights/analytics/big-data-analytics .html (accessed November 15, 2015).
2. Z. Budryk, "5 Health IT Terms Every Hospital CEO Must Know" (June 24, 2015). www .fiercehealthcare.com/healthcare/5-health-it-terms-every-hospital-ceo-must-know (accessed September 17, 2016).
3. D. Hillblom, A. Schueth, S. M. Robertson, L. Topor, and G. Low, "The Impact of Information Technology on Managed Care Pharmacy: Today and Tomorrow," *Journal of Managed Care & Specialty Pharmacy,* 20 (2014): 1076.
4. Institute for Health Technology Transformation (IHTT), "Transforming Health Care Through Big Data: Strategies for Leveraging Big Data in the Health Care Industry," 2013, http://c4fd63cb482ce6861463-bc6183f1c18e748a49b87a25911a0555.r93.cf2.rackcdn .com/iHT2_BigData_2013.pdf
5. What's a Byte? http://www.whatsabyte.com/P1/byteconverter_App.htm (accessed February 17, 2016).
6. W. Raghupathi and V. Raghupathi, "Big Data Analytics in Healthcare: Promise and Potential," *Health Information Science and Systems,* 2 (2014): 3, http://www.hissjournal .com/content/2/1/3
7. A. Bickmore, "Prospective Analytics: The Next Thing in Healthcare Analytics," www.healthcatalyst.com/using-prospective-analytics-to-improve-outcomes (accessed February 17, 2016).
8. *Healthcare Finance News,* June 6, 2015.
9. D. Peck, "They're Watching You at Work: What Happens When Big Data Meets Human Resources?" *The Atlantic,* December 2013.
10. http://www.mentorhealth.com/control/category/~category_id=W_ HOSPITAL/~status=live (accessed December 16, 2016).
11. Express Scripts, "INFOGRAPHIC: Prescription Drug Fraud and Abuse," http://lab.express-scripts.com/insights/drug-safety-and-abuse/infographic-prescription-drug-fraud-and-abuse (accessed February 16, 2016).
12. Ibid.
13. Express Scripts, "Rx Addiction: One Family's 7,000 Pills," http://lab.express-scrpts .com/insights/drug-safety-and-abuse/rx-addiction-one-faily's-7000-pills/ (accessed February 16, 2016).

14. Ibid.

15. E. Kiesler, "Tumor Sequencing Test Brings Personalized Treatment Options to More Patients," Memorial Sloan Kettering Cancer Center News, June 12, 2014, https://www.mskcc.org/blog/new-tumor-sequencing-test-will-bring-personalized-options-more-patients (accessed February 2015).

16. M. Stempniak, "Big Data Applied to Patient Safety in Children's Hospitals," Hospitals and Health Networks, July 14, 2015, http://www.hhnmag.com/articles/3335-big-data-applied-to-patient-safety-in-children-s-hospitals

17. Institute for Health Technology Transformation, "Transforming Health Care Through Big Data: Strategies for Leveraging Big Data in the Health Care Industry," http://c4fd-63cb482ce6861463-bc6183f1c18e748a49b87a25911a0555.r93.cf2.rackcdn.com/iHT2_BigData_2013.pdf

18. Ibid.

19. S. Lohr, "IBM Buys Truven for $ 2.6 Billion, Adding to Trove of Patient Data," *New York Times*, February 18, 2016, http://www.nytimes.com/2016/02/19/technology/ibm-buys-truven-adding-to-growing-trove-of-patient-data-at-watson-health.html

20. J. Shaw, "Why 'Big Data' Is a Big Deal," *Harvard Magazine*, March–April 2014, http://harvardmagazine.com/2014/03/why-big-data-is-a-big-deal

21. N. D. Shah and J. Pathak, "Why Health Care May Finally Be Ready for Big Data," *Harvard Business Review*, December 3, 2014, https://hbr.org/2014/12/why-health-care-may-finally-be-ready-for-big-data

22. Q. Hardy, "AT&T's New Line: Adapt, or Else," *New York Times*, December 16, 2016, www.nytimes.com/2016/02/14/technology/gearing-up-for-the-cloud-att-tells-its-workers-adapt-or-else.html?_r=0

PART

VIII

Financial Terms, Costs, and Choices

Understanding Investment and Statistical Terms Used in Finance

© LFor/Shutterstock

INVESTMENT OVERVIEW

The language of investment is an integral part of the finance world. Being knowledgeable about the meaning that lies behind investment terms allows you a wider view of finance transactions. This chapter concerns a selection of common investment terms. We will briefly explore investment terminology and related meanings for cash equivalents, long-term investments in bonds, investments in stocks, and company ownership (public or private) in the context of investing, along with investment indicators.

Investments should be recorded as either current assets or long-term assets on the balance sheet of the organization. You will recall from a previous chapter that current assets involve cash and cash equivalents, along with short-term securities (those that will mature in one year or less). These items should all appear as current assets on the balance sheet. Long-term investments, on the other hand, involve longer-term securities that will mature in more than one year. These investments should appear as long-term items on the balance sheet.

CASH EQUIVALENTS

Cash equivalents are termed liquid assets; that is, they can be liquidated and turned into cash on short notice when needed. Healthcare organizations need to keep operating monies on hand. But it is not usually practical to hold those monies in a non-interest-bearing checking account. Instead, the chief financial officer will probably decide to temporarily place the monies in some type of liquid asset (a cash equivalent) in order to earn a little interest.

Actual cash includes not just currency (the dollar bills in your wallet), but also monies held in bank checking

Progress Notes

After completing this chapter, you should be able to

1. Define cash equivalents.
2. Understand what the FDIC does and does not insure.
3. Understand the difference between municipal bonds and mortgage bonds.
4. Understand the difference between privately held companies and public companies.
5. Define Gross Domestic Product (GDP).
6. Understand the difference between deciles and quartiles.
7. Describe the differences among mean, median, and mode.

245

accounts and savings accounts, plus coins, checks, and money orders. Cash equivalents include the following:

- Certificates of deposit (CDs) from banks
- Government securities (including both Treasury bills and Treasury notes)
- Money market funds

All of these short-term investments should be not only very liquid, but low risk. (A prudent chief financial officer should, of course, seek low-risk investments.)

Certificates of deposit can be purchased for various short periods of time (30 days, 60 days, 90 days, etc.). The certificates earn interest and can be withdrawn (cashed) after the short period, or term, expires, without paying a penalty.

Government securities that rank as cash equivalents include both Treasury bills and Treasury notes. Treasury bills are typically issued with maturities of 3, 6, or 12 months. There is a minimum dollar amount to purchase. A Treasury bill pays the full amount invested if redeemed at maturity. If the bill is redeemed prior to maturity, however, the amount received may be either higher or lower than your cost, depending upon the current market.

Treasury notes are typically issued with longer maturities—years instead of months. The shortest maturity period for a Treasury note is one year. A one-year note would be classified as short-term and could be recorded as a current asset.

Money market funds are supposed to invest in conservative instruments such as commercial bank CDs and Treasury bills. A money market fund should invest in an assortment of such conservative instruments. Portfolio managers, who are expected to manage responsibly and thus select only low-risk investments, manage these funds. Money market funds are somewhat of a hybrid, as these funds typically allow check-writing privileges. Thus, the investor is able to withdraw funds by writing what is actually a draft against the fund, although most everyone thinks of this draft as a check.

GOVERNMENTAL GUARANTOR: THE FDIC

In the United States, the Federal Deposit Insurance Corporation (FDIC) "preserves and promotes public confidence in the U.S. financial system by insuring deposits in banks and thrift institutions ... by identifying and monitoring and addressing risks to the deposit insurance funds; and by limiting the effect on the economy and the financial system when a bank or thrift institution fails."[1] The FDIC insured deposits in banks and thrift institutions for at least $250,000 through December 31, 2009. However, this was supposed to be a temporary increase and the FDIC deposit insurance was supposed to be restored to its usual limit of $100,000 after that date. Savings, checking, and other deposit accounts are combined to reach the deposit insurance limit. "Deposits held in different categories of ownership—such as single or joint accounts—may be separately insured. Also, the FDIC generally provides separate coverage for retirement accounts, such as individual retirement accounts (IRAs) and Keoghs."[2] It is important to note that not all institutions—and thus not all funds—are insured by the FDIC. **Exhibit 21–1** sets out these facts.

LONG-TERM INVESTMENTS IN BONDS

A bond is a long-term debt instrument under which a borrower agrees to make payments of interest and principal on particular dates to the holder of the debt (the bond). We have titled

Exhibit 21–1 The FDIC: Insured or Not Insured?

FDIC-Insured

- Checking Accounts (including money market deposit accounts)
- Savings Accounts (including passbook accounts)
- Certificates of Deposit

Not FDIC-Insured

- Investments in mutual funds (stock, bond, or money market mutual funds), whether purchased from a bank, brokerage, or dealer
- Annuities (underwritten by insurance companies, but sold at some banks)
- Stocks, bonds, Treasury securities or other investment products, whether purchased through a bank or a broker/dealer

Reproduced from the Federal Deposit Insurance Corporation. "The FDIC: Insured or Not Insured?: A Guide to What Is and Is Not Protected" (April 2011).

---

this section "long-term investments in bonds," but in actuality the bondholder is a creditor, because bonds are liabilities to the issuing company.

Because these are long-term contracts, bonds typically mature in 20 to 30 years, although there are exceptions. In general, interest is paid throughout the term, or life, of the bonds, and the principal is paid at maturity. (Although there are exceptions to this rule of thumb, too.) Three types of bonds are discussed below.

Municipal Bonds

Municipal bonds are long-term obligations that are typically used to finance capital projects. Municipal bonds are issued by states and also by political subdivisions. The political subdivision might be, for example, a county, a bridge authority, or the authority for a toll road project.

General Obligation Bonds

General obligation bonds are backed, or secured, by the "full faith and credit" of the municipality that issues them. This means the bonds are backed by the full taxing authority of the municipality that issues them.

Revenue Bonds

Revenue bonds, as their name implies, are backed, or secured, by revenues of their particular project. Eligible healthcare organizations that are not-for-profit can sometimes issue revenue bonds through a local healthcare financing authority.

Mortgage Bonds

Mortgage bonds, as their name implies, are backed, or secured, by certain real property. When first mortgage bonds are issued, this means the first mortgage bondholders have first claim to the real property that has been pledged to secure the mortgage. If second mortgage bonds are also issued, this means the second mortgage bondholders will not have a claim against the real property until the claims of the first mortgage bondholders have been paid.

Debentures

Debentures are bonds that are unsecured. Instead of being backed by real property, debentures are backed by revenues that the issuing organization can earn. Unlike bondholders, holders of debentures are unsecured. Subordinated debentures are even further unsecured, in that these debentures cannot be paid until any and all debt obligations that are senior to the subordinated debentures have been paid.

INVESTMENTS IN STOCKS

Stocks represent equity, or net worth, in a company. This is in contrast to bonds. Generally speaking, a bondholder is a creditor, because bonds are liabilities to the issuing company. On the other hand, an individual or organization that buys stock in that company becomes an investor, not a creditor.

Common Stock

A purchaser of common stock expects to receive a portion of net income of the company who issues the stock. The proportionate share of net income will be paid out as a dividend. (Note that start-up companies that do not pay dividends are not part of this discussion about investments in stocks.)

Preferred Stock

Preferred stock, as its name implies, has preference over common stock in certain issues such as payment of dividends. In actual fact, preferred stock is a type of hybrid, in that it generally has a fixed-rate dividend payment, much like a bond's interest payment. But like common stock, it also expects to receive a portion of net income of the company who issues the stock, up to the amount of the fixed-rate dividend payment. (Also note that the preferred stock dividends are paid before the common stock dividends.)

Convertible preferred stock is a type of preferred stock that can be exchanged for common shares. The exchange is usually at a particular time and price, and the exchange ratio of preferred-to-common is also stipulated.

Stock Warrants

Stock warrants allow the owner of the warrant to purchase additional shares of stock in the company, generally at a particular price and prior to an expiration date. Warrants do not pay dividends. They are often part of the compensation package awarded to executives.

PRIVATELY HELD COMPANIES VERSUS PUBLIC COMPANIES

Whether a stock is listed on a stock exchange or not is a function of ownership and size of the organization. These distinctions are described here.

Privately Held Companies

A small company with common stock that is not traded is known as a "privately held" company. Its stock is termed "closely held" stock.

Public Companies

Companies with publicly owned common stock are known as "public companies." The stocks of many larger public companies may be listed on one of several stock exchanges. Stock exchanges exist to trade the stock of publicly held companies. At the time of this writing, besides multiple regional exchanges such as the Chicago Stock Exchange, there is the American Stock Exchange, known as AMEX, along with the New York Stock Exchange, known as the NYSE. (At the time of this writing it is probable that the New York Stock Exchange will be acquired by the Intercontinental Exchange [ICE]. If so, the NYSE acronym may be changed to reflect the new ownership.)[3]

Smaller public companies, however, may not be listed on a stock exchange. The stock of these companies is considered to be unlisted; instead, their stock is traded "over the counter," or OTC. The National Association of Securities Dealers (NASD) oversees this market. The OTC stock market uses a computerized trading network called NASDAQ, which stands for the "NASD Automated Quotation system."

Published stock tables typically reflect the composite regular trading on the stock exchanges as of closing. A stock table will generally contain four columns: the first column is an abbreviation of the public company's name, the second column is the company's symbol (an alpha symbol), the third column is the stock's price as of closing for that day, and the fourth column is the net change of the stock price when compared to close of the previous day. Using healthcare organizations as examples, Johnson & Johnson's symbol is "JNJ," while Humana, Inc.'s symbol is "HUM."

Governmental Agency as Overseer

At the time of this writing, the overseer of the stock market in the United States is the U.S. Securities and Exchange Commission (SEC). (It is possible that in the future the SEC may be reorganized as a somewhat different entity with somewhat different responsibilities.) The mission of the SEC is to "protect investors, maintain fair, orderly, and efficient markets, and facilitate capital formation."[4] The SEC oversees "the key participants in the securities world, including securities exchanges, securities brokers and dealers, investment advisors, and mutual funds. Here, the SEC is concerned primarily with promoting the disclosure of important market-related information, maintaining fair dealing, and protecting against fraud."[5]

INVESTMENT INDICATORS

The annual rate of inflation (or deflation) is a typical investment indicator, as is the gross domestic product measure. Both are discussed here.

Inflation Versus Deflation

Inflation means "an increase in the volume of money and credit relative to available goods and services resulting in a continuing rise in the general price level."[6]

"Indexed to inflation" means these monies will rise in accordance with an inflationary increase. For example, Social Security payments are indexed to inflation. Excessive inflation is feared because it reduces or devalues the spending power of the dollars you possess.

Deflation, on the other hand, means "a contraction in the volume of available money and credit that results in a general decline in prices."[7] Deflation is feared because the contraction in volume of available money and credit generally results in a fall in prices that limits and/or reduces the country's economic activity.

Gross Domestic Product (GDP)

The GDP measures "the output of goods and services produced by labor and property located in the United States."[8] Investors watch the GDP because this measure is considered to be the "gold standard" measure of the country's overall economic fitness. The Bureau of Economic Analysis (BEA), located within the U.S. Department of Commerce, releases quarterly estimates of the GDP. The BEA is also responsible for the price index for gross domestic purchases. The price index measures "prices paid by U.S. residents,"[9] and is also released on a quarterly basis.

STATISTICS OVERVIEW

This overview provides an introduction to statistics, along with a discussion of mathematics versus statistics.

Introduction

This section contains general definitions of statistical and other terms that may commonly be used within the finance department. It is important to understand that our usage of statistical terms in the world of healthcare finance is a specialized view. (For instance, in the case of one example, we are concerned with how statistical analysis is used to score performance measures.) In other words, we need enough information to understand the general process and what the terms mean in general usage. As such, the following definitions are not technical, but instead are intentionally generalized.

The Field of Mathematics Versus the Discipline of Statistics

The field of mathematics is broad and varied. The National Council of Teachers of Mathematics (NCTM) has developed a set of mathematical standards for teaching and learning mathematics. These standards are important because they help to understand the breadth and depth of mathematics.

The NCTM has set two categories of standards: thinking math and content math. Thinking math standards are problem solving, communication, reasoning, and connections. Content math standards are statistics and probability, fractions and decimals, estimation, number sense, geometry and spatial sense, measurement, and patterns and relationships.[10] As you can see, the field of mathematics includes, among other disciplines, those of statistics and probability as well as that of basic arithmetic.

- Statistics is the branch of mathematics that deals with collecting, summarizing, and analyzing numerical data, along with estimating probability and interpreting analytical results.
- Arithmetic, on the other hand, is the branch of mathematics that covers the basic functions of multiplication, division, addition, subtraction, and so on.

In other words, statistics often provides sophisticated analytical results, while arithmetic provides the results of basic calculations.

COMMONLY USED STATISTICAL AND OTHER MATHEMATICAL TERMS

This section includes a variety of mathematical terms that are commonly used in finance departments.

Mean, Median, and Mode

Mean, median, and mode are basic statistical concepts, but they are often confused for one another. The following descriptions are intended to clarify the differences among them.

In order to begin our description of mean, median, and mode, first imagine a set of numbers that are arranged, or ranked, in order. They can be arranged either from the highest to the lowest, or vice versa. Now visualize this set of numbers as they apply to the following three descriptions.

Mean: The mean is the average of numbers, or values. To obtain the average, all the values are added together to obtain the total. Then the total is divided by the number of line items to obtain the average, or mean. This method is known as the "arithmetic mean" and is the most commonly used. (Two other analytical methods, known as the geometric mean and the harmonic mean, are obtained through statistical formulas.)

Median: The median occupies a position in a ranked series of values (numbers) in which the same number of values appear above the median as appear below it. Or, to put it another way, there are an equal number of values (numbers) above and below the median. (In a situation where there is no one middle number [as in the case of an even number of values], the median instead is the average of the two middle numbers within the ranked series of values.)

Mode: The mode is the number, or value, that appears for the most times (is the most frequent) within a series of numbers or values.

Illustrating the Difference

We show these differences in **Table 21–1**. Here you see a series of physicians' scores. Their scores represent a set of numbers, ranked from high to low as previously described. Within the table you can see the mean, the median, and the mode each indicated within the ranked data set of scores.

Other Statistical Analysis Terms

These descriptions pertain to other types of statistical analysis terminology.

Algorithm: A problem-solving, step-by-step process, or a set of formulas used in calculations, particularly in computer programs.

Domain: A subgroup of a whole group that is of particular interest for research or for measurement purposes. For example, the domain of safety is one subgroup of an entire patient care grouping.

Table 21–1 Illustration of Mean, Median, and Mode

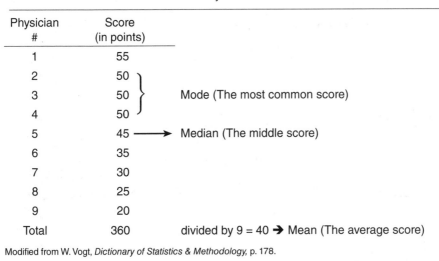

Physicians' CPIA Scores

Physician #	Score (in points)	
1	55	
2	50	
3	50	Mode (The most common score)
4	50	
5	45	→ Median (The middle score)
6	35	
7	30	
8	25	
9	20	
Total	360	divided by 9 = 40 → Mean (The average score)

Modified from W. Vogt, *Dictionary of Statistics & Methodology*, p. 178.

Measure: A unit of analysis, such as a measurement standard.

Measurement: The process of assigning numbers to something, such as to variables. (In other words, measurement is how we get the numbers we analyze using statistical methods.)

Standard Deviation: Measures the average amount that a set of data within a distribution may deviate from the mean. The further apart the values are, the larger the standard deviation will be. A formula is used to compute the standard deviation (SD).

Standardized Measure or Scale: A statistical method that can compare data measured on different scales or instruments. (For example, the method of comparison could be a score or a percentage.)

Statistically Significant: In general terms, a result or relationship is found to be reliable, and thus statistically significant, if it is either bigger or smaller than if the equivalent result could be attributed to chance alone. In other words, the finding is a result that is not merely attributable to random chance alone.

Variable: A finding or quantity that can vary, or is apt to vary. Examples of variables include just about anything that is capable of being measured. (Note that a constant is the opposite of a variable, because it does not vary [and thus is constant].)

Variance: The difference between a standard value and an actual value. The difference is typically arrived at through statistical analysis.

Terms About Distributions

These descriptions pertain to distribution terms, such as those used to explain scoring methodology.

Frequency Distribution: A count of how many times (how frequently) a number appears in a group of numbers.

Decile: A distribution into 10 classes, each of which contains one-tenth of the whole; any one of the 10 classes is a decile.

Quartile: A distribution into four classes, each of which contains one-quarter of the whole; any one of the four classes is a quartile.

Terms Used in Mathematical (Arithmetic) Computations

These descriptions pertain to computation terms, such as those sometimes used to explain reporting-measures methods.

Decimal: The decimal system subdivides into tenth or hundredth units. A decimal point number is typically expressed with a decimal point to show units that have a value of less than one. For example, one dollar is equal to 100 cents. Thus, 30 cents can be expressed as a decimal (0.30) because it has a value (30) that is less than the 100 cents that represents 1. Thus, the 30 that is shown to the right of the decimal point has a value of less than 1 (1 dollar, in this example).

Fraction: Indicates both part of a whole (the numerator, which is the top part) and the entire whole (the denominator, which is the total number of parts to be divided). For example, 30 cents can be written as a fraction (30/100) because the numerator is the part (30) and the denominator is the whole (100 cents, or 1 dollar).

Numerator: The top part of a fraction. The numerator indicates the portion of the total under consideration. See also *Denominator.*

Denominator: The bottom part of a fraction. The denominator indicates all the values under consideration. See also *Numerator.*

Percent (Percentage): Typically 1 part or unit in every 100 parts or units. For example, 50% means 50 parts per 100.

Terms About Data

These descriptions pertain to data. Note that the word "data" is plural. (This means that we should say "The data are showing" instead of "The data is showing.")

Data: The factual information being analyzed. This information is typically used to measure and/or calculate, although it may also be used for reasoning and/or discussion.

Data Base (also Database): A particular set of computerized data organized in a manner designed for efficient retrieval.

Data Entry: The process of recording data, generally by electronic means.

Data Mining: A process used by organizations to turn raw data into useful information.

Data Processing: Generally speaking, taking raw data and converting it into a form that can be readily used by computer software (processing). The processing can take place in magnetic, optical, or mechanical form.

Data Set: A group of data (a set) gathered together for a like purpose.

Data Standardization: The process that converts data into a standard, such as the creation of standard scores.

Big Data: Large data sets that are analyzed for patterns or trends.

Terms About Time Measurements

These descriptions pertain to terms about time measurements.

Period: A unit of time.

Baseline Period: A unit of time (period) used as a basis for comparison.

Base Year: A 12-month unit of time (year) used as a basis for comparison.

Performance Period: A unit of time during which performance is measured.

Illustrating Analytical Results

Graphics summarize and assist in interpreting statistical results. In fact, "graphing is another way to show and see information mathematically."[11] There are multiple types of graphics available for this task. The most common types include the following:

Pie Chart: Presents data as portions of a circle

Bar chart: Presents data as horizontal bars

Line chart: Presents data as multiple lines that track along a grid

Column chart or table: Presents data as columns

Scatterplot: Shows the relationship between two data sets via a graph that plots points along both the horizontal and vertical axes

Venn diagram: Shows the relationships between data points as a series of overlapping circles

Illustrated examples of a pie chart, bar chart, and line chart are found in the chapter, "Using Comparative Data."

To summarize, we may not tend to design a graphic for its particular use. Instead we may rely on two or three formats that are used over and over. However, we should try to design a graphic that communicates results that are often complex in a precise, clear and efficient manner.[12]

INFORMATION CHECKPOINT

What is needed?	A copy of the *Wall Street Journal.*
Where is it found?	At a newsstand or possibly within the offices of your own organization.
How is it used?	Locate the "Stock Tables" section of the *Journal.* Review the column headings in the tables and locate the names of various stock exchanges that are included in the findings.

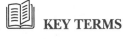 KEY TERMS

Common Stock	Deflation	Federal Deposit Insurance
Debentures	Denominator	Corporation (FDIC)
Decile		

Gross Domestic Product (GDP)

Inflation

Mean

Median

Mode

Money Market Funds

Municipal Bonds

Numerator

Quartile

Preferred Stock

Securities and Exchange Commission (SEC)

Stock Warrants

DISCUSSION QUESTIONS

1. Do you know if your own monies on deposit are FDIC insured? If you do not know, how would you go about finding out?
2. Do you know of a healthcare company whose stock is publicly held? If you do not know, how would you go about finding out?
3. Do you know if any healthcare company that you have worked for (now or previously) had issued revenue bonds that were purchased by investors? If you do not know, how would you go about finding out?
4. Do you agree with the distinction between thinking math and content math? What type(s) of mathematics have you ever studied?

NOTES

1. Federal Deposit Insurance Corporation, "Who Is the FDIC?" Federal Deposit Insurance Corporation, http://www.fdic.gov/about/index.html
2. Ibid.
3. Wall Street Journal Opinion, "ICE Buys NYSE," *Wall Street Journal*, December 21, 2012, A18.
4. U.S. Securities and Exchange Commission, "The Investor's Advocate: How the SEC Protects Investors, Maintains Market Integrity, and Facilitates Capital Formation." Last modified June 10, 2013, www.sec.gov/about/whatwedo.shtml
5. Ibid.
6. *Merriam Webster's Collegiate Dictionary*, 10th ed., s.v. "Inflation."
7. Ibid., "Deflation."
8. U.S. Department of Commerce, Bureau of Economic Analysis (BEA). News Release: Gross Domestic Product: Fourth Quarter 2008 (Final), http://bea.gov/newsreleases/national/gdp/gdpnewsrelease.htm
9. Ibid.
10. "What Is Mathematics?" p. 1, www.2.ed.gov/pubs/EarlyMath/whatis.html (accessed July 12, 2016).
11. Ibid., p. 7.
12. R. Hawkins and J. J. Baker. *Management Accounting for Health Care Organizations: Tools and Techniques for Decision Support*. (Boston: Jones & Bartlett Publishers, 2004). p. 376.

Business Loans and Financing Costs

Business loans, as the term implies, represent debts incurred to assist in running a business. Whether to take on debt and how much to take on are common and necessary parts of financial planning. This type of planning involves the organization's capital structure, as discussed in the following section.

OVERVIEW OF CAPITAL STRUCTURE

"Capital" represents the financial resources of the organization and is generally considered to be a combination of debt and equity.

"Capital structure" means the proportion of debt versus equity within the organization. The phrase "capital structure" actually refers to the debt–equity relationship. For example, if a physician practice partnership owed $500,000 in debt and also had $500,000 in partner's equity, the partnership capital structure, or debt–equity relationship, would be 50–50.

Different industries typically have different debt–equity relationships. In the case of health care, the chief financial officer of the organization is usually responsible for guiding decisions about the proportion of debt. The chief financial officer will take into account various sources of capital, as discussed in the next section.

SOURCES OF CAPITAL

Sources of capital traditionally include four methods of obtaining funds:

- Borrowing from a lending institution
- Borrowing from investors
- Retaining the excess of revenues over expenses
- Selling an additional interest in the organization

Progress Notes

After completing this chapter, you should be able to

1. Understand what capital structure means.
2. Recognize four sources of capital.
3. Explain an amortization schedule.
4. Understand loan costs.

Borrowing from a lending institution is generally classified by the length of the loan. Short-term borrowing is commonly expected to be repaid within a 12-month period. Long-term borrowing is usually to finance land, buildings, and/or equipment. Long-term borrowing for these purposes is usually accomplished by obtaining a mortgage from the lending institution.

Borrowing from investors assumes the organization is big enough and has the proper legal structure to do so. A common example of borrowing from investors is that of selling bonds. Bonds represent the company's promise to pay at a future date. When bonds are sold, the purchaser expects to receive a certain amount of annual interest and also expects that the bonds will be redeemed on a certain date, several years in the future.

Retaining the excess of revenues over expenses represents retaining operating profits to a proprietary, or for-profit, company. (Of course this assumes there is an excess of funds to retain.) A not-for-profit organization may be bound by legal limitations on the retention of its funds. However, the not-for-profit organization can also sometimes rely on a different income stream. Church-affiliated not-for-profits, for example, may be able to solicit donations. This example represents a unique method of raising capital.

Selling an additional interest in the organization depends on its legal structure. Typically, this method involves a for-profit corporation selling additional shares of common stock to raise funds. Not-for-profit organizations are bound by legal limitations and may not be able to follow this route.

THE COSTS OF FINANCING

Financing costs typically involve interest expense and usually also involve loan costs, as described in this section.

Interest Expense

Payments on a business loan typically consist of two parts: principal and interest expense. The principal portion of the loan payment reduces the loan itself, while the rest of the payment is made up of interest on the remaining balance due on the loan.

The amount of principal and the amount of interest contained in each payment are illustrated in an "amortization schedule." For example, assume the purchase of equipment for $60,000. Monthly payments will be made over a 3-year period, and the annual, or per-year, interest rate will be 12%. The first 6 months of the amortization schedule for this loan is illustrated in **Table 22–1**. The entire 36-month amortization schedule is found in Appendix 22-A at the end of this chapter.

The interest expense for each monthly payment is computed on the principal balance remaining after the principal portion of the previous payment has been subtracted. The "Remaining Principal Balance" column shows the declining balance of the principal. Now refer to the "Remaining Principal Balance" column and compare it with the "Interest Expense Portion of Payment" column. Remember that the 12% annual interest rate in this example amounts to 1% per month. You can see how 10% of $60,000.00 amounts to a $600.00 interest payment for month 1; 10% of $58,607.14 amounts to a $586.07 interest payment for month 2; and so on. The remainder of the payment amount—after interest expense—is then deducted from the principal amount due, as shown in Table 22–1. Thus, of the $1,992.86 monthly payment 1, if $600.00 is interest, then $1,392.86 is the principal portion, and of the $1,992.86 monthly payment 2, if $586.07 is interest, then $1,406.79 is the principal portion, and so on.

Table 22–1 Loan Amortization Schedule

Payment Number	Total Payment	Principal Portion of Payment	Interest Expense Portion of Payment	Remaining Principal Balance
Beginning balance = $60,000.00				
1	$1,992.86	$1,392.86	$600.00	$58,607.14
2	1,992.86	1,406.79	586.07	57,200.35
3	1,992.86	1,435.07	572.00	55,779.49
4	1,992.86	1,449.42	557.79	54,344.42
5	1,992.86	1,463.91	543.44	52,895.00
6	1,992.86	1,478.55	528.95	51,431.09

Not all amortization schedules are set up in the same configuration. The columns that are shown can vary. For example, the entire 36-month amortization schedule for the Table 22–1 loan is contained in Appendix 22-A. Refer to this appendix to see how the columns are different from Table 22–1. While the basic information necessary for computation is shown, the layout of the schedule is different.

Loan Costs

The term "loan costs" covers expenses necessary to close the loan. Loan closing costs generally include some expenses that would be reported in the current year and some other expenses that should be spread over several years.

Suppose, for example, the Great Lakes Home Health Agency bought a tract of land for expansion purposes. The home health agency paid a 20% down payment and obtained mortgage financing from a local bank for the remainder of the purchase price. When the loan was closed, meaning the transaction was completed, the statement that lists closing costs included prorated real estate taxes and "points" on the loan. Points represent a certain percentage of the loan amount paid, in this case to the bank, to cover costs of the financing.

The prorated real estate taxes represent an expense to be reported in the current year by the HHA. The points, however, would be spread over several years. How would this multiple-year reporting be handled? The total would first be placed on the balance sheet as an amount not yet recognized as expense. Each year a certain portion of that amount would be charged to current operations as an "amortized expense." Amortization expense is a noncash expense that is assigned to multiple reporting periods. It works much the same way as depreciation expense.

MANAGEMENT CONSIDERATIONS ABOUT REAL ESTATE FINANCING

Real estate financing typically occurs in the form of real estate mortgages. Management must take several important considerations into account when contemplating a real estate purchase that involves a mortgage. These considerations include the following:

- What would the return on investment (ROI) be for this purchase?
- What is the cost of money (i.e., the interest rate) for this mortgage?
- What would the return of capital (equity) computation amount to?
- What is the liquidity prospect (i.e., the ability to sell this property)?

- What is the potential risk factor (if any) involved in the purchase and/or the mortgage financing?
- Is there an income tax factor to be considered? If so, what is the impact?

Repayment of a mortgage is typically a long-term liability, and this fact is yet another element in management's decision-making process.

MANAGEMENT DECISIONS ABOUT BUSINESS LOANS

Decisions concerning how to obtain capital are an important part of financial management decision making. The chapter on capital expenditures budgets discussed how new capital often has to be rationed within an organization. Repaying long-term loan obligations will impact the facility's cash flow for years to come, and decisions to undertake a large debt load should not be made lightly. Therefore, most institutions and/or companies have put a formal approval process into place that generally begins with the chief financial officer and his or her staff and progresses upward all the way to board of trustees' approval, depending on the amount of the debt proposed.

Because of the implications, management decisions about business loans are often interwoven with strategic planning.

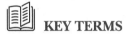 **INFORMATION CHECKPOINT**

What is needed?   An example of the details of a loan.
Where is it found?   In the department responsible for the organization's finances.
How is it used?   Loan information is used by your financial decision makers.

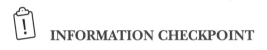 **KEY TERMS**

Amortization Schedule	Capital Structure	Long-Term Borrowing
Bonds	Equity Ratio	Short-Term Borrowing
Capital	Loan Costs	

 DISCUSSION QUESTIONS

1. Have you ever been informed of details about business loans in your unit or division?
2. If so, did you receive the information in the context of a new project (a new business loan that was made for purposes of the new project)?
3. Do the operating reports you receive contain information about loan costs, such as interest expense?
4. If so, do you think the interest expense seems reasonable for the operation? Why?

Sample Amortization Schedule 22-A

© LFor/Shutterstock

Principal borrowed: $60,000.00

Annual payments: 12

Total payments: 36

Annual interest rate: 12.00%

Periodic interest rate: 1.0000%

Regular payment amount: $1,992.86[*]

Final balloon payment: $0.00

The following results are estimates that do not account for values being rounded to the nearest cent. See the amortization schedule for more accurate values.

Total repaid: $71,742.96[**]

Total interest paid: $11,742.96

Interest as percentage of principal: 19.572%

---

[*]Take any line item on the next page. If you add the amount in the principal column and the amount in the interest column together, the total will amount a payment of $1,992.86.
[**]($60,000 principal plus $11,742.96 equals $71,742.96.)

Table 22-A–1 36-Month Sample Amortization Schedule

Payment Number	Principal	Interest	Cumulative Principal	Cumulative Interest	Principal Balance
1	$1,392.86	$600.00	$1,392.86	$600.00	$58,607.14
2	$1,406.79	$586.07	$2,799.65	$1,186.07	$57,200.35
3	$1,420.86	$572.00	$4,220.51	$1,758.07	$55,779.49
4	$1,435.07	$557.79	$5,655.58	$2,315.86	$54,344.42
5	$1,449.42	$543.44	$7,105.00	$2,859.30	$52,895.00
6	$1,463.91	$528.95	$8,568.91	$3,388.25	$51,431.09
7	$1,478.55	$514.31	$10,047.46	$3,902.56	$49,952.54
8	$1,493.33	$499.53	$11,540.79	$4,402.09	$48,459.21
9	$1,508.27	$484.59	$13,049.06	$4,886.68	$46,950.94
10	$1,523.35	$469.51	$14,572.41	$5,356.19	$45,427.59
11	$1,538.58	$454.28	$16,110.99	$5,810.47	$43,889.01
12	$1,553.97	$438.89	$17,664.96	$6,249.36	$42,335.04
13	$1,569.51	$423.35	$19,234.47	$6,672.71	$40,765.53
14	$1,585.20	$407.66	$20,819.67	$7,080.37	$39,180.33
15	$1,601.06	$391.80	$22,420.73	$7,472.17	$37,579.27
16	$1,617.07	$375.79	$24,037.80	$7,847.96	$35,962.20
17	$1,633.24	$359.62	$25,671.04	$8,207.58	$34,328.96
18	$1,649.57	$343.29	$27,320.61	$8,550.87	$32,679.39
19	$1,666.07	$326.79	$28,986.68	$8,877.66	$31,013.32
20	$1,682.73	$310.13	$30,669.41	$9,187.79	$29,330.59
21	$1,699.55	$293.31	$32,368.96	$9,481.10	$27,631.04
22	$1,716.55	$276.31	$34,085.51	$9,757.41	$25,914.49
23	$1,733.72	$259.14	$35,819.23	$10,016.55	$24,180.77
24	$1,751.05	$241.81	$37,570.28	$10,258.36	$22,429.72
25	$1,768.56	$224.30	$39,338.84	$10,482.66	$20,661.16
26	$1,786.25	$206.61	$41,125.09	$10,689.27	$18,874.91
27	$1,804.11	$188.75	$42,929.20	$10,878.02	$17,070.80
28	$1,822.15	$170.71	$44,751.35	$11,048.73	$15,248.65
29	$1,840.37	$152.49	$46,591.72	$11,201.22	$13,408.28
30	$1,858.78	$134.08	$48,450.50	$11,335.30	$11,549.50
31	$1,877.37	$115.49	$50,327.87	$11,450.79	$9,672.13
32	$1,896.14	$96.72	$52,224.01	$11,547.51	$7,775.99
33	$1,915.10	$77.76	$54,139.11	$11,625.27	$5,860.89
34	$1,934.25	$58.61	$56,073.36	$11,683.88	$3,926.64
35	$1,953.59	$39.27	$58,026.95	$11,723.15	$1,973.05
36	*$1,973.05	$19.73	$60,000.00	$11,742.88	$0.00

*The final payment has been adjusted to account for payments having been rounded to the nearest cent.

Choices: Owning Versus Leasing Equipment

23

PURCHASING EQUIPMENT

Purchasing equipment means taking title to, or assuming ownership of, the item. In this case, the asset representing the equipment is recorded on the organization's balance sheet. The purchase could take place by paying cash from the organization's cash reserves, or the organization could finance all or part of the purchase. If financing occurs, the resulting liability is also recorded on the balance sheet.

LEASING EQUIPMENT

When is a lease not a lease? When it is a lease-purchase, also known as a financial lease. This is a very real question that affects business decisions. The financial lease is described in the next section, and it is followed by a description of the operating lease.

Financial Lease

The lease-purchase is a formal agreement that may be called a lease, but it is really a contract to purchase. This contract-to-purchase transaction is also called a financial lease. The important difference is this: the equipment must be recorded on the books of the organization as a purchase. This process is called "capitalizing" the lease.

A financial lease is considered a contract to purchase. Generally speaking, a lease must be capitalized and thus placed on the balance sheet as an asset, with a corresponding liability, if the lease contract meets any one of the following criteria:

1. The lessee can buy the asset at the end of the lease term for a bargain price.

Progress Notes

After completing this chapter, you should be able to

1. Understand what purchasing equipment involves.
2. Understand what leasing equipment involves.
3. Recognize a for-profit organization.
4. Recognize a not-for-profit organization.

2. The lease transfers ownership to the lessee before the lease expires.
3. The lease lasts for 75% or more of the asset's estimated useful life.
4. The present value of the lease payments is 90% or more of the asset's value.

Operating Lease

The cost of an operating lease is considered an operating expense. It does not have to be capitalized and placed on the balance sheet because it does not meet the criteria just described.

An operating lease is treated as an expense of current operations. This is in contrast to the financial lease just described that is treated as an asset and a liability. A payment on an operating lease becomes an operating expense within the time period when the payment is made.

BUY-OR-LEASE MANAGEMENT DECISIONS

Leasing is an alternative to other means of financing. When analyzing lease-versus-purchase decisions, it is usually assumed that the money to purchase the equipment will be borrowed. In some cases, however, this is not true. The organization might decide to use cash from its own funds to make the purchase. This decision would, of course, change certain assumptions in the comparative analysis.

Another differential in comparative analysis concerns service agreements. Sometimes the service contracts or service agreements (to service and/or repair the equipment) are made a part of the lease agreement. This feature would need to be deleted from the total agreement before the comparison between leasing and purchasing can occur. Why? Because the service agreement would be an expense, regardless of whether the equipment would be leased or purchased.

An Example

The question for our example is whether a clinic should purchase or lease equipment. We examine two clinics: Northside Clinic, a for-profit corporation, and Southside Clinic, a not-for-profit corporation.

For both Northside and Southside, assume that the equipment's cost will be $50,000 if it is purchased. Likewise, assume for both Northside and Southside that if the equipment is leased, the lease will amount to $11,000 per year for five years.

We also need to make assumptions about depreciation expense for the purchased equipment. We further assume straight-line depreciation in the amount of $10,000 for years 2 through 4. For the initial year of acquisition (year 0), we assume the half-year method of depreciation, whereby the amount will be one-half of $10,000, or $5,000. We will further assume the purchased equipment will be sold for its salvage value of 10%, or $5,000, on the first day of year 5. (Therefore, the full amount of [prior] year 4's depreciation can be taken.)

The difference between the for-profit Northside and the not-for-profit Southside is that the for-profit is subject to income tax. We assume the federal and state income taxes will amount to a total of 25%. Thus, the depreciation taken as an expense results in a tax savings amounting to one-quarter of the total expense in each year. The depreciation expense and its equivalent tax savings are shown by year in **Table 23–1**. Also, the same rationale is applicable for the leasing expense in the for-profit organization.

In the following section, we compare two financial situations that affect the way the analysis is performed: a for-profit, or proprietary, clinic and a not-for-profit clinic. For purposes of this analysis, what is the major difference? As we have previously stated, the for-profit practice realizes tax savings on expense items such as depreciation. The not-for-profit clinic does not realize such tax savings because it does not pay taxes. Consequently, one analysis later here (the for-profit) includes the effect of tax savings on depreciation, and the other analysis (the not-for-profit) does not.

Computing the Comparative Net Cash Flow Effects of Owning Versus Leasing

This description results in computation of the net cash flow for owned equipment versus leased equipment in a for-profit organization compared with that of a not-for-profit organization. **Table 23–2–A.1** and **Table 23–2–A.2** first illustrate the comparative net cash flow effects of owning versus leasing in a for-profit organization. Table 23–2–A.1 illustrates the cost of owning. The equipment purchase price of $50,000 in year 0 (line 1) and the salvage value of $5,000 in year 5

Table 23–1 Depreciation Expense Computation

	Year 0	Year 1	Year 2	Year 3	Year 4	Year 5
Depreciation expense	$5,000	$10,000	$10,000	$10,000	$10,000	—
Depreciation expense tax savings	$1,250	$2,500	$2,500	$2,500	$2,500	—

Table 23–2–A.1 Cost of Owning—Northside Clinic (For-Profit)—Comparative Cash Flow

Line Number		Year 0	Year 1	Year 2	Year 3	Year 4	Year 5
1	Equipment purchase price	($50,000)					
2	Depreciation expense tax savings	$1,250	$2,500	$2,500	$2,500	$2,500	—
3	Salvage value	—	—	—	—	—	$5,000
4	Net cash flow	($48,750)	$2,500	$2,500	$2,500	$2,500	$5,000

Table 23–2–A.2 Cost of Leasing—Northside Clinic (For-Profit)—Comparative Cash Flow

Line Number		Year 0	Year 1	Year 2	Year 3	Year 4	Year 5
5	Equipment lease (rental) payments	($11,000)	($11,000)	($11,000)	($11,000)	($11,000)	—
6	Lease expense tax savings	$2,750	$2,750	$2,750	$2,750	$2,750	—
7	Net cash flow	($8,250)	($8,250)	($8,250)	($8,250)	($8,250)	—

(line 3) are shown. The for-profit's net cash flow is also affected by tax savings from depreciation expense, as was previously explained and as is shown on line 2. The resulting net cash flow by year is shown on line 4.

Table 23–2–A.2 illustrates the cost of leasing in the for-profit organization. The equipment lease or rental payments are shown on line 5. The for-profit's net cash flow is affected by tax savings from the lease payments, as is shown on line 6. The resulting net cash flow by year is shown on line 7.

Table 23–2–B.1 and **Table 23–2–B.2** now illustrate the comparative net cash flow effects of owning versus leasing for the not-for-profit organization. Table 23–2–B.1 illustrates the cost of owning. The equipment purchase price of $50,000 in year 0 (line 8) and the salvage value of $5,000 in year 5 (line 10) are shown. The not-for-profit's net cash flow is not affected by tax savings from depreciation expense because it is exempt from such income taxes. Therefore, the depreciation expense tax savings entry on line 9 is shown as not applicable, or "n/a." The resulting net cash flow by year is then shown on line 11.

Table 23–2–B.2 illustrates the cost of leasing in the not-for-profit organization. The equipment lease or rental payments are shown on line 12. The not-for-profit's net cash flow is not affected by tax savings from the lease payments because it is exempt from such income taxes. Therefore, the lease expense tax savings entry on line 13 is shown as not applicable, or "n/a." The resulting net cash flow by year is then shown on line 14.

Computing the Comparative Present Value Cost of Owning Versus Cost of Leasing

This continuing description results in computation of the present value cost of owning versus leasing equipment in a for-profit organization compared with that of a not-for-profit organization.

Table 23–2–B.1 Cost of Owning—Southside Clinic (Not-for-Profit)—Comparative Cash Flow

Line Number		Year 0	Year 1	Year 2	Year 3	Year 4	Year 5
8	Equipment purchase price	($50,000)					
9	Depreciation expense tax savings	n/a	n/a	n/a	n/a	n/a	—
10	Salvage value	—	—	—	—	—	$5,000
11	Net cash flow	($50,000)	—	—	—	—	$5,000

Table 23–2–B.2 Cost of Leasing—Southside Clinic (Not-for-Profit)—Comparative Cash Flow

Line Number		Year 0	Year 1	Year 2	Year 3	Year 4	Year 5
12	Equipment lease (rental) payments	($11,000)	($11,000)	($11,000)	($11,000)	($11,000)	—
13	Lease expense tax savings	n/a	n/a	n/a	n/a	n/a	—
14	Net cash flow	($11,000)	($11,000)	($11,000)	($11,000)	($11,000)	—

Table 23–2–C.1 and **Table 23–2–C.2** now illustrate the present value cost of owning versus leasing for the for-profit organization. Table 23–2–C.1 first carries forward (on line 15) the net cash flow computed on line 4. Line 16 then shows the present value factor for each year at 8%, which is the assumed cost of capital in this example. Line 17 contains the present value answers, which result from multiplying line 15 times line 16. The overall present value cost of owning (derived by adding all items on line 17) is shown on line 18.

Table 23–2–C.2 illustrates the present value cost of leasing in the for-profit organization. Table 23–2–C.2 first carries forward (on line 19) the net cash flow computed on line 7. Line 20 then shows the present value factor for each year at 8%, which is the assumed cost of capital in this example. Line 21 contains the present value answers, which result from multiplying line 19 times line 20. The overall present value cost of owning (derived by adding all items on line 21) is shown on line 22.

Finally, **Table 23–2–C.3** compares the for-profit organization's cost of owning to its cost of leasing. In the case of the for-profit, the net advantage is to leasing by a net amount of $1,489. The tables now illustrate the present value cost of owning versus leasing for the not-for-profit organization. **Table 23–2–D.1** illustrates the present value cost of owning. It first carries forward (on line 24) the net cash flow computed on line 11. Line 25 then shows the present value factor for each year at 8%, which is the assumed cost of capital in this example. Line 26 contains the present value answers, which result from multiplying line 24 times line 25. The overall present value cost of owning (derived by adding all items on line 26) is shown on line 27.

Table 23–2–C.1 Cost of Owning—Northside Clinic (For-Profit)—Comparative Present Value

Line Number	For-Profit Cost of Owning	Year 0	Year 1	Year 2	Year 3	Year 4	Year 5
15	Net cash flow (from line 4)	($48,750)	$2,500	$2,500	$2,500	$2,500	$5,000
16	Present value factor (at 8%)	n/a	0.926	0.857	0.794	0.735	0.681
17	Present value answers =	($48,750)	$2,315	$2,143	$1,985	$1,838	$3,405
18	Present value cost of owning = ($37,064)						

Table 23–2–C.2 Cost of Leasing—Northside Clinic (For-Profit)—Comparative Present Value

Line Number	For-Profit Cost of Leasing	Year 0	Year 1	Year 2	Year 3	Year 4	Year 5
19	Net cash flow (from line 7)	($8,250)	($8,250)	($8,250)	($8,250)	($8,250)	—
20	Present value factor (at 8%)	n/a	0.926	0.857	0.794	0.735	—
21	Present value answers =	($8,250)	($7,640)	($7,070)	($6,551)	($6,064)	—
22	Present value cost of leasing = ($35,575)						

Table 23–2–C.3 Comparison of Costs—Northside Clinic (For-Profit)

Line Number	Computation of Difference
23 Net advantage to leasing = $1,489	(37,064) (line 18) less (35,575) (line 22) equals 1,489

Table 23–2–D.1 Cost of Owning—Southside Clinic (Not-for-Profit)—Comparative Present Value

Line Number	Not-for-Profit Cost of Owning	Year 0	Year 1	Year 2	Year 3	Year 4	Year 5
24	Net cash flow (from line 11)	($50,000)	—	—	—	—	$5,000
25	Present value factor (at 8%)	n/a	—	—	—	—	0.681
26	Present value answer =	($50,000)	—	—	—	—	$3,405
27	Present value cost of owning = ($46,595)						

Table 23–2–D.2 Cost of Leasing—Southside Clinic (Not-for-Profit)—Comparative Present Value

Line Number	Not-for-Profit Cost of Leasing	Year 0	Year 1	Year 2	Year 3	Year 4	Year 5
28	Net cash flow (from line 14)	($11,000)	($11,000)	($11,000)	($11,000)	($11,000)	—
29	Present value factor (at 8%)	n/a	0.926	0.857	0.794	0.735	
30	Present value answer =	($11,000)	($10,186)	($9,427)	($8,573)	($8,085)	—
31	Present value cost of leasing = ($47,271)						

Table 23–2–D.3 Comparison of Costs—Southside Clinic (Not-for-Profit)

Line Number	Computation of Difference
32 Net Advantage to Owning = $676	(47,271) (line 31) less (46,595) (line 27) equals 676

Table 23–2–D.2 illustrates the present value cost of leasing in the not-for-profit organization. It first carries forward (on line 28) the net cash flow computed on line 14. Line 29 then shows the present value factor for each year at 8%, which is the assumed cost of capital in this example. Line 30 contains the present value answers, which result from multiplying line 28 times line 29. The overall present value cost of owning (derived by adding all items on line 30) is shown on line 31.

Finally, **Table 23–2–D.3** compares the not-for-profit organization's cost of owning to its cost of leasing. In the case of the not-for-profit, the net advantage is to owning by a net amount of $676. It might be noted that the net difference of $676 is so small that it might be disregarded and considered as a nearly neutral comparison between the two methods of financing.

In summary, the tax effect on cash flow of for-profit versus not-for-profit will generally (but not always) be taken into account in comparative proposals for funding.

ACCOUNTING PRINCIPLES REGARDING LEASES

As previously explained, financial statements used for external purposes in the United States must follow generally accepted accounting principles, or GAAP. The treatment of equipment leases for such accounting purposes would, of course, fall under GAAP, and the technical aspects of such reporting are beyond the scope of this text. Be aware, however, that sometime in the near future, U.S. publicly held companies may be required to adopt certain international accounting standards as produced by the International Accounting Standards Board (IASB).[1] The treatment of leases is a particular issue within these potential adoption requirements and is, of course, beyond the scope of this text.

INFORMATION CHECKPOINT

What is needed?	An example of a buy-or-lease management decision analysis.
Where is it found?	Probably with your manager or your departmental director.
How is it used?	Study the way the analysis is laid out and the method of comparison used.

KEY TERMS

Buy-or-Lease Decisions	Financial Lease	Not-for-Profit Organization
Depreciation	For-Profit Organization	Operating Lease
Equipment Purchase	Lease-Purchase	Present Value

DISCUSSION QUESTIONS

1. In the examples given in the chapter, there is not much monetary difference between owning versus leasing. In these circumstances, which method would you recommend? Why?
2. Have you ever been involved in a lease-or-buy decision in business? In your personal life?
3. If so, was the decision made in a formal reporting format, or as an informal decision?
4. Do you think this was the best way to make the decision? If not, what would you change? Why?

NOTE

1. K. Tysiac, "Still in Flux: Future of IFRS in U.S. Remains Unclear After SEC report," *Journal of Accountancy*, p.4 (September 2012). www.journalofaccountancy.com/Issues/2012/Sep/20126059.htm

PART

IX

Strategic Planning: A Powerful Tool

Strategic Planning and the Healthcare Financial Manager

MAJOR COMPONENTS OF THE STRATEGIC PLAN: OVERVIEW

This chapter will cover the six major components of planning and their process flows, along with various examples of mission, value, and vision statement types. A federal governmental agency planning example will be presented. The chapter also discusses strategic planning tools, including situational analysis and financial projections.

INTRODUCTION

Strategic planning is vital for any organization. There are multiple approaches to accomplish such planning, and there is often confusion about the terminology used in these different approaches. In this section we will describe the typical components of strategic planning. We will also discuss the confusion about differences in approach and related terminology.

SIX MAJOR COMPONENTS

The ultimate result of strategic planning is an actual plan, presented in report form. The major components of a strategic plan include the following:

- Mission Statement
- Vision Statement
- Organizational Values
- Goals
- Objectives
- Action Plans and/or Performance Plans and/or Initiatives

These components are illustrated in **Figure 24–1** and are further described as follows.

273

Progress Notes

After completing this chapter, you should be able to

1. Describe the six major components of strategic planning.
2. Understand the purpose and relationship between mission, vision, and value statements.
3. Describe the strategic planning cycle and its process flow.
4. Understand why the governmental planning requirements are important.
5. Identify the four components of a SWOT analysis.
6. Recognize the difference between a financial forecast and a financial projection.

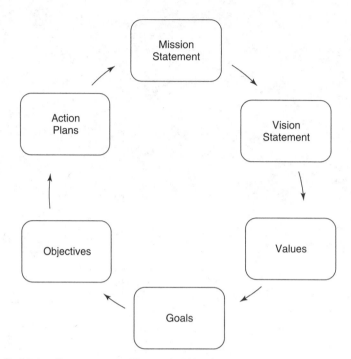

Figure 24–1 The Six Major Components of Strategic Planning.
Courtesy of J.J. Baker and R.W. Baker, Dallas, Texas.

Mission Statement

The mission statement explains the purpose of the organization. In other words, it explains "what we are now." Generally speaking, the mission statement will cover a near-future period, usually three to five years.

Vision Statement

The vision statement explains "what we want to be" or perhaps "what we aspire to be." It is a look further into the future, perhaps 10 years from now. Not all organizations publicize a vision statement.

Organizational Values

Values express the philosophy of the organization. There seems to be two approaches to expressing values: either they are summarized into just a few meaningful phrases or they are quite lengthy and "wordy."

Goals

A goal is "…a statement of aim or purpose included in a strategic plan."[1] Goals support the mission statement. While strategic goals are necessarily broad in nature, nevertheless each goal should tie directly into an element of the mission statement. Every goal should be considered an outcome that can be accomplished in the future.

Objectives

A strategic objective further defines intended outcomes in order to achieve a goal. Each objective must support—and thus tie directly into—a particular strategic goal. There are typically several objectives associated with each goal.

Action Plans

An Action Plan is a detailed plan of operations that shows how one part of a particular objective will be accomplished. It supports a subcomponent of the overall objective. It is a short-term plan that provides details (actions) about how a specific area of a particular objective will be carried out. Action plans are often called by other names, such as "Operational Plans," "Performance Plans" or "Initiatives." They may also be called "Targets."

VARIED APPROACHES TO STRATEGIC PLANNING

How strategic planning is approached may be affected by the organization type and/or the program or project type.

Governmental Versus Nongovernmental

Governmental entities are guided by regulatory restrictions. Among these restrictions are federal regulations that mandate strategic planning. These regulations apply to federal governmental organizations and specify the format, contents, and timing of the required strategic plans. On the other hand, nongovernmental entities are not covered under these mandated requirements.

For-Profit Versus Not-For-Profit

A for-profit company is in business to make a profit (supposedly, anyway) and is answerable to its owners. Its owner may be shareholders (for corporations) or partners (for partnerships) or possibly sole proprietors. This company's mission will generally be proprietary in nature.

A not-for-profit organization, on the other hand, is expected to have a mission that is broadly charitable in nature. It is typically answerable to the stakeholders who are impacted in one way or another by its mission.

Specific Programs or Projects

In some cases the type of program or project or initiative will define the basic approach to strategic planning. Funding sources and/or regulations may also make such demands. For example, in some states construction of healthcare facilities is controlled by a regulatory Certificate of Need process. In these states, then, strategic planning for a new facility would be a specific project. The outcome would be uncertain—because there is competition, success would be unknown—so the project would be specially treated within the plan.

EXAMPLES OF MISSION, VISION, AND VALUE STATEMENTS

This section introduces various types of mission, vision, and value statements. The organization and the length of statements can vary. Their terminology and their emphasis can also vary. One set of examples that follow recognizes a special status or focus, another recognizes a financial emphasis, and a third shows how the message is relayed.

RECOGNIZING A SPECIAL STATUS OR FOCUS WITHIN THE STATEMENTS

The following five examples each recognize a special status or focus within the statements.

Recognizing Non-Profit Status: Sutter Health

Sutter Health is a network of doctors and hospitals located in Northern California. Sutter's mission statement specifically points out its not-for-profit commitment.

Mission

We enhance the well-being of people in the communities we serve through a not-for-profit commitment to compassion and excellence in healthcare services.

Vision

Sutter Health leads the transformation of health care to achieve the highest levels of quality, access and affordability.

Values

- Excellence and Quality
- Innovation
- Affordability
- Teamwork
- Compassion and Caring
- Community
- Honesty and Integrity[2]

[Note: Sutter's values are arranged in a circular graphic, with "Honesty & Integrity" in the middle of the circle.]

Recognizing For-Profit Status: Tenet Healthcare Corporation

Tenet Healthcare Corporation is a publicly held corporation that is listed on the New York Stock Exchange (NYSE:THC). As a for-profit corporation operating a healthcare delivery system, Tenet specifically mentions providing a return to its shareholders.

Mission

At Tenet, our business is health care. Our mission is to improve the quality of life of every patient who enters our doors. Our approach makes us unique and defines our future.

Values

As we seek to improve the quality of our patients' lives, to serve our communities, to provide an exceptional environment for our employees and affiliated physicians, and to provide an attractive return to our shareholders, we are guided by five core values.[3]

Recognizing Hospital Taxing-District Status: Parkland Hospital

Parkland Hospital is the tax-supported hospital serving Dallas County, Texas. As such, Parkland first states its mandate from the taxpayers.

Mandate

To furnish medical aid and hospital care to indigent and needy persons residing in the hospital district.

Mission

Dedicated to the health and well-being of individuals and communities entrusted to our care.

Vision

By our actions, we will define the standards of excellence for public academic health systems.

Guiding Principles

Our values and principles reflect our shared responsibility to achieve healthcare excellence for our patients and communities.[4]

Recognizing the Vision and Intent of Their Founders: Mayo Clinic

The Mayo Clinic, a large nonprofit organization with a long history, provides medical care, research, and education at locations including the Midwest, Arizona, and Florida. The Mayo Clinic is research oriented and is known for treating difficult cases.

Mission

To inspire hope and contribute to health and well-being by providing the best care to every patient through integrated clinical practice, education, and research.

Primary Value

The needs of the patient come first.

Value Statements

These values, which guide Mayo Clinic's mission to this day, are an expression of the vision and intent of our founders, the original Mayo physicians and the Sisters of Saint Francis.[5]

♭ Recognizing Patient and Community Commitment: Regions Hospital

Regions Hospital is a private not-for-profit hospital in St. Paul, Minnesota, that is over 100 years old. Regions' commitment to both patients and community is very clear.

Mission

Our mission is to improve the health of our patients and community by providing high quality health care, which meets the needs of all people.

Vision

Our vision is to be the patient-centered hospital of choice of our community.[6]

FINANCIAL EMPHASIS WITHIN THE STATEMENTS

This section presents two examples of financial emphasis within the statements, as follows.

A Foundation's Financial Responsibility: Saint Barnabas Medical Center Foundation

A healthcare foundation typically exists to receive and manage charitable gifts. This foundation exists to support a specific hospital: Saint Barnabas Medical Center, a major teaching hospital located in Livingston, New Jersey.

Mission

The Saint Barnabas Medical Center Foundation is a charitable organization dedicated to nurturing philanthropic support for the programs and services of Saint Barnabas Medical Center.

These programs provide the communities we serve with the highest quality, most compassionate health care. To accomplish our mission, the Foundation will:

- Ensure that charitable gifts are used effectively, responsibly, and as directed by the donor; and
- Carefully manage the endowed funds entrusted to us.[7]

A Medical Practice Network Emphasizes Financial Structure: Texas Oncology

Texas Oncology specializes in oncology patients through a network of physicians that covers the state of Texas. This organization places its vision first and mission second, as follows. Note also that evidence-based, or scientific, care is contained within the mission statement.

Vision

To be the first choice for cancer care.

Mission

To provide excellent, evidence-based care for each patient we serve, while advancing cancer care for tomorrow.

Texas Oncology has three Core Values, consisting of Patient Care, Culture, and Business. The Business Core Value is of particular interest to us. At the time of this writing, it reads as follows: Business—Our practice values professional management that:

- Promotes convenient access at rural and urban sites.
- Provides leadership in efficient care delivery and improves all aspects of cancer care.
- Provides a financial structure to expand services to our patients.
- Is competitive in all aspects of our business.[8]

These values clearly recognize the fact that an organization must have the financial structure and resources to endure and to succeed.

RELAYING THE MESSAGE

The results of strategic planning as expressed in the mission statement, vision, and values are of little use unless people know about them and what they say. This section focuses upon relaying that message.

Introducing the Message

This section presents three examples of introducing the message within the statements, as follows.

An Overall Title for the Message: Aetna Insurance Company

Aetna is a national insurance company over 150 years old that offers health insurance plans. This company has wrapped their mission, values, and goals together under one overall title called The Aetna Way, as follows:

Our company's mission, values and goals are expressed through The Aetna Way. The Aetna Way, comprising the elements below, encompasses our shared sense of purpose and provides clarity as we pursue our operational and strategic goals.[9]

Emphasizing Areas of Focus: American Medical Association

The American Medical Association (AMA) is, according to its website, "…the largest physician organization in the nation."[10] It provides a wide variety of resources and support for its members.

The AMA has created a five-year strategic plan, "…which aims to ensure that enhancements to health care in the United States are physician-led, advance the physician-patient relationship, and ensure that health care costs can be prudently managed."[11]

This plan places emphasis on three particular "core areas of focus," which include the following:

- Improving health outcomes
- Accelerating change in medical education
- Enhancing physician satisfaction and practice sustainability by shaping delivery and payment models[12]

The plan was posted electronically, and an AMA member could click on any of the three focus areas to read more. The AMA also provided a members-only feedback form in order to receive input.

Explaining the Terms: Good Samaritan Society

The Good Samaritan Society is the largest not-for-profit provider of senior care and services in the United States.

There is an important paragraph that appears before Good Samaritan's Strategic statements. That paragraph explains the purpose of each term contained with the statements, as follows:

- Our Mission states why the Society exists.
- Our Vision defines the desired outcome of our work.
- Our Strategic Direction defines where we want to be as an organization.
- And our Hallmark Values and related Core Principles identify the values that we strive to integrate into all aspects of our work.[13]

Mission Expressed as a Motto

Mottos are an effective way to communicate the organization's mission. However, composing such a short piece is much more difficult than it seems at first. Two examples follow.

A Six-Word Motto: Good Samaritan Society

The Good Samaritan Society has also created a pithy concise motto consisting of only six words.

Grounded in Mission
Centered in Values[14]

A Three-Phrase Motto: Providence Healthcare Network

Providence Healthcare Network is a member of Ascension Health, "…the nation's largest Catholic and largest nonprofit health system."

A mission of compassion.
Compassion is perfected by excellence.

Because excellence goes beyond the will to help others by providing the determination and tools to succeed where the heart takes you.[15]

The Message Available as Website Downloads

Website downloads make the information available to anyone who has access to a computer. This section presents two examples of making the message available as a website download.

Downloadable Summaries from Duke Medicine

The umbrella term "Duke Medicine" actually covers three components—the Duke University Health System, the Duke University School of Medicine, and the Duke University School of Nursing, all based in the Raleigh-Durham, North Carolina area. Duke Medicine has created both a mission and a vision that encompasses all these components. Then each component also has its own strategic plan that feeds in turn into the combined plan.

At the time of this writing an overview of these plans was available in booklet form. The booklet, entitled "Thinking Big" could be downloaded from the Duke Medicine website as a

PDF file.[16] Summaries of each strategic plan could also be downloaded. Thus Duke provides transparency and useful summaries in a readily accessible electronic format.

Downloadable Visuals from Johns Hopkins Medicine

Johns Hopkins also uses a single name—John Hopkins Medicine—for its overall medical enterprise. This enterprise, based in Baltimore, Maryland, includes the Johns Hopkins Health System along with the John Hopkins University School of Medicine.

Johns Hopkins Medicine has created a mission, vision, and core values for the entire enterprise. At the time of this writing it was possible to download and print out the Johns Hopkins Medicine mission, vision, and core values in one of three ways:

- A Wall-Mounted Poster (large)—24" × 36"
- A Framed Desk-top Poster (small)—8" × 10"
- A Pocket Card—2.5" × 3.5"[17]

Thus the message is definitely relayed, and in three possible forms, for three different display purposes. It keeps the message visible as a reminder.

THE STRATEGIC PLANNING CYCLE AND ITS PROCESS FLOW

The basic elements of strategic planning can be visualized as a series of process flows. Thus by visualizing the process involved, the planning function can be broken into its various manageable components.

PROCESS FLOW FOR CREATING GOALS, OBJECTIVES, AND ACTION PLANS

Figure 24–2 illustrates these initial three components of the strategic plan.

Establishing Goals

You will recall that a goal is a statement of aim or purpose. In order to establish such a goal, it is important to define how it will accomplish a particular segment of the mission statement. Establishing the actual goal involves the following:

- Define the goal.
- Determine that there is a clear and distinct connection to the mission statement.
- Decide how long it will take to accomplish this goal; that is, will it take one year, two years, three years?
- Compose and condense final wording of the goal to properly express it in a concise manner.

Broad Goals Become Narrower Objectives

A strategic objective further defines a particular strategic goal. Thus a single broad goal is segmented into several narrower and more defined objectives, as illustrated in Figure 24–2.

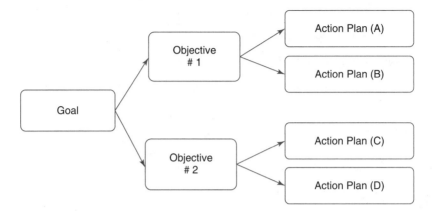

Figure 24–2 Process Flow for Creating Goals, Objectives, and Action Plans.
Courtesy of J.J. Baker and R.W. Baker, Dallas, Texas.

Narrower Objectives Become Detailed Action Plans

You will also recall that an action plan provides a detailed plan of operations that shows how to achieve one part of a particular objective. Thus a single defined objective is segmented into a number of even more detailed action plans. This step shows how part of the objective will actually be accomplished. The action plan's relationship to objectives and to goals is also illustrated in Figure 24–2.

PROCESS FLOW FOR CREATING ACTION PLANS AND THEIR PERFORMANCE MEASURES

Figure 24–3 illustrates the multiple performance measures that make each action plan operational.

The Action Plan Must Relate to Its Objective

As previously discussed, an action plan should always directly relate to the relevant component of its specific strategic objective. Details will be organized into subcomponents as necessary and, as its title implies, the action plan will demonstrate how actions will be accomplished.

Detailed Action Plans Will Contain Multiple Performance Measures

So how will the action plan demonstrate that its actions will be accomplished? The required actions, or operations, will be linked to a series of performance measures, as illustrated in Figure 24–3. The performance measures provide accountability.

When these measures are properly designed, performance can be reported as outcomes. This achieves desired accountability and one cycle of the planning process flow is thus complete.

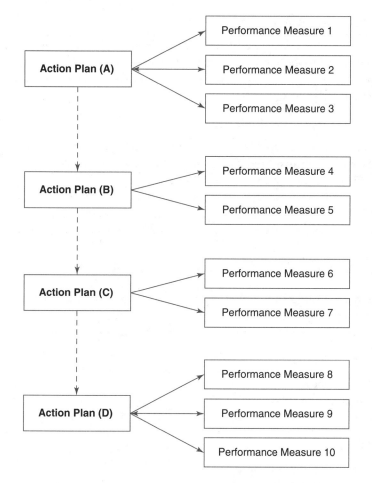

Figure 24–3 Process Flow for Creating Action Plans and Their Performance Measures.
Courtesy of J.J. Baker and R.W. Baker, Dallas, Texas.

THE PLANNING CYCLE OVER TIME

We visualize the ideal strategic planning cycle itself as a never-ending process. In other words, a completed plan is not set in stone, never to change. Instead, there should be a "refresh and renew" approach to such planning. Incidentally, planning cycle segments may be called by different names, but they are still in a cycle. Look past the names to see the "skeleton" of the overall process.

Goals, Objectives, and Action Plans Interact and Repeat

The interaction of goals, objectives, and action plans should take feedback into account. This feedback should be obtained as is appropriate from all levels of management within the organization. However, internal managers are not the only stakeholders involved with the strategic plan.

Planning Revisions and Updates Are Necessary

The capability for planning revisions and updates should ideally be built into the plan itself. Unanticipated events can occur—both internally and externally—that require major revisions if the plan is to be kept operational. Updates, on the other hand, are to be expected and allowance should be made for them in order to keep the plan.

Stakeholders Provide Input Within the Cycle

Stakeholders can be both internal and external. In order to maintain a manageable planning cycle, questions need to be answered. For example, how many external stakeholders need input into the plan? Who, specifically are they? How will they provide this input?

Likewise, how many internal stakeholders need to provide input and/or feedback to the plan? Who, specifically, are they? What departments or divisions do they represent within the organization? Is this representation a good balance? And how will they provide this input?

Programming and Budgets Support the Planning Cycle

It makes sense that planning should be supported by budgets and the related funding. It is also logical that programming should in turn support these budgets. We can then ask: "What goal and what objective does this particular program and this budget support?"

Financial Aspects of the Plan

A plan must, above all, be operational. And to be operational, it must have financial support. How will this financial support be provided? Will another division or project be cut in order for this to happen? Can the consequences be predicted? If so, what will they be?

Related Timeframes

Necessary timeframes are appropriate for the particular portion of strategic planning. For example, the plan itself typically covers a period of 4 to 5 years. If there is a vision statement, it should be much further into the future, perhaps out to 10 years. Yet the managers' accountability should be at least annually, and in fact may be quarterly.

MANAGERS' RESPONSIBILITIES

Responsibility for the various segments can be assigned. The manager's responsibility will generally rest in one of three management areas as follows.

Planning

The manager may contribute to planning by gathering data or by analyzing the data to provide specific information that is desired and necessary for the plan. In other words, the manager is participating in the planning function by doing his/her part in the preliminary segment of the process.

Decision Making

The manager may or may not be able to participate in the actual decision making for the plan, depending upon his/her staff level within the organization. However, he/she may be assigned to work on a planning committee or a task force that contributes directly to the decision makers in the organization. This type of assignment is an important responsibility.

Providing Accountability

The manager can definitely contribute in suggesting criteria for performance measures. The action plan will require performance measures in order to provide the necessary accountability. And the manager is the best person to understand what measures are needed within his/her department or division.

A well-designed planning process will also include milestones. The milestones signify the completion of plan segments within a designated timeframe for completion of the entire plan. The manager can and should be responsible for assisting in reaching certain milestones on a timely basis. This function (one hospital CEO called it "ramrodding") is another type of accountability responsibility.

FEDERAL GOVERNMENTAL AGENCIES MUST PREPARE STRATEGIC PLANS

Agencies in the federal government are required by law to prepare strategic plans. They are also required by law to provide reports on performance that tie to the strategic plans. This section explains the importance of the federal planning cycle and describes its planning and performance requirements. It also provides an example of an agency strategic planning cycle.

WHY ARE FEDERAL PLANNING REQUIREMENTS IMPORTANT TO US?

The federal government's planning requirements are important to us because they provide guidance in the form of well-thought-out and time-tested regulated concepts and a framework for strategic planning.

INTRODUCTION: REQUIREMENTS, PLANS, AND PERFORMANCE

Legislative requirements for strategic planning and related performance reporting are discussed as follows.

Legislative Requirements: Overview

Congress has enacted a law that provided for the establishment of strategic planning and performance measurement in the federal government. This law, known as the Government Performance and Results Act (GPRA) of 1993, required each agency of the federal government to prepare a strategic plan for program activities. These strategic plans were then to be submitted to Congress and to the Director of the Office of Management and Budget (OMB).[18]

Legislative Requirements for Strategic Planning

Each agency's strategic plan must contain the following:

- A comprehensive mission statement
- General goals and objectives for major functions and operations

- A description of how these goals and objectives are to be achieved
- Key factors external to the agency and beyond its control that might significantly affect achieving these goals and objectives[19]

Strategic Plan Timeframes

The original 1993 Act required that the strategic plan cover a period of not less than five years forward from the fiscal year in which it would be submitted. (You will recall that the federal government's fiscal year is not a calendar year. Instead it begins on October 1st and ends on September 30th.) In addition the plan was to be updated and revised at least every three years.[20]

The plan's timeframe has been subsequently revised to four years by the GPRA Modernization Act of 2010. At the time of this writing, the specific requirement is as follows: "…The plan shall cover a period of not less than four years following the fiscal year in which the plan is submitted."[21]

Plans' Impacts on Budgets and Funding

Governmental managers must reconcile their budget requests with their applicable part of the strategic plan. The projects for which they are responsible can't (usually) be funded if they are not approved in the budget.

A common problem involves maintaining a project's carry forward over sequential annual budgets. In other words, a multi-year project will need to be recognized for funding in each annual budget as the project progresses. This can be a real problem, considering the multiple levels of bureaucracy within the government that hinder the approval process.

We can also turn the concept of "impact" around the other way. Instead of asking "What is the impact of the plan on budgets and funding," we can ask the opposite questions. They include, "Does the intent of the plan actually get funded? And stay funded?"

How Agency Strategic Plans Are Tied to Performance

This section describes performance reporting requirements for federal agencies.

Legislative Requirements for Performance Reporting

The 1993 Act actually had three elements: besides requiring strategic plans that covered multiple years, it also required that performance plans and program performance reports be submitted. These requirements actually make the strategic plan itself operational because they hold the agencies accountable.

Agency Performance Plans Are Required

The GPRA Modernization Act of 2010 legislation requires the agency performance plans to be submitted annually. The performance plans are to be posted on the Agency's website.[22]

Agency Performance Reports Are Also Required

The Agency is also required to prepare an update report that compares actual performance achieved with performance goals as established in the performance plan. This report is also to be posted on the Agency's website.[23]

Unmet Goals May Require a Performance Improvement Plan

Each fiscal year the Office of Management and Budget (OMB) is supposed to determine whether the Agency has met the performance goals and objectives of the performance plan. The OMB produces a review report. If goals are not met according to the OMB report, the Agency must then prepare and submit a Performance Improvement Plan to increase program effectiveness for each unmet goal. The plan must include measurable milestones.[24]

Strategic Mission Statements: Two Federal Departmental Examples

Two departmental examples of governmental strategic mission statement appear in this section. The first example belongs to the Department of Health and Human Services (HHS). This mission statement is of interest because the Centers for Medicare and Medicaid Services (CMS) is an agency within the HHS department. The Medicare and Medicaid programs administered by CMS are frequent subjects of interest in this book.

The second example belongs to the Department of Veterans Affairs (VA). We include this example as background information because the VA's Office of Information Technology is the subject of the governmental planning cycle example that appears in the next section of this chapter. Note the necessarily broad wording within both of these departmental mission statements.

Department of Health and Human Services (HHS)

The Department of Health and Human Services (HHS) is "...the United States government's principal agency for protecting the health of all Americans and providing essential human services, especially for those who are least able to help themselves."[25]

There are more than 300 programs within HHS, including both the Medicare and the Medicaid programs.

Department of Health and Human Services (HHS) Mission Statement

The mission of the U.S. Department of Health and Human Services (HHS) is to enhance the health and well-being of Americans by providing for effective health and human services and by fostering sound, sustained advances in the sciences underlying medicine, public health, and social services.

HHS accomplishes its mission through several hundred programs and initiatives that cover a wide spectrum of activities, serving the American public at every stage of life.[26]

Department of Veterans Affairs (VA)

The Department of Veterans Affairs (VA) oversees benefits and services, including health care, for the nation's veterans. There are three VA sub-agencies within the Department as follows. The Veterans Health Administration (VHA) manages veterans' health care and services. The Veterans Benefits Administration (VBA) manages veterans' benefits, including life insurance and pensions. The National Cemetery Administration (NCA) oversees both burials and memorials for veterans.[27]

Department of Veterans Affairs (VA) Mission Statement

"Our mission at VA is to serve Veterans by increasing their access to our benefits and services, to provide them the highest quality of health care available, and to control costs to the best of our abilities."[28]

AN EXAMPLE: THE VA OFFICE OF INFORMATION TECHNOLOGY IT STRATEGIC PLANNING CYCLE

This section contains a governmental planning cycle example. Elements of the cycle are then defined and discussed. The section concludes with a summary of management responsibilities.

INTRODUCTION

You will recall that federal planning requirements are especially important to us because these requirements provide guidance through a time-tested and regulated framework for strategic planning. We are about to provide a real-life illustration of the planning cycle.

We present the illustrated cycle as an excellent example of the planning process. This example is drawn from a VA Directive concerning strategic planning. The entire scope of the Directive's requirements is, of course, well beyond the scope of this text. We have had to generalize the required process in order to provide this example. In generalizing, we are forced to disregard additional explanations, terminology, and background details contained in the Directive. Please refer to it as a source for further details.

The elements within this VA illustrated example include components that we have described earlier in this chapter. The components include the following:

- Set Broad Goals and Narrower Objectives for Programs
- Set Performance Measures to Achieve the Goals and the Objectives
- Determine External Key Factors That Are Significant
- Prepare Annual Performance Plan
- Prepare Periodic Performance Reports
- Revise and Update as Needed

THE VA OFFICE OF INFORMATION TECHNOLOGY IT STRATEGIC PLANNING CYCLE: AN EXAMPLE

Figure 24–4 illustrates the planning cycle in accordance with VA Directive 6052. The Directive's version used here is dated 2009. While there will inevitably be future updates and revisions, this example of the planning cycle process serves our purpose very well.[29]

THE VA PLANNING CYCLE'S PROCESS FLOW

Figure 24–4 shows the overall VA Strategic Plan and Goals at the top of the visual. This overall plan and its goals then flow to four "administrative strategic plans." The four plans include one apiece for the three subagencies (VHA, VBA, and NCA), plus a fourth plan for the VA Staff Office.

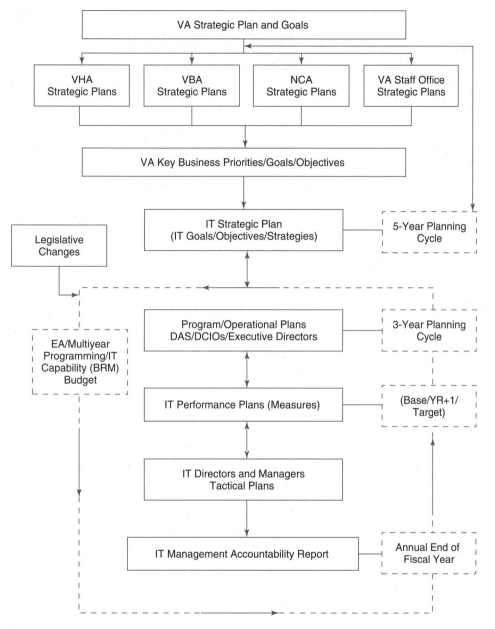

Figure 24–4 VA Office of Information Technology IT Strategic Planning Cycle.
Reproduced from the Department of Veterans Affairs. VA Directive 6052 Appendix A (April 23, 2009).

Each of the four plans flow to, and relate to, VA key business priorities, goals, and objects. The Information Technology (IT) Strategic Plan contains IT goals, objectives, and strategies. Its multi-year planning cycle (shown on Figure 24–4 as a five-year cycle) flows back in and out of the four Administrative Strategic Plans, as indicated by the two-way arrows.

Program and Operational Plans that support the IT Strategic Plan are the responsibility of the Deputy Assistant Secretary (DAS), the Deputy Chief Information Officers (DCIOs) and the Executive Directors. These plans are shown on a three-year planning cycle.

IT Performance Plans and their related Performance Measures are an outgrowth of the Program and Operational Plans. They are on a shorter cycle that we interpret as the base year plus one target.

The Tactical Plans that will carry out the Performance Plans are the responsibility of the IT Directors and Managers. Finally, an IT Management Accountability Report is required annually at the end of each fiscal year.

The Legislative Changes (an external factor that influences the process) are shown in a box on the left-hand side of the visual. Their influence feeds into and impacts the overall process.

Finally, the box on the dotted line to the left reads "EA/Multiyear Programming/IT Capability (BRM) Budget." We understand this is a budget that contains multi-year programming. We further understand it references IT Capability. The remaining portion of the acronym references the "One VA EA Business Reference Model," or BRM. The BRM was developed in part to provide a common set of process definitions. It thus assists in making "…the complex integration between business processes transparent."[30]

PLANNING CYCLE DEFINITIONS FOR THIS EXAMPLE

The following definitions are contained in the Office of Information Technology IT Planning Directive. While they are specific to the Directive's purpose, they provide greater depth to an overall understanding of the illustrated cycle and its process flow.

Strategic Planning

Strategic planning is a continuous process by which IT determines direction and operational focus over the next three to five years consistent with priorities established by the Secretary of Veterans Affairs as expressed in the Departmental Strategic Plan. There is one IT Strategic Plan; however, strategic planning involves all parts of VA Administrations and Staff Offices.

IT Mission

A mission statement is brief, defines the basic purpose of the organization, and corresponds directly with the organization's core programs and activities. An organization's program goals should flow from the mission statement. The mission defines the approach and means IT will take to fulfill the mission of VA as a whole.

IT Vision

The vision defines the ideal state for IT. (It is) what an organization desires to accomplish in the future.

IT Strategic Goals

A goal is a statement of aim or purpose included in a strategic plan (required under GPRA). The strategic goal defines how an agency will carry out a major segment of its mission over a period of time. The goal is expressed in a manner that allows a future assessment to be made of whether the goal was or is being achieved. Most strategic goals will be outcomes and are long-term in nature. IT goals define the forward-thinking and transformational outcomes IT pursues to achieve its mission over a period of time.

IT Strategic Objectives

Strategic objectives are strategy components or continuous improvement activities that are needed to create value for the customers. IT objectives further define intended program outcomes to achieve IT goals.

Program Plans

A program plan consists of planned activities or related projects managed in a coordinated way to include an element of ongoing work products or projects. A program plan is designed to accomplish a predetermined objective or set of objectives.

Operational Plans

An operational plan is a detailed action plan to accomplish the specific objectives. The plan is a derivative of the strategic plan describing short-term business strategies, showing how the strategic plan will be put into operation and serving as a basis for an annual operating budget. An operational plan may comprise a three-year rolling plan to be completed by a small subgroup of people with expertise and/or a stake relating to a major goal.

Performance Measures

Performance measures are valid and reliable metrics for evaluating the extent to which goals and objectives are achieved. The measures should be SMART (Specific, Measurable, Achievable, Results-oriented, Time-limited).

IT Management Accountability Report

The IT management accountability report (IT MAR) is an annual report that provides OI&T performance information (i.e., strategic goals, objectives, fiscal year performance goals, and outcomes). The IT MAR is a management tool that will provide a basis for assessing the organization's effectiveness.

Environmental Scan: Feedback and Assessment

An environment scan is an ongoing internal and external customer feedback and assessment process conducted at all levels of the organization for use in developing vision, goals, and objectives.[31]

MANAGEMENT RESPONSIBILITIES WITHIN THE PLANNING CYCLE

This section concludes with a generalized view of planning responsibilities by three levels of management. **Figure 24–5** illustrates the three levels. Any planning cycle should reflect these levels, as does the previous example.

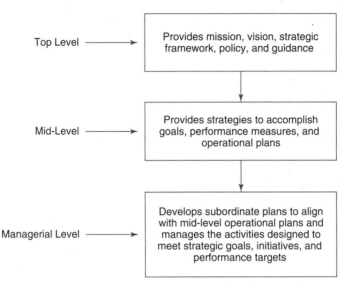

Figure 24–5 Primary Planning Responsibilities by Management Levels.

Upper-Level Responsibilities

Top-level management represents those individuals at the top of the organization chart. These upper-level individuals should provide overall direction for the organization's mission, vision, and strategic framework. They should be responsible for policymaking and supervisory guidance issues.

Mid-Level Responsibilities

Mid-level individuals are basically accountable to those above, while they operate in a supervisory mode to those below them in the organization chart. Mid-level management should typically provide the strategies to accomplish goals, performance measures, and operational plans.

Managerial-Level Responsibilities

The managers, meanwhile, are accountable to all those above them on the organization chart. The managerial level should typically develop the subordinate plans that will align with mid-level operational plans. Other responsibilities include managing the activities that are designed to meet strategic goals, initiatives, and performance targets.

TOOLS FOR STRATEGIC PLANNING: SITUATIONAL ANALYSIS AND FINANCIAL PROJECTIONS

Situational analysis and feasibility studies are discussed in this section, with an emphasis on their roles in strategic planning.

SITUATIONAL ANALYSIS

This section defines situational analysis (SWOT) and discusses its components.

Definition

A situational analysis does two things. It reviews the organization's internal operations for strengths and weaknesses and it explores the organization's external environment for opportunities and threats. (Thus SWOT: strengths-weaknesses-opportunities-threats.) A situational analysis allows management to, literally, analyze the organization's situation.

SWOT Analysis as a Strategic Tool

A SWOT analysis, properly performed, can be an excellent strategic tool. The four components of a SWOT analysis include the following:

- Strengths
- Weaknesses
- Opportunities
- Threats

The basic SWOT analysis format is illustrated in **Figure 24–6**. Here we see that the "Strengths" and "Weaknesses" sectors of the matrix are labeled "Internal," while the "Opportunities" and "Threats" sectors are labeled "External."

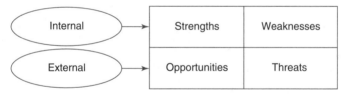

Figure 24–6 Basic SWOT Analysis Format.

Sample SWOT Worksheets Are Contained in Appendix 24-A

Appendix 24-A contains Sample SWOT Worksheets. The worksheets and their supplemental Question Guides concern Electronic Health Records (EHR) adoption and implementation. These worksheets can, however, be easily adopted for other purposes.

Appendix 24-A contains three "Internal Worksheets" for analyzing strengths and weaknesses, and an "External Worksheet" for analyzing external opportunities and threats. Supplemental Question Guides are also included for each worksheet. A Scoring Summary Sheet is included to complete the analysis.

Sequential Steps in the SWOT Analysis Project

The following steps pertain to both the internal and external components of the analysis:

1. First, decide if the sample worksheets and the supplemental question guides need to be customized; if so, do so.

2. Gather necessary information.
3. Fill in the worksheets, utilizing the question guides as needed.
4. Reach agreement, or consensus, on the final score for each line item on the worksheets.
5. Summarize the scores.
6. Enter the final net scores on the Scoring Summary Sheet.
7. Report the results.

Commencing the SWOT Analysis Project Process

In order to commence the SWOT analysis project's process, a number of decisions must be made. They include the following:

1. What type of task force or committee does the project need?
2. Who will be appointed to this task force?
3. What types of data/information should be gathered for this project?
4. Who will gather the information that is needed?
5. Will the scoring process be subjective or objective? (This may depend on the amount and type of available data.)
6. Will the same task force members that are involved in recording the worksheet information also be involved in the scoring process, or will a separate group be appointed to carry out the scoring function?
7. Who prepares the final report?
8. Who receives the report?
9. Who is responsible for taking appropriate action after the analysis and its report are completed?

Conclusion

Situational analysis is particularly appropriate for the analysis of electronic records implementation because such implementation requires the collaboration of multiple knowledge areas. A meeting of the minds can better occur with the discipline that a situational analysis can impose. It is a powerful tool when properly applied.

We should also acknowledge that there are a variety of approaches to performing a situational analysis, and this brief discussion features only a single approach. No matter what approach is utilized, the results of the situational analysis are what count.

FINANCIAL PROJECTIONS FOR STRATEGIC PLANNING

The type of financial projection that we discuss is this section is produced internally. These projections are intended for internal use during the planning process, and are thus not intended for any use outside the organization.

Definition

Projections are views into the future. We "project" future events, projects, or operations using a set of presumed, or hypothetical, assumptions.

Projections are different than forecasts, although both are considered to be "prospective" (thus "future") financial statements. Forecasts are based on assumptions that are expected to exist, and that reflect actions that are expected to occur.[32]

Projections, on the other hand, are often prepared to answer a "what-if" question, such as "what if … this service/program/initiative were to be adopted?" In these "what-if" situations several projections may be prepared, each based on a different set of hypothetical assumptions and each reflecting the actions that might occur, based on such assumptions.[33]

Build a Planner's Projection

An eight-step process for building a financial projection to be used internally for planning purposes is described as follows. The process is also illustrated in **Figure 24–7**.

Determine the Future Timeframe

What should the future start and end dates be for this projection? Is the time period to be covered long enough? Or is it too long for reasonable assumptions to be made?

Determine the Focus

Focus on what the plan (or planner) needs to know in order to go forward. Let that focus determine the direction your search for information will take. (Also note that sometimes a different agenda can redirect the focus.)

Gather Enough Information

You will need enough information to make informed decisions about your projection. The range of subjects may vary, but the information should be as up-to-date as possible.

Make Reasonable Assumptions

By "reasonable assumptions" we mean no wildly unattainable assumptions. For example, in most instances "we will increase revenue by 200% in the fourth quarter of next year" is an assumption that will not be accomplished thus is not reasonable.

Document the Assumptions

Assumptions used for the projection are key to its success. Documenting the assumptions is an indication of a well-constructed projection. The documentation adds validity to the final product. It also provides a record of the overall process of information-gathering that underlies the assumptions themselves.

Prepare the Projected Statements

Projected financial statements are then assembled using the documented assumptions. In accountant's terminology this is known as "compiling" the projections.

1)	Determine the future time frame
2)	Determine the focus
3)	Gather enough information
4)	Make reasonable assumptions
5)	Document the assumptions
6)	Prepare the projected statements
7)	Review for reasonableness
8)	Create alternative scenarios

Figure 24–7   Build a Planner's Financial Projection. Courtesy of J.J. Baker and R.W. Baker, Dallas, Texas.

Review for Reasonableness

For example, ask: "Is this assumption reasonable for an organization of my type and size?" This type of review may be subjective, but it is a logical part of the process. Appropriate members of the organization may also perform a review in order to highlight any weak spots within the assumptions.

Create Alternative Scenarios

It is often helpful to produce multiple versions of the projections ("Model A," "Model B," etc.). In this case, certain key assumptions are changed for each model. Thus the "what if" question is answered in several different ways.

Financial Projections as Strategic Tools

These internal planning projects may be used to better make informed decisions. If properly constructed, they can provide information that is laid out in a logical format, supported by assumptions that are properly explained for the knowledgeable reader. To summarize, projections can be an important tool to inform and support the planning process.

CASE STUDY: STRATEGIC FINANCIAL PLANNING IN LONG-TERM CARE

Chapter 32, "Case Study: Strategic Financial Planning in Long-Term Care" later in this volume involves a case study about strategic financial planning in long-term care. The case study is authored by Dr. Neil R. Dworkin, Emeritus Associate Professor of Management at Western Connecticut State University. His case study merits your close attention, as it will utilize planning concepts that have been discussed within this chapter.

APPENDIX 24-A: SAMPLE SWOT WORKSHEETS AND QUESTION GUIDES

Appendix 24-A contains four Sample SWOT Worksheets (three internal and one external) concerning EHR adoption and implementation, along with a Scoring Summary Sheet. A Question Guide is also included for each Worksheet. Electronic medical records adoption is a good subject for situational analysis. The sample worksheets in this Appendix can assist in beginning such a project.

INFORMATION CHECKPOINT

What is needed?	A "set" of an organization's mission statement, vision statement, and values.
Where is it found?	In the planning and policy division or within the administration office.
How is it used?	These documents are used to guide the organization.

📖 KEY TERMS

Action Plan	Innovation	SWOT Analysis
Financial Forecast	Mission Statement	Values Statement
Financial Projection	Situational Analysis	Vision Statement
Goal	Strategic Objective	

❓ DISCUSSION QUESTIONS

1. Do you know if your organization has a mission statement and a vision statement? If so, how are they communicated? Are they printed, posted on a website, or available in some other format? Please describe.

2. Have you ever been involved in a strategic planning session? If so, please describe how the group and the session were structured (but without revealing proprietary information).

3. Have you ever been involved in (or have observed) the process of a situational analysis (SWOT)? If so, please describe how the group went about performing the analysis (but again without revealing proprietary information).

NOTES

1. Department of Veterans Affairs (VA), VA Directive 6052 Appendix A (April 23, 2009).
2. Sutter Health, www.sutterhealth.org/about/mission (accessed May 31, 2012).
3. Tenet Health, www.tenethealth.com/about/pages/missionandvalues.aspx (accessed July 30, 2012).
4. Parkland, www.parklandhospital.com/whoweare/mission_vision.html (accessed June 7, 2012).
5. Mayo Clinic, www.mayoclinic.org/about/missionvalues.html (accessed July 30, 2012).
6. Regions Hospital, www.regionshospital.com/rh/about/index.html (accessed May 31, 2012).
7. Saint Barnabas Medical Center, www.saintbarnabasfoundation.org/about/mission.html (accessed July 30, 2012).
8. Texas Oncology, www.texasoncology.com/about-txo/vision-mission-history.aspx (accessed December 3, 2012).
9. Aetna, www.aetna.com/about-aetna-insurance/aetna-corporate-profile/aetna_mission_statement (accessed July 30, 2012).
10. AMA Press Release November 26, 2012, www.ama-assn.org (accessed January 16, 2013).
11. American Medical Association, www.ama-assn.org/ana/pub/about-ama/strategic-focus.page? (accessed October 17, 2012).
12. Ibid.

13. Good Samaritan Society, www.good-sam.com/index.php/about_us/ (accessed July 30, 2012).

14. Ibid.

15. Providence Healthcare Network, http://www.providence.net/about/ (accessed January 16, 2013).

16. Duke Health, www.dukemedicine.org/AboutUs (accessed July 30, 2012).

17. John Hopkins Medicine, www.hopkinsmedicine.org/se/util/display_mod.cfm? MODULE=/se-server/mod/mod (accessed July 30, 2012).

18. Public Law 103-62. 103 P.L. 62; 107 Stat. 285—Section 3(a), The language of the Act says "every agency," but in fact certain Executive agencies were excluded, including the Central Intelligence Agency, the General Accounting Office, the Panama Canal Commission, the United States Postal Service, and the Postal Rate Commission. [See 103 P.L. 62 Section 3(f).]

19. P.L. 62—Section 3(a) (1), (2), (3), (5).

20. P.L. 62—Section 3(a) (6b).

21. P.L. 111-352 Section 2(b).

22. Ibid. Section 3(b)(1).

23. Ibid. Section 4(b).

24. Ibid. Section 4(g).

25. U.S. Department of Health & Human Services (HHS), HHS Agencies & Offices, http://www.hhs.gov/about/whatwedo.html (accessed December 4, 2012).

26. U.S. Department of Health & Human Services (HHS), HHS Strategic Plan, http://www.hhs.gov/secretary/about/introduction.html (accessed May 25, 2012).

27. Administrative Law Review, www.administrativelawreview.org/publicresources/ index.php?option=com_content&view=article&id=21&Itemid=28 (accessed February 2, 2013).

28. Department of Veterans Affairs, Strategic Plan: Refresh, FY 2011–2015, http://www.amvets.org/pdfs/legislative_pdfs/2012/VA-Strategic-Plan-Refresh-FY-2011-2015.pdf (accessed November 21, 2016).

29. Department of Veterans Affairs (VA), "VA Directive 6052, Information Technology Strategic Planning" (April 23, 2009), http://www.itstrategy.oit.va.gov/docs/directive_6052.pdf, p. 6 (accessed December 4, 2012).

30. M Powered Strategies, www.mpoweredstrategies.com/news/2011/12/one-va-ea-business-reference-model/ (accessed February 2, 2013).

31. Ibid.

32. American Institute of Certified Public Accountants (AICPA), "Financial Forecasts and Projections" AT Section 301 (c)(d), http://www.aicpa.org/Research/Standards/AuditAttest/DownloadableDocuments/AT-00301.pdf

33. Ibid. AT Section 301 (d)(f).

Sample SWOT Worksheets and Question Guides 24-A

The following Sample SWOT Worksheets and their supplemental Question Guides concern Electronic Health Records (EHR) adoption and implementation. However, the worksheets and question guides can be readily adapted for other purposes.

INTRODUCTION

Situational analysis explores an organization's internal operation for strengths and weakness and observes the organization's external environment for opportunities and threats. The analysis process is often called "SWOT," for strengths-weaknesses-opportunities-threats. To be effective, the analysis must be objective and realistic.

Electronic medical records adoption is a good subject for situational analysis. The sample worksheets in this Appendix provide assistance in commencing such a project.

This Appendix contains four Sample SWOT Worksheets (three internal and one external) concerning EHR adoption and implementation, along with a Scoring Summary Sheet. A Question Guide is also included for each Worksheet. The Guides are intended to commence the process of analysis. Other questions may be added to customize the analysis for a particular process, situation, or department.

SCORING SUMMARY SHEET FOR EHR ADOPTION AND IMPLEMENTATION

Exhibit 24-A–1 collects and summarizes the SWOT analysis scores. Both the internal and external worksheets are to be scored for each item appearing on that particular worksheet. The scores range from 1 to 5, as follows: 1 = very good; 2 = good; 3 = fair; 4 = poor; and 5 = very poor. These scores are then summarized and the final net score is entered on the Exhibit 24-A–1.

THREE INTERNAL WORKSHEETS FOR STRENGTHS AND WEAKNESSES

Three internal worksheets present the results of the SWOT strengths and weaknesses internal analysis. These worksheets represent four important subjects that are relevant to EHR. The first two worksheets concern staff members involved in some capacity with EHR. The third worksheet addresses both technology and capital funding. These subjects are, of course, separate from the staffing issues. Each worksheet is described below.

Exhibit 24-A–1 SWOT Scoring Summary Sheet for EHR Adoption and Implementation

	1	2	3	4	5
INTERNAL STRENGTHS SCORES					
IT Department Staff	☐	☐	☐	☐	☐
Financial, Clinical, and Administrative Staff	☐	☐	☐	☐	☐
EHR Technology	☐	☐	☐	☐	☐
Capital Funding	☐	☐	☐	☐	☐
INTERNAL WEAKNESSES SCORES					
IT Department Staff	☐	☐	☐	☐	☐
Financial, Clinical, and Administrative Staff	☐	☐	☐	☐	☐
EHR Technology	☐	☐	☐	☐	☐
Capital Funding	☐	☐	☐	☐	☐
EXTERNAL OPPORTUNITIES SCORES					
Government	☐	☐	☐	☐	☐
Economy	☐	☐	☐	☐	☐
Competition	☐	☐	☐	☐	☐
Other Funding Sources	☐	☐	☐	☐	☐
EXTERNAL THREATS SCORES					
Government	☐	☐	☐	☐	☐
Economy	☐	☐	☐	☐	☐
Competition	☐	☐	☐	☐	☐
Other Funding Sources	☐	☐	☐	☐	☐

Score 1 to 5 with 1 being very good and 5 being very poor

Courtesy of J.J. Baker and R.W. Baker, Dallas, Texas.

INTERNAL WORKSHEET FOR EHR INFORMATION TECHNOLOGY (IT) STAFF

Exhibit 24-A–2 specifically addresses the information technology staffing. These staff members are the ones who must make electronic health records implementation work. The responsible staff are divided into three levels, depending upon the type of work they are expected to perform. The three levels represent "IT operations staff," who are the most directly involved; the "hands-on managers," who manage the operations staff day-to-day; and the "upper-level supervisory IT management," who manage from afar, but who are responsible for results.

Question Guide for EHR Information Technology Staff

Exhibit 24-A–3 contains 10 questions about IT staff. The questions are to be answered as is appropriate for the various staff levels described in the preceding paragraph.

Exhibit 24-A–2 EHR Internal Operations Analysis: Worksheet for Information Technology (IT) Department Staff

IT OPERATIONS STAFF (for each type of position listed)
Overall Computer Skills
Strengths _____
Weaknesses _____

Specific EHR Skills
Strengths _____
Weaknesses _____

Staffing Capacity
Strengths _____
Weaknesses _____

HANDS-ON IT MANAGERS
Background and Experience
Strengths _____
Weaknesses _____

EHR Proficiency and Support
Strengths _____
Weaknesses _____

Coverage (Man Hours Available)
Strengths _____
Weaknesses _____

UPPER-LEVEL SUPERVISORY IT MANAGEMENT
Background and Experience
Strengths _____
Weaknesses _____

EHR Proficiency and Support
Strengths _____
Weaknesses _____

Coverage (Man Hours Available)
Strengths _____
Weaknesses _____

Attach sheets to document the additional information used for this analysis.

Courtesy of J.J. Baker and R.W. Baker, Dallas, Texas.

Exhibit 24-A–3 Question Guide for EHR Internal Operations Analysis: Information Technology (IT) Department Staff

---

Staff questions (Answer the questions about IT staff as appropriate for the various staff levels: IT operations staff, hands-on IT managers, and upper-level supervisory IT management.)

- ☐ Possess advanced computer operations concepts?
- ☐ Possess basic computer operations concepts?
- ☐ Understand EHR technical computer applications in depth?
- ☐ Understand basic EHR technical computer applications?
- ☐ Understand the concept of EHR calculations?
- ☐ Cooperate/support multidisciplinary EHR adoption and implementation efforts?
- ☐ Resist/ignore EHR process and procedures?
- ☐ Sufficient IT staffing for EHR implementation?
- ☐ Sufficient IT staffing for EHR ongoing support?
- ☐ Acceptable productivity for EHR implementation?

Attach sheets to document the additional information used for this analysis.

Courtesy of J.J. Baker and R.W. Baker, Dallas, Texas.

INTERNAL WORKSHEET FOR OTHER STAFF INVOLVED IN EHR

Exhibit 24-A–4 addresses responsible staff in three other departments of the organization. These staff members are the ones who must make electronic health records implementation work within their own departments. The responsible staff members in each of these three departments (financial, clinical, and administrative) are again divided into three levels, depending upon the type of work they are expected to perform. The three levels represent "Staff responsible for some aspect of EHR," who are the most directly involved; the "hands-on managers," who are responsible for some aspect of EHR; and the "upper-level supervisory management," who manage from afar, but who are responsible for results.

Question Guide for Financial, Clinical, and Administrative Staff

Exhibit 24-A–5 contains 14 questions about relevant staff members within these three departments. This guide and its accompanying worksheet would, of course, be reproduced with as many copies as would be necessary in order to answer these questions for each department.

INTERNAL WORKSHEET FOR TECHNOLOGY AND CAPITAL FUNDING

Exhibit 24-A–6 addresses two subjects: computer technology and capital funding resources. The computer technology section concerns hardware, software, space requirements, and vendors. The section is then divided into two parts: one for overall computer systems and one for specific EHR computer resources.

Exhibit 24-A–4 Worksheet for EHR Internal Operations Analysis: Financial, Clinical, and Administrative Staff

---

STAFF RESPONSIBLE FOR SOME ASPECT OF EHR
Overall Computer Skills
Strengths _____
Weaknesses _____

Specific EHR Skills
Strengths _____
Weaknesses _____

Staffing Capacity
Strengths _____
Weaknesses _____

HANDS-ON MANAGERS RESPONSIBLE FOR SOME ASPECT OF EHR
Background and Experience
Strengths _____
Weaknesses _____

EHR Proficiency and Support
Strengths _____
Weaknesses _____

Coverage (Man Hours Available)
Strengths _____
Weaknesses _____

UPPER-LEVEL SUPERVISORY MANAGEMENT RESPONSIBLE FOR SOME ASPECT OF EHR
Background and Experience
Strengths _____
Weaknesses _____

EHR Proficiency and Support
Strengths _____
Weaknesses _____

Coverage (Man Hours Available)
Strengths _____
Weaknesses _____

Attach sheets to document the additional information used for this analysis.

Courtesy of J.J. Baker and R.W. Baker, Dallas, Texas.

Exhibit 24-A–5 Question Guide for EHR Internal Operations Analysis: Financial, Clinical, and Administrative Staff

---

Staff questions (Answer the questions about staff as appropriate for the various financial, clinical, and administrative staff levels: workers; hands-on managers, and upper-level supervisory management.)

☐ Possess advanced financial management concepts?
☐ Possess basic financial management concepts?
☐ Possess advanced clinical management concepts?
☐ Possess basic clinical management concepts?
☐ Understand EHR technical applications in depth from the financial view?
☐ Understand basic EHR technical applications from the financial view?
☐ Understand EHR technical applications in depth from the clinical view?
☐ Understand basic EHR technical applications from the clinical view?
☐ Understand the concept of EHR calculations?
☐ Cooperate/support multidisciplinary EHR adoption and implementation efforts?
☐ Resist/ignore EHR process and procedures?
☐ Sufficient relevant staffing for EHR implementation?
☐ Sufficient relevant staffing for EHR ongoing support?
☐ Acceptable productivity for EHR implementation?

Attach sheets to document the additional information used for this analysis.

Courtesy of J.J. Baker and R.W. Baker, Dallas, Texas.

The capital funding section of the worksheet addresses both short-term and long-term funding resources. The short-term funding requirement concerns EHR transition cash flow. The long-term funding requirement concerns what fixed capital may be specified for EHR implementation. Both are important to success.

Question Guide for Technology and Capital Funding Resources

Exhibit 24-A–7 contains eight questions about computer systems and four questions about capital funding resources. Additional customized questions may supplement this initial guide's content.

EXTERNAL WORKSHEET FOR OPPORTUNITIES AND THREATS

Exhibit 24-A–8 addresses four external environment subjects, including Government, Economy, Competition, and Funding Sources Other than Patient Revenue. Other subjects may, of course, be added as desired.

Exhibit 24-A–6 Worksheet for EHR Internal Operations Analysis: Resources Other than Staff

---

OVERALL COMPUTER SYSTEMS

Hardware and Software
Strengths _____
Weaknesses _____

Space Requirements
Strengths _____
Weaknesses _____

Vendor Contractual Agreements (if applicable)
Strengths _____
Weaknesses _____

Vendor Performance (if applicable)
Strengths _____
Weaknesses _____

SPECIFIC EHR COMPUTER RESOURCES

Hardware and Software
Strengths _____
Weaknesses _____

Additional Space Requirements (if applicable)
Strengths _____
Weaknesses _____

Vendor Contractual Agreements (if applicable)
Strengths _____
Weaknesses _____

Vendor Performance (if applicable)
Strengths _____
Weaknesses _____

CAPITAL FUNDING

Short-Term EHR Transition Cash Flow Requirements
Strengths _____
Weaknesses _____

Long-term Fixed Capital Specified for EHR Implementation
Strengths _____
Weaknesses _____

Attach sheets to document the additional information used for this analysis.

Courtesy of J.J. Baker and R.W. Baker, Dallas, Texas.

Exhibit 24-A–7 Question Guide for EHR Internal Operations Analysis: Resources Other than Staff

---

OVERALL COMPUTER SYSTEMS
   ☐ Sufficient equipment (hardware and software) for general operations?

SPECIFIC EHR COMPUTER RESOURCES
   ☐ Sufficient equipment (hardware and software) for EHR implementation?
   ☐ Sufficient equipment (hardware and software) for EHR ongoing support?
   ☐ Equipment operates adequately?
   ☐ Equipment costly to maintain? To operate?
   ☐ If applicable, are vendor contracts costly to maintain (updates, add-ons, etc.)?
   ☐ Does the equipment produce desired results? Timely results?
   ☐ If applicable, does the vendor produce desired results? Timely results?

CAPITAL FUNDING
   ☐ Have the short-term EHR transition cash flow requirements been accurately projected?
   ☐ Are these cash flow requirements accurately presented in the organization's budget?
   ☐ Are the long-term fixed capital specified for EHR implementation accurately projected?
   ☐ Are these long-term fixed capital requirements acknowledged in the strategic plan?

Attach sheets to document the additional information used for this analysis

Courtesy of J.J. Baker and R.W. Baker, Dallas, Texas.

Question Guide for EHR External Environment Analysis

Exhibit 24-A–9 contains a total of 22 questions about various components of the external environment. This guide may also be augmented with customized questions that relate to issues within the specific organization under analysis.

Exhibit 24-A–8 Worksheet for EHR External Environment Analysis

GOVERNMENT (EHR impact for each governmental element listed)
Medicare Program
Opportunities _____
Threats _____

Medicaid Program
Opportunities _____
Threats _____

Regulations About Electronic Standards (Version 5010 and ongoing versions)
Opportunities _____
Threats _____

Other Federal/State Regulations
Opportunities _____
Threats _____

ECONOMY (as to continuing need for and impact of EHR)
Opportunities _____
Threats _____

COMPETITION (relevant to EHR)
Opportunities _____
Threats _____

FUNDING SOURCES OTHER THAN PATIENT REVENUE (impact, if any, on EHR)
Opportunities _____
Threats _____

Attach sheets to document the additional information used for this analysis.

Courtesy of J.J. Baker and R.W. Baker, Dallas, Texas.

Exhibit 24-A–9 Question Guide for EHR External Environment Analysis

---

GOVERNMENT (EHR impact for each governmental element listed)
Medicare Program

☐ What EHR implementation costs are related to this program initiative?
☐ What revenues from EHR governmental sources are related to this program initiative?
☐ What savings in work flow or processes are related to adopting EHR?
☐ Additional changes to the EHR Medicare Initiative are scheduled to occur at various points in the future. How will these initiative changes impact the organization?

Medicaid Program

☐ What EHR implementation costs are related to this program initiative?
☐ What revenues from EHR governmental sources are related to this program initiative?
☐ What savings in work flow or processes are related to adopting EHR?
☐ Additional changes to the EHR Medicaid Initiative are scheduled to occur at various points in the future. How will these initiative changes impact the organization?

Regulations About Electronic Standards (Version 5010 and ongoing versions)

☐ What EHR implementation costs are related to these requirements?
☐ What savings in work flow or processes are related to adopting these standards?
☐ Additional changes to the regulatory electronic standards are scheduled to occur at various points in the future. How will these initiative changes impact the organization?

Other Federal/State Regulations

☐ What other federal and/or state regulations affect EHR implementation?
☐ How do these regulations impact the organization?

ECONOMY (as to continuing need for and impact of EHR)

☐ Will EHR affect continuing need for medical services? If so, how?
☐ What impact is EHR implementation projected to have on the medical services economy nationally? Regionally?

COMPETITION (relevant to EHR)

☐ What are your three biggest competitors?
☐ How do the services they provide compare to your services?
☐ What do you predict the impact of EHR adoption will be on each?
☐ How have they prepared for EHR initial implementation?
☐ How does their preparation and impact affect your own organization?

OTHER FUNDING SOURCES (impact, if any, on EHR)

☐ Does your organization have such funding sources?
☐ If so, what impact, if any, will EHR adoption have on such sources?

Attach sheets to document the additional information used for this analysis.

Courtesy of J.J. Baker and R.W. Baker, Dallas, Texas.

Putting It All Together: Creating a Business Plan That Is Strategic

OVERVIEW

A business plan is a document typically prepared in order to obtain funding and/or financing. A traditional business plan typically contains information about three major elements: the proposed project's organization, marketing, and financial aspects. However, the actual business plan is generally constructed in a series of segments, each involving a particular type of information. The overall business plan is built up as these individual segments are completed. The segments are described in this chapter.

ELEMENTS OF THE BUSINESS PLAN

A traditional business plan typically contains three major elements:

- Organization plan
- Marketing plan
- Financial plan

The organization segment should describe the management team. The marketing segment should discuss who may use the service and/or product. The financial segment should contain the numbers that illustrate how the project is expected to operate over an initial period of time. We believe that it is also important to begin the business plan with an executive summary that outlines key points, plus a clear and concise description of the service and/or product that is the subject of the plan.

Progress Notes

After completing this chapter, you should be able to

1. Understand the construction of a business plan.
2. Describe the organization segment of a business plan.
3. Describe the marketing segment of a business plan.
4. Describe the financial segment of a business plan.

PREPARING TO CONSTRUCT THE BUSINESS PLAN

The planning stage will shape a business plan's content. The initial decisions, such as those shown in **Exhibit 25–1**, will determine your approach to the plan. For example, if your organization requires a certain type of format and preexisting blank spreadsheets, many of the initial decisions have already been made for you. Otherwise, the checklist contained in Exhibit 25–1 will assist you in making initial decisions for the business plan's approach.

It is important to note that the level of sophistication for the overall plan should be based on the decision makers who will be the primary audience. Another practical consideration involves creating a grid or matrix to assist in gathering all necessary information. The grid or matrix could also include which individuals are responsible for helping to create or collect the required information. Finally, it is important to create a file at the beginning of the project in which all computations, backup information, dates, and sources are kept together in an organized fashion.

Exhibit 25–1   Initial Decisions for the Business Plan

> **Business Plan Initial Decisions**
>
> - Outline necessary format
> - Decide on length
> - Decide on level of sophistication
> - Determine what information is needed
> - Determine who will provide each piece of information
>
> Courtesy of J.J. Baker and R.W. Baker, Dallas, Texas.

Exhibit 25–2   Basic Information for the Service or Equipment Description

> **Service or Equipment Description**
> - What the service specifically provides
> - Why this service is different and/or special
> - What the equipment specifically does
> - Why this equipment is different and/or special
> - Required training, if applicable
> - Regulatory requirements and/or impact, if any
>
> Courtesy of J.J. Baker and R.W. Baker, Dallas, Texas.

THE SERVICE OR EQUIPMENT DESCRIPTION

The service and/or equipment description should do a good job of describing what the heart of the business plan is about. If the business plan is for a project or a new service line, then this description would expand to include the entire project or the overall service line. Information that should always be included in the description is contained in **Exhibit 25–2**.

The test of a good description is whether an individual who has never been involved in your planning can read the description and understand it without additional questions being raised.

THE ORGANIZATION SEGMENT

The organization segment should describe the management team. But it should also describe how the proposed service or equipment fits into the organization. Who will be charged with the new budget? Who will be responsible for the controls and reporting for this proposal? It is important to provide a clear picture that informs decision makers about how the proposed acquisition will be managed. Basic facts to explain are included in **Exhibit 25–3**. Visual depictions of the chain of authority and supervisory responsibilities provide helpful illustrations for this segment.

THE MARKETING SEGMENT

The marketing segment should describe the available market, that portion of the market your service or equipment should attract, and that portion of the market occupied by the competition. This segment should achieve a balance between describing those individuals who will be availing themselves of the service or equipment and a description of the competition. A description of who will be responsible for the marketing is also valuable information for the decision makers. Strive for a realistic and objective appraisal of the situation. Basic facts to include are illustrated in **Exhibit 25–4**.

Of all areas of the business plan, the marketing segment is most likely to be overoptimistic in its assumptions. It is wise to be conservative about estimations of physician and patient acceptance and usage. And it is equally wise to be realistic when assessing the competition and its likely impact.

THE FINANCIAL ANALYSIS SEGMENT

The financial segment should contain the numbers that illustrate how the project is expected to operate over an initial period of time. Financial plans may range from a projected period of 1 year to as much as 10 years. A 1-year projection is often too short to show true outcomes, whereas a 10-year projection may be too long to meaningfully forecast. Your organization will usually have a standard length of time that is accepted for these projections. The standard forecasted periods for high-tech equipment, for example, often range from 3 to 5 years. Why? Because advances in technology may render them obsolete in 5 years or less. Therefore, the forecast is set for a realistically short time period.

The financial analysis for a business plan should contain a forecast of operations. The forecast may be simple, such as a cash flow statement, or it may be more extensive. A more extensive forecast would also require a balance sheet and an income statement. The required statements and schedules will depend on two factors: the size and complexity of the project and the usual procedure for a business plan presentation that is expected in your organization.

Exhibit 25–3 Basic Information for the Organization Segment

Organization Segment Information

- Physical location where service will be provided
- Physical location of the equipment
- The department responsible for the budget
- The division responsible for operations
- The directly responsible supervisor
- Composition of the overall management team

Courtesy of J.J. Baker and R.W. Baker, Dallas, Texas.

Exhibit 25–4 Basic Information for the Marketing Segment

Marketing Segment Information

- Physicians who will use the service or equipment
- New patients who will use the service or equipment
- Established patients who will use the service or equipment
- Estimated portion of the market to be captured
- Competition and its impact

Courtesy of J.J. Baker and R.W. Baker, Dallas, Texas.

The Projected Cash Flow Statement

As we have just stated, it is possible that the forecast of operations may simply consist of the cash flow statement. In any case, the statement can be complex, with many detailed line items, or it can be condensed. The condensed type of statement is most often found in a business plan. Keep in mind, however, that a detailed worksheet—the source of the information on the condensed statement—may well be filed in the supporting work papers for the project. Necessary cash flow assumptions are illustrated in **Exhibit 25–5**.

Exhibit 25–5 Basic Assumptions for Business Plan Cash Flow Statement Projections

---

Cash Flow Statement Assumptions

- Number of years in the future to forecast
- Capital asset purchase or lease information
- Capital asset salvage value (if any)
- Cash inflow
- Cash outflow
- Cost of capital (if applicable)

Courtesy of J.J. Baker and R.W. Baker, Dallas, Texas.

Exhibit 25–6 Basic Assumptions for Business Plan Income Statement Projections

---

Income Statement Assumptions

- Revenue type
- Revenue source(s) *Universities, fed funding - grant, Donations/federal.*
- Revenue amount
- Expenses:
  - Labor
  - Supplies
  - Cost of drug or device (if applicable)
  - Equipment
  - Space occupancy
  - Overhead

Courtesy of J.J. Baker and R.W. Baker, Dallas, Texas.

---

fed funding?

The Projected Income Statement

What income statement assumptions will your business plan's financial analysis require? The basic assumptions for a healthcare project's income statement are illustrated in **Exhibit 25–6**.

The "revenue type" in Exhibit 25–6 refers to whether, for example, the revenue is derived entirely from services or whether part of the revenue is derived from drugs and devices. The "revenue sources" refers to how many payers will pay for the service and/or drug and device, and in what proportion (such as Medicare 60%, Medicaid 15%, and commercial payers 25%). The "revenue amount" refers to how much each payer is expected to pay for the service and/or drug and device. The total amount of revenue can then be determined by multiplying each payer's expected payment rate times the percentage of the total represented by that payer.

In regard to the "expenses" in Exhibit 25–6, the labor cost will usually be determined by staffing assumptions. The required staffing should be set out by type of employee and the pay rate for each type of employee. The number of full-time equivalents (FTEs) for each type of employee will then be established. The FTEs will be multiplied times the assumed pay rate to arrive at the labor cost assumption.

"Supplies" refers to the necessary supplies required to perform the procedure or service. "Cost of drug or device" refers to the cost to the organization of purchasing the drug or device (if a drug or device is necessary to the service). The labor, supplies, and cost of drug or device are costs that can be directly attributed to the service that is the subject of the business plan. Likewise, the "equipment" cost refers to the annual depreciation expense of any equipment that is directly attributed to the service that is the subject of the business plan.

"Space occupancy" refers to the overall cost of occupying the space required for the service or procedure. "Space occupancy" is a catchall phrase. It includes either annual depreciation expense (if the building is owned) or annual rent expense (if the building is leased) of the square footage required for the service. Space occupancy also includes other related costs such as utilities, maintenance, housekeeping, and insurance. Security might also be included in this category. The actual forecast might group these expense items into one line item, or the forecast might show each individual expense (depreciation, housekeeping, etc.) on a separate line. If the expenses are grouped, a footnote or a supplemental schedule should show the actual detail that makes up the total amount.

"Overhead" refers to the remaining expenses of operation that are necessary to produce the service but that are not directly attributable to that service. Examples of such overhead in a physician's office might include items such as postage and copy paper. This amount of indirect overhead may be expressed as a percentage; for example, "overhead equals 10%." Whether the "space occupancy" example or the "overhead" example discussed previously here are grouped or detailed in the forecast will probably depend on how large the amount is in relation to the other expenses, or it might depend instead on the usual format that your organization expects to see in a typical business plan that is presented to management.

The Projected Balance Sheet

What balance sheet assumptions will your business plan's financial analysis require? The basic assumptions for a healthcare project's balance sheet are illustrated in **Exhibit 25–7**.

The elements of a balance sheet (assets, liabilities, and equity) are described in a previous chapter. If a full projected set of statements is required for the business plan, the balance sheet entries will in large part be a function of the income statement projections discussed in the preceding section of this chapter. For example, accounts receivable would be primarily determined by the revenue assumptions, while accounts payable would be primarily determined by the expense assumptions. Likewise, acquisition of equipment or other capital assets will affect capital assets (property and equipment), while their funding assumptions will affect either or both liability and equity totals on the projected balance sheet.

THE "KNOWLEDGEABLE READER" APPROACH TO YOUR BUSINESS PLAN

We believe a good business plan should answer the questions that occur to a knowledgeable reader. Thus, the information you include in the business plan should reflect

Exhibit 25–7 Basic Assumptions for Business Plan Balance Sheet Projections

Balance Sheet Assumptions

- Cash
- Accounts Receivable
- Inventories
- Property and Equipment
- Accounts Payable
- Accrued Current Liabilities
- Long-Term Liabilities
- Equity

Courtesy of J.J. Baker and R.W. Baker, Dallas, Texas.

Exhibit 25–8 Considerations for Forecasting Equipment Acquisition

Considerations for Forecasting Equipment Acquisition

- Only one location?
- Equipment single purpose or multi-purpose?
- Technology: new, middle-aged, old (obsolete vs. untested)?
- Equipment compatibility?
- Medical supply cost?
- High or low capital investment?
- Buy new or used (refurbished)?
- Buy or lease?
- Lease for number of years or lease on a pay-per-procedure deal?
- How much staff training is required?
- Certification required?
- Square footage required for equipment?
- Is the required square footage available?
- Cleaning methods and equipment (and staff level required)?
- Repairs and maintenance expense (high, medium, low)?

Courtesy of J.J. Baker and R.W. Baker, Dallas, Texas.

Exhibit 25–9 Sample Format for a Business Plan

A Sample Business Plan Format

- Title Page
- Table of Contents
- Executive Summary
- Service and/or Equipment Description
- The Organizational Plan
- The Marketing Plan
- The Financial Plan
- Appendix (optional)

Courtesy of J.J. Baker and R.W. Baker, Dallas, Texas.

the choices that you made in selecting the assumptions for your financial analysis. For instance, an example of considerations for forecasting an equipment acquisition is presented in **Exhibit 25–8**. The content of the final business plan should touch upon these points in describing your assumptions that underlie the financial analysis.

THE EXECUTIVE SUMMARY

The executive summary should contain a well-written and concise summary of the entire plan. It should not be longer than two pages; many decision makers consider one page desirable. Some people like to write the executive summary first. They tend to use it as an outline to guide the rest of the content. Other people like to write the executive summary last, when they know what all the detailed content contains. In either instance, the executive summary should tell the entire story in a compelling manner.

ASSEMBLING THE BUSINESS PLAN

The business plan should be assembled into a suitable report format that is determined by many of your initial decisions, such as length and level of sophistication. A sample format appears in **Exhibit 25–9**.

If an appendix is desired, it should contain detail to support certain contents in the main part of the business plan. In preparing the final report, certain other logistics are important. It is expected, for example, that the pages should be numbered. (You might also want to add the date in the footer and perhaps a version number as well.) Although the report may or may not be bound, it should have all pages firmly secured.

PRESENTING THE BUSINESS PLAN

You may be asked to present more than once. Sometimes you will have to prepare a short form and a long form of the plan, depending on the audience. Tips on presenting your business plan are presented in **Exhibit 25–10**.

It is especially important to practice your presentation in advance. When you leave time for questions and for discussion, you also want to be well prepared for anticipated questions. By constructing a well-thought-out business plan, you have substantially increased your chances for a successful outcome.

STRATEGIC ASPECTS OF YOUR BUSINESS PLAN

Your business plan must fit into your organization's strategic plan. To begin to do so, you might answer the following questions:

- How does my business plan fit into the overall strategic plan (the "master plan") for my organization?
- How does my business plan specifically fit into my department or division's segment of the organization's overall strategic plan/master plan?
- Does the proposed timing of my business plan coincide with the strategic plan's time frames?
- Does the proposed funding of my business plan fit into available funding resources mentioned in the strategic plan?
- What competition will my business plan face, strategically speaking, within my organization? Does my plan provide a good defense against this competition?
- Are there external competition and/or legislative aspects mentioned in my business plan that are also addressed within the strategic plan? If so, does my plan's treatment of these external aspects coordinate with that of the strategic plan? If not, have I explained why not?

The previous chapter explored Strategic Planning in some depth. Other aspects contained in that chapter may also be applicable to your business plan.

Exhibit 25–10 Tips on Presentation of the Business Plan

> **Tips on Presenting Your Business Plan**
>
> - Determine who will be attending ahead of time
> - Determine how long you will have for the presentation
> - Be sure you have a copy for each attendee
> - Decide upon whether to use audio/visual aids
>   - LCD projector and PowerPoint slides?
>   - Flip chart and markers?
>   - Other methods?
> - Practice your presentation in advance
> - Leave time for questions and for discussion
>
> Courtesy of J.J. Baker and R.W. Baker, Dallas, Texas.

INFORMATION CHECKPOINT

What is needed?	A sample of a business plan.
Where is it found?	Probably with your manager or the departmental director.
How is it used?	Study the way the business plan was distributed. Who received it? What did they do with it? What was the result?

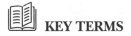

KEY TERMS

Business Plan	Revenue Sources	Space Occupancy
Overhead	Revenue Type	Supplies
Revenue Amount		

DISCUSSION QUESTIONS

1. Have you ever been involved in the creation of a business plan?
2. If so, did the plan include all three segments (organizational, marketing, and finance)? If not, why do you think one or more of the segments was missing?
3. Have you ever attended the formal presentation of a business plan? If so, was it successful in obtaining the desired funding?
4. Was the plan that was presented similar to what we have described in this chapter? What would you have changed in the presentation? Why?

Understanding Strategic Relationships: Health Delivery Systems, Finance, and Reimbursement

© LFor/Shutterstock

INTRODUCTION

We begin this chapter by defining three areas: health delivery systems, finance, and reimbursement. We include these definitions in order to illustrate where finance and reimbursement fit into the overall system. We will then describe the various strategic relationships that are involved.

By its very nature, the complexion and purpose of a health delivery system cannot be considered separately from the range of values and issues surrounding finance and reimbursement, including the magnitude of government involvement. Healthcare finance is the linchpin of the United States healthcare delivery system. While there are some similarities to corporate finance (i.e., budgeting; financial planning), there are major differences.

DEFINING HEALTH DELIVERY SYSTEMS

This section defines the health delivery system before observing its strategic relationships within an overall system.

What Is a Health Delivery System?

A health delivery system typically contains different levels of patient care and different sites of service, all operating under one integrated system for the delivery of health care.

A more formal definition is as follows:

> A delivery system which "provides or aims to provide a coordinated continuum of services to a defined population and are willing to be held clinically and fiscally accountable for the outcomes and the health status of the population served."[1]

Progress Notes

After completing this chapter, you should be able to

1. Define health delivery systems.
2. Define the area of healthcare finance.
3. Understand the strategic relationship between healthcare delivery systems and finance.
4. Understand the strategic relationship between finance and reimbursement.
5. Recognize the strategic relationship between third-party reimbursement and government expenditures.
6. Recognize a new focus on the relationship between finance and healthcare delivery.

A successful health system that functions properly needs the six following elements:

- Trained health workers who are motivated
- A well-managed infrastructure
- A reliable supply of medicines and technologies
- Adequate funding
- Evidence-based policies
- Strong health plans, including strong updated strategic plans[2]

Who Are the Stakeholders in Health Delivery Systems?

Stakeholders in health delivery systems can be divided into two categories: internal and external. The internal stakeholders consist of those delivering care (clinicians), those who support the care deliverers (administrators), and those receiving care (the patients).

External stakeholders are varied and numerous. Their motivations may vary, but their interests still center upon the delivery of care within the internal system. **Figure 26–1** illustrates 12 different types of external stakeholders. They include the following:

- Insurance providers
- Government providers
- Government policy makers
- Government overseers
- The pharmaceutical industry
- The medical device industry
- Other health industry suppliers
- Professional organizations
- Educators

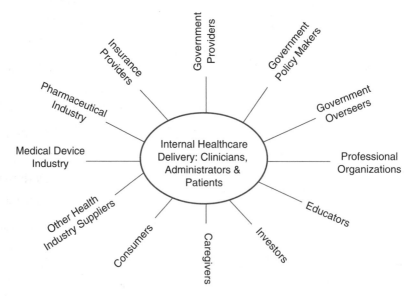

Figure 26–1 Stakeholders in Health Delivery Systems.

- Investors
- Caregivers
- Consumers

Insurance company providers include such organizations as Aetna, United Health, etc. Government providers include federal agencies such as Medicare, Medicaid, and TRICARE, along with state agencies. Government policy makers include Congress and many supporting federal agencies such as the Office of Management and Budget (OMB), while individual states also determine relevant health policy. Other government agencies oversee various elements of our public health; they include the Centers for Disease Control and Prevention (CDC), the National Institute of Health (NIH), and various others.

Health care is a huge industry in the United States. Figure 26–1 highlights three types of industry: pharmaceutical, medical device, and all other health industry suppliers. The "all other" includes both services and supplies, as varied as computer services to food and cleaning supplies.

Numerous professional organizations provide support for both clinicians and administrators; examples include the American Hospital Association (AHA) and the American Medical Association (AMA), though there are many more and they play an important supporting role. Academia is a stakeholder for its educational role in both medical schools and business schools.

Investors play an important stakeholder role, as they provide funding. Caregivers have a personal interest in the health delivery system. And consumers are stakeholders because they are impacted by rising costs of the healthcare industry as a whole.

DEFINING THE AREA OF HEALTHCARE FINANCE

This section defines the area of healthcare finance within the overall system.

What Are the Responsibilities Associated with Finance?

There are four major responsibilities typically associated with healthcare finance. They include:

- Planning
- Controlling
- Organizing and directing
- Decision making[3]

One of our colleagues, a nurse, talks about the area of healthcare finance as "a method of getting money in and out of the business." It is not a bad description, because the Finance Department is primarily responsible for achieving the most beneficial financial outcome for the organization.

What Are the Duties Associated with Finance?

The duties associated with healthcare finance revolve around the successful management of planning, controlling, organizing and directing, and decision making. Specific duties for a financial officer will depend upon the type of organizational structure where he or she works.

For example, is the organization large and consolidated, with a head office? If so, some (or all) of the planning and decision making around planning will probably be handled in the head office. The onsite financial officer's duties will then center mostly upon operational matters such as controlling and organizing and directing. Such a large organization may have a treasurer in addition to a chief financial officer. Or is the organization smaller, without a head office? If so, the financial officer may have to direct all financial matters. He or she would have to direct planning and related decision making in addition to the day-to-day operational matters.

The individual performing these duties may have one of several different job titles. A description of three such titles follows.

Chief Financial Officer: Responsible for operations (administrative, financial, and risk management), including both financial and operational strategies; determining the metrics that are related to the strategies; and developing and monitoring internal control systems.[4]
Controller: Responsible for the organization's accounting functions; includes producing accurate financial reports that adhere to appropriate standards, maintaining the accounting system, and overseeing controls and budgets.[5]
Treasurer: Responsible for a higher level of the organization's financial activities, mainly centering upon financial liquidity, investments, and risk management.[6]

DEFINING THE AREA OF HEALTHCARE REIMBURSEMENT

This section defines the area of healthcare reimbursement within the overall system. The term "reimbursement" basically means a method of paying (reimbursing) a healthcare provider for services or procedures provided. Payment is made upon receipt of a claim (bill) from the service provider. This claim typically contains codes for specific procedures and services that tie to relevant payment amounts. Payment of the claim may be made by a third-party payer or by the patient directly.[7]

What Are the Responsibilities Associated with Reimbursement?

Simply put, there are three major responsibilities associated with reimbursement:

- Prepare correct and complete claims
- Get these claims to the correct payer(s) in a timely manner
- Collect the proper payment that is due in a timely manner

In addition, the reimbursement personnel are responsible for carrying out any directives received from the Finance Department, including those of strategic planning.

What Are the Duties Associated with Reimbursement?

Reimbursement duties within the system may be split up into different positions. For example, the following job titles may typically be responsible for these duties. (Note: other job titles also exist that describe these same duties.)

- Data entry clerk: Enters codes and insurance information
- Medical coder: Enters service and procedure codes onto a claim
- Medical biller: Verifies the patient's insurance coverage; prepares the bill (claim form); reviews unpaid claims and/or appeals those that are denied

- Billing supervisor or coordinator: Oversees scheduling, monitoring, and training of personnel
- Medical claims specialist or examiner: Reviews samples of claims for accuracy; documents information for legal actions; provides legal support when required (this position functions outside the regular day-to-day operations and may work directly from the Finance Department)

Other reimbursement duties involve management of monies received (or not received). Incoming payments of claims must be reconciled and matched to the organization's records of billings. And nonpayments (past-due bills) must have collection efforts made. These payment duties are typically handled by different personnel.

It is also possible that the billing and collection duties may be performed by an outside contractor. One specialist physician that we know uses such an outside contractor.

Both medical information and billing information can now be generated in real time. For example, the doctor may have a data entry person right in the exam room with him. (Sometimes this is a nurse who has many other duties as well, but other doctors may use a "scribe" whose only job is the data entry.) The doctor dictates medical notes as he performs his examination and the assistant enters the information into the computer. At the end of the visit, he refers to his super bill. (The super bill is a customized form that contains procedure and diagnosis codes specific to a particular practice and/or specialty. A super bill allows information to be recorded quickly and efficiently). He calls off the codes to be billed for this examination, including any lab work ordered, etc. The data entry assistant also enters this coding information into the computer. The billing codes are then transmitted electronically, either to the internal billing department or to the outside billing service. And if transmitted externally, the outside billing service is then typically responsible for all billing and collection—for a fee, of course.

While the above encapsulates the essence of healthcare reimbursement, two caveats are worth mentioning. When healthcare reimbursement involves a third party, consumers may be largely unconcerned with the costs of their care, knowing that their bills are paid by another party. Moreover, third-party transactions may also remove providers from concerns about the cost of care, as they may not need to confront a patient covered by insurance with the actual charges, no matter how high. One may assume that these third-party concerns should be mitigated by the further implementation of value-based purchasing.

STRATEGIC RELATIONSHIP BETWEEN THE HEALTHCARE DELIVERY SYSTEM AND FINANCE

This section discusses strategic relationships and their impacts across the system.

Relationship Cause-and-Effect: An Example

This relationship can be described as a circular cause-and-effect. That is, finance department actions often affect the overall delivery system, and the overall delivery system in turn often affects the finance department. We illustrate this cause-and-effect with an example. In this example, particular elements of the overall delivery system will affect the strategic positioning of the finance department.

Value-based programs are an important current trend in payment for U.S. healthcare services. Briefly, the programs rely upon digitally recorded performance measures, including

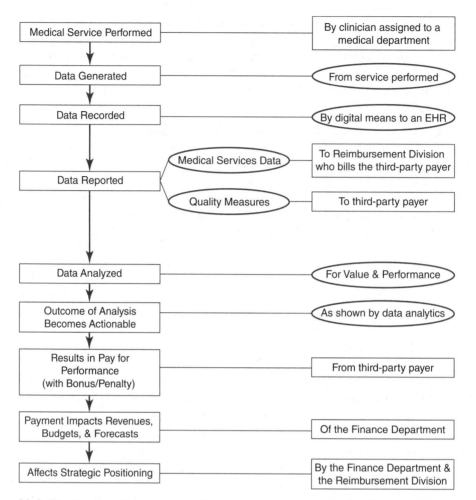

Figure 26–2 The Strategic Relationship of Value-Based Programs, Quality Measures, Finance, and Reimbursement.

certain quality measures, to reflect value provided by the system. That value is then basically rewarded by a bonus payment or penalized by a negative payment.

It follows, then, that accurate and timely recording of such quality measures will ultimately affect total payments, which will affect the finance department's financial strategic planning. But the finance department has no control over how (or when) these measures are recorded. They happen elsewhere within the system. This strategic relationship is illustrated step-by-step in **Figure 26–2**.

Note that the information generated in this example is used both internally and externally. Steps are as follows:

Step 1: A medical service is performed by a clinician. This professional is assigned to a medical department somewhere within the system.

Step 2: The data generated from this service is recorded within an electronic health record (EHR). It includes the service itself plus specific quality information (quality measures).

Step 3.1: The data is reported in two parts. First, the medical service portion is transmitted to the Reimbursement Division, who then bills the third-party payer.

Step 3.2: In the second part of this step, the quality measures portion of the data is transmitted to the third-party payer, who accumulates it for future analysis.

Step 4: At a future point in time, the third-party payer analyzes the accumulated quality measure data.

Step 5: The outcome of this analysis becomes actionable by the payer, as shown by the data analytics.

Step 6: The resulting action is a pay-for-performance bonus or penalty from the third-party payer.

Step 7: This payment result impacts the finance department's revenues, budgets, and forecasts.

Step 8: The resulting financial impact affects strategic positioning by the finance department.

The resulting financial impact also, of course, impacts the financial position of the overall system. Thus, the strategic relationship of the entire system versus the finance department is cause-and-effect. Accurate reporting of good quality measures by an entirely separate department trickles down to affect dollars received (or not received), which in turn affects both the finance department and the entire system.

Strategic Analysis Relationships Within the System

The previous example illustrated a relationship that resulted in payment impacts from a payer outside the health delivery system itself. However, the same data can and should be analyzed for internal strategic uses. **Figure 26–3** illustrates this type of analysis as follows:

a. The medical service data is generated and recorded via EHRs, using software installed by the organization.

b. The accumulated data is analyzed for value-based purposes. This analysis may be performed internally by the IT department or by an outside contractor.

c. The outcome of such analysis, as shown by data analytics, becomes actionable. This is an internal analysis, generated for internal use.

d. The strategic action plan is then revised. Revisions are undertaken by the personnel who are responsible for strategic planning within the system.

e. Strategic positioning results from plan revisions.

Such analysis highlights strategic relationships between and among the various departments within the system. While the positioning in this example may be most likely to affect the Finance Department and its Reimbursement Division, as shown, that might not always be the case. The result of the internal strategic analysis may reveal faults in the process and workflow at the clinical level. Strategic relationships should then be activated to remedy the faults, wherever they may lie.

THE STRATEGIC RELATIONSHIP BETWEEN FINANCE AND REIMBURSEMENT

At first glance, the strategic relationship between finance and reimbursement seems like a one-way street. That is, finance personnel provide the lead in strategy and reimbursement personnel must follow.

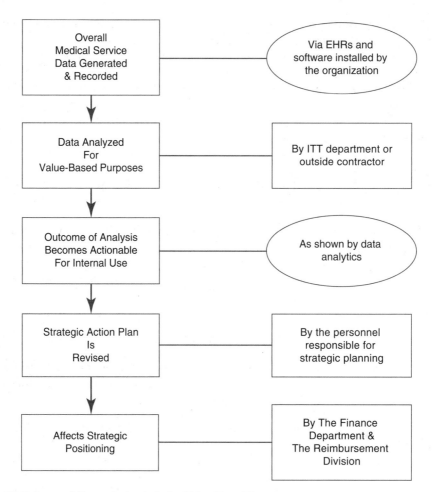

Figure 26–3 Internal Strategic Analysis for Value-Based Programs.

However, what happens if the reimbursement division fails in its responsibilities? Answer: Cash flow for the organization is reduced. (And, in some cases, the reduction in cash flow can be significant.) In this case, finance must react to the reimbursement situation instead of providing the lead. Finance personnel will have to find funding to make up the cash shortfall. Strategic planning must be revised while remedial action is taken.

Inasmuch as the Chief Financial Officer (or Vice President of Finance in a larger organization) is responsible for all finance activities within the organization, it is incumbent upon that person to raise the necessary funds and to ensure that those funds are effectively used. Specific applications may include the acquisition of capital, cash and debt management, and lease financing among strategic alternatives.

It is worth noting that some things are beyond the organization's control. A case-in-point is the Centers for Medicare and Medicaid Services' (CMS's) Readmission Reduction Program. Penalties are levied against hospitals for excessive readmissions within 30 days of discharge.[8]

THIRD-PARTY REIMBURSEMENT AND GOVERNMENT EXPENDITURES: ANOTHER STRATEGIC RELATIONSHIP

This section discusses third-party reimbursement and government expenditure relationships.

Reliance on Third-Party Reimbursement

Reliance on third-party reimbursement sets healthcare finance apart from its corporate brethren. It plays the dominant role in the configuration of finance flow in the healthcare industry. Without third-party reimbursement, inclusive of private insurance carriers, healthcare finance and the delivery system that it supports would take on a very different complexion, one that would not be sustainable.

Reimbursement Methods Have Evolved

Historically, different methods of reimbursement have had attendant risks and incentives associated with them. They have gone through an evolution of sorts, beginning with the retrospective cost-based or cost-plus method, moving on to charge-based methods (using negotiated rates that sometimes reflect discounts), and evolving into the prospective payment system that pays a predetermined, fixed amount.[9] (The retrospective system pays after the service is provided, while the prospective payment system pays before the service is provided.) These three types of reimbursement mechanisms are indicative of a fee-for-service framework.

Two additional types of reimbursement that are relevant to the interplay between health delivery systems and finance are capitation and pay-for-performance (P4P). In the former, the provider is typically paid a fixed per-member-per-month payment for each covered participant. This payment is to cover all medical services that have been contracted for the period.[10] In P4P, providers receive payment incentives when they meet specific performance measures that show they are delivering high-quality, efficient care. Thus, pay-for-performance is also referred to as value-based purchasing (VBP), in that it "...connects reimbursement to the quality of patient care rather than just the quantity of services received."[11]

Government Support in Healthcare Spending

The magnitude of government support, of which third-party reimbursement is a central feature, is illustrated by the following data. Healthcare spending in the United States grew 5.3% in 2014, reaching $3 trillion or $9,523 per person. As a share of the nation's Gross Domestic Product (GDP), health spending accounted for 17.5%, up from 17.3% in 2013.[12] See **Figure 26–4** for a visual representation of these data.

The CMS predicts annual healthcare costs will be $4.64 trillion by 2020, which would be nearly 20% of the U.S. GDP. Moreover, Medicare's major role in the health delivery system is illustrated by its accounting for 20% of total health spending in 2014, the majority of which was spent on hospital care (27%) and physician services (23%).[13] In fiscal year 2014, Medicaid accounted for 16% of national health expenditures, comprised of acute care (68.2%), long-term care (28.1%), and Disproportionate Share Hospital (DSH) payments (3.7%).[14] **Figure 26–5** illustrates these health-spending percentages.

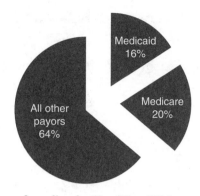

Figure 26–4 Total U.S. Healthcare Spending for Fiscal Year 2014.
Data from CMS. NHE Fact Sheet (12-03-15).

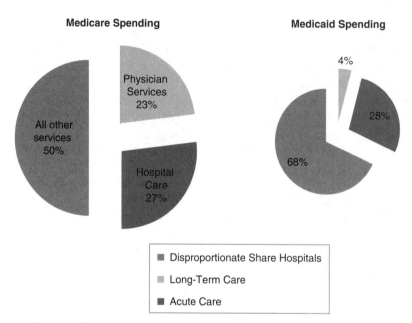

Figure 26–5 Medicare and Medicaid Spending for Fiscal Year 2014.
Data from CMS. NHE 2014 Highlights.

In the latter context, federal law requires that state Medicaid programs make DSH payments to qualifying hospitals that serve a larger number of Medicaid and uninsured individuals. Although there has been a noticeable slowing in the rate of increase in annual healthcare expenditures, the largest spending increase in 2014 was registered for prescription drugs (12.2%, compared to 2.4% growth in 2013).[15]

A NEW FOCUS ON THE RELATIONSHIP BETWEEN FINANCE AND HEALTHCARE DELIVERY

This section describes a new relationship focus.

Trending Forward Toward the Future

Medicare and Medicaid just turned 50. No statutes have had more of an impact on American health care and well-being. That said, it should be noted that the Affordable Care Act, signed into law in March 2010, created new areas of focus between the relationship of finance to delivery. It is the largest change in healthcare financing and accessibility to health care since 1965.

CMS unveiled its Accountable Care Organization (ACO) program in 2012. The ACO model stresses primary care coordination, primarily for the chronically ill, and beneficiary engagement opportunities, as well as advancing the managed care concept by rewarding providers for measurably improving care quality and efficiency rather than simply for saving money.[16] The groups of providers who are integral to ACOs come together voluntarily. Recent revisions are designed to test whether stronger incentives can improve outcomes and cut costs for Medicare beneficiaries. As of July 2015, there were over 750 ACOs.[17]

The New Finance–Delivery Link Is a Challenge

As such, this new focus on the finance–delivery link reflects the ongoing challenge for healthcare leaders to integrate clinical and business data. It's the shift to value-based care that is making this integration an imperative. An important part of this shift entails at-risk payments, such as those that characterize the aforementioned ACOs, both upside risk (sharing in savings) and downside risk (reimbursement penalties).[18] The presence of risk causes providers, such as physician organizations, to increase their dependence on analytics modules. We need to know the cost of care if we're going to be at risk.

REIMBURSEMENT AND PHYSICIANS: AN ONGOING STRATEGIC CHALLENGE

This section discusses a particularly important strategic challenge.

The Sustainable Growth Rate and Physician Reimbursement

Healthcare finance and reimbursement is anathema to many physicians. Aspects of Medicare illustrate the complexity that many physicians contend with. An ongoing feature of the program has been the Sustainable Growth Rate (SGR), which was used by CMS to control growth in Medicare physician service expenditures. Generally, this was a method to ensure that the yearly increase in expense per Medicare beneficiary did not exceed the growth in the GDP.[19]

On March 1 of each year, the physician fee schedule was updated accordingly. This has been euphemistically known as a "doc fix." Physician groups, including the AMA and the American Osteopathic Association (AOA) have lobbied for a permanent reform to the SGR so that physician payment rates are not subject to annual cuts; a permanent doc fix.

The SGR Has Been Replaced

A 1.5% or less annual update in payment rates has been common over the last 10 years.[20] Predictably, these low increases in Medicare payments have consequences: while fewer physicians may take on new Medicare patients, other physicians may withdraw entirely from the program. On April 14, 2015, Congress ended the doc fix by passing the Medicare Access and Children's Health Insurance Program (CHIP) Reauthorization Act (MACRA). This Act put an end to the SGR physician payment formula. Providers would have seen Medicare reimbursement rates drop by 21% starting on April 15, 2015, had this legislation not been enacted. The Act establishes an automatic 0.5% raise annually in provider reimbursement rates from 2015 through 2019.[21]

The New Performance-for-Payment Reimbursement Method Presents Different Physician Challenges

From 2019 on, payments to providers are adjusted based on performance under a two-part Quality Payment Program (QPP). The QPP thus includes certain payment adjustments under the Merit-Based Incentive Payment System (MIPS). The program also provides certain payment adjustments for "Advanced" Alternative Payment Model (APM) entities. What QPP underscores, potentially further vexing physicians, is CMS's objective to tie the majority of reimbursement to quality outcomes and increased beneficiary access to quality care.

The program may also present practice management challenges to providers and their business partners. For example, starting in 2019, MIPS mandates negative payment adjustments for providers who fall below certain performance thresholds. By 2022, some providers may see payments cut by up to 9%. (For more detail about QPP, see the chapter entitled "New Payment Methods and Measures: MIPS & APMs for Eligible Professionals.")

Physician Leadership Is Needed

Concurrent with the change to value-based payment and the resulting value-focused organization should be a shift in leadership roles that involves more physicians. Physicians should be employed as leaders. They have unique insight into the needs of the patient population. Their knowledge of optimal patient outcomes and how to achieve them are critical to effectively adopting to the new reimbursement climate based on value. Building an effective "Physician Enterprise" wherein new management structures are physician directed and led requires that the resulting organization be both flexible and transparent enough to achieve both cost reduction and better outcomes.[22]

In conclusion, CMS's attempt to remake the nation's heathcare finance system based upon value-based payments is a "sea change". Strategic relationships are very much affected by this sea change. Recognizing the importance of such change and how it impacts various areas of the organization is an important step in revising the strategic plan.

INFORMATION CHECKPOINT

| What is needed? | A description of your organization's health delivery system, finance department, or reimbursement division. |

Where is it found?	This information may be present on your organization's website or within a brochure prepared for the public. In the case of the health delivery system, it may even be found within a PowerPoint presentation, but be careful about proprietary use if that is the case.
How is it used?	Use will depend upon the item you find. Typically, it could be used for marketing, for training, or even for recruitment purposes.

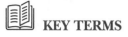

KEY TERMS

Capitation
Electronic Health Record
Finance
Gross Domestic Product
 (GDP)

Health Delivery System
Information Technology
 (IT)
Pay-for-Performance (P4P)
Reimbursement

Super Bill
Stakeholder
Sustainable Growth Rate
 (SGR)

OTHER ACRONYMS

ACO: Accountable Care Organization
AHA: American Hospital Association
AMA: American Medical Association
AOA: American Osteopathic Association
APM: Alternative Payment Model
CDC: Centers for Disease Control and Prevention
CHIP: Children's Health Insurance Program
MACRA: Medicare Access and CHIP Reauthorization Act
MIPS: Merit-Based Incentive Payment System
NIH: National Institutes of Health
OMB: Office of Management and Budget
QPP: Quality Payment Program
WHO: World Health Organization

DISCUSSION QUESTIONS

1. If you work in a healthcare organization, do you know how your finance operation is organized? Please describe.
2. Discuss the essence of the relationship between the healthcare delivery system and third-party reimbursement.
3. Do you think that the transition from fee-for-service payment to value-based payment is feasible?
4. If you work in a healthcare organization, what percentage of your revenue is derived from third-party reimbursement?

NOTES

1. F. Lega, "Organizational Design for Health Integrated Delivery Systems: Theory and Practice," *Health Policy*, 81 (2007): 258–279.

2. World Health Organization (WHO), "Health Systems Service Delivery," www.who.int /healthsystems/topics/delivery/en/, accessed December 15, 2016.

3. Note that these areas of responsibility are more fully discussed under "The Elements of Financial Management" in the introductory chapter of this text.)

4. Accounting Tools, "Chief Financial Officer (CFO) Job Description," www.accountingtools .com/job-description-cfo, accessed March 1, 2016.

5. Ibid.

6. Ibid.

7. Note: The term "reimbursement" implies that a claim is being paid, or reimbursed, for services already rendered. We now have prospective reimbursement whereby payment may be made for services that will be rendered in the future. Nevertheless, "reimbursement" is still being used as a descriptive term even though the payment method may be prospective.

8. CMS, Hospital Readmissions Reduction Program, www.medicare.gov/hospitalcompare /readmission-reduction-program.html, accessed September 17, 2016.

9. Health Care Financing & Organization (HCFO) & Robert Wood Johnson Foundation (RWJF), "Learning from Medicare: Prospective Payment," May 2011; also: CMS, "Hospital Value-Based Purchasing," www.cms.gov/Medicare /Quality-Initiatives-Patient-Assessment-Instruments/hospital-value-based-purchasing/, accessed June 28, 2016.

10. J. McCally, *Capitation for Physicians* (Chicago: Irwin Professional Publishing, 1996), 176.

11. HCFO & RWJF, "Learning from Medicare."

12. CMS, "National Health Expenditures 2014 Highlights," https://www.cms.gov/research -statistics-data-and-systems/statistics-trends-and-reports/nationalhealthexpenddata /downloads/highlights.pdf, accessed February 7, 2016.

13. Ibid.

14. Ibid.

15. Ibid.

16. H. Larkin, "ACO or No?" *Hospitals & Health Networks*, 88, no. 5 (2014): 26–31.

17. S. Shortell, "The Next Frontier: Creating Accountable Communities for Health," *Hospitals & Health Networks*, 89, no. 7 (2015): 12.

18. M. Zeis, "The Certainty of Analytics," *HealthLeaders*, 18, no. 3 (2015): 32–36.

19. CMS, "Estimated Sustainable Growth Rate and Conversion Factor, for Medicare Payments to Physicians in 2015," p. 1, www.cms.gov/medicare/medicare-fee-for-service-payment/sustainablegratesconfact/downloads/sgr2015.pdf, accessed September 17, 2016.

20. Ibid., Table 6, p. 8.

21. Medicare Access and CHIP Reauthorization Act of 2015, Pub. L. No. 114-10 (2015).

22. P. Betbeze, "Building an Effective Physician Enterprise," *HealthLeaders*, 18, no. 3 (2015): 38–42.

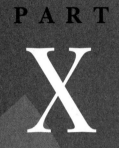

Information Technology as a Financial and Strategic Tool

Understanding Value-Based Health Care and Its Financial and Digital Outcomes

THE VALUE-BASED CONCEPT: INTRODUCTION

To many financial managers, the term "value-based" has come to mean a combination of both quality and cost. If you are shopping, whether for a box of cereal or a car, you will probably consider this combination. In the case of low-cost items, like the cereal, you might first consider quality (taste and so on) and then its cost; with larger purchases, such as a car, you may consider the cost first and then its quality. Either way, both cost and quality will usually enter into your equation.

Healthcare organizations have used a variety of methods to determine cost and to measure the quality of care delivery over the years. However, in the past few years, the concept of value-based health care has come about. A primary feature of a "value-based" approach is to recognize both quality and cost, just as you might in your personal life.

Meanwhile, in today's healthcare world, the term "value-based" actually has come to have multiple definitions. The particular definition depends upon the particular focus. For purposes of healthcare finance, value-based concepts can be, and are, applied to value-based purchasing (as with your car and the cereal), payment adjustments, pricing, strategy, and patient care. When we speak of value-based healthcare financial management, we may be referring to different aspects of all these concepts. We can even view the broad span of value-based population health and the role that financial management can play.

This chapter, therefore, addresses different facets of the value-based concept in healthcare finance and related financial management. We have divided the chapter into several parts, and each part builds upon your understanding

Progress Notes

After completing this chapter, you should be able to

1. Describe value-based progress and programs in the private and public sector.
2. Distinguish among different types of value-based education efforts.
3. Understand the basics of value-based legislative reform.
4. Describe quality measurement in the public and private sectors.
5. Recognize various possible digital outcomes.
6. Identify types of financial outcomes.
7. Describe elements of strategic planning in the public and private sectors.

of the value-based concept. The remainder of the chapter will discuss the following value-based health concepts:

- Progress in the private sector
- Progress in the public sector
- Education efforts
- Legislative reform
- Quality measurement concept
- Public reporting efforts
- Financial and digital outcomes
- Strategic planning approaches

VALUE-BASED PROGRESS IN THE PRIVATE SECTOR

Leaders in innovation within the private sector have adopted a variety of value and quality efforts. This section discusses value-based progress in implementing, research, and collaboration.

Implementing Value-Based Approaches

Two examples appear below.

An Organizational System Approach

The Mayo Clinic's "Value Creation System" and Office of Value Creation are the direct result of this improvement strategy. The Office of Value Creation was originally tasked with owning the various value-based projects. As time went on, however, responsibility and accountability for quality and value efforts shifted to operational levels. This left the Office of Value Creation available to monitor quality and value within the organization. Thus, Mayo's system has been in place long enough that progress has moved to a second, higher value-based level.[1]

A Data-Driven Approach

The Geisinger Health System has implemented an approach to health care that is data driven. As a *Wall Street Journal* article commented, Geisinger's "...decades of investment in technology and integration have made it a pioneer in the use of electronic medical records and other data."[2] And that is a true statement: Geisinger is indeed a pioneer. The system utilizes data-driven management and achieves value through standardization and care coordination.

Value-Based Research Centers

Two examples appear below.

A Center for Value-Based Care Research

The Cleveland Clinic supports its own Center for Value-Based Care Research. The Center's researchers focus on not only identifying high-value health care, but also disseminating the information obtained. That focus is reflected in the Center's mission statement: "to make quality healthcare possible for all Americans by conducting research to identify value in healthcare."[3]

A Comparative Effectiveness Research Center

The Brigham and Women's Hospital has established its own Patient-Centered Comparative Effectiveness Research Center (PCERC). As its name suggests, the Center focuses upon comparative effective research (CER) and patient-centered outcomes research (PCOR) at the hospital. This Center provides value in that it studies both the comparable effectiveness of treatment options for individual patients and the outcomes of healthcare practices. The Center's overall approach is to improve the quality of health care.[4]

Value-Based Collaboration and Affiliation

A definite effort toward both collaboration and affiliation among organizations is underway. Two examples follow.

The High Value Healthcare Collaborative

This collaboration actually began in late 2010 with four organizations: the Mayo Clinic, Denver Health, Intermountain Healthcare, and the Dartmouth Institute for Health Policy and Clinical Practice (TDI). The group wanted to achieve high value by improving health care and lowering costs. They also wanted to "move best practices out to the national provider community."[5] Since its formation, the collaborative has expanded to almost 20 health systems.

Network Affiliations

The National Comprehensive Cancer Network (NCCN) is a "not-for-profit alliance of 27 of the world's leading cancer centers devoted to patient care, research and education." The NCCN is dedicated to "improving the quality, effectiveness and efficiency of cancer care so that patients can live better lives."[6] Network membership such as this is a type of affiliation that can provide significant value-based benefits, especially in the areas of evidence-based treatment and quality of care.

VALUE-BASED PROGRESS IN THE PUBLIC SECTOR

At the time of writing, the Centers for Medicare and Medicaid Services (CMS) have a total of seven value-based programs (VBPs): Five programs are already implemented and two are in the planning and development stages. The seven programs are illustrated in **Exhibit 27–1.** These programs tie payment to value (thus "value-based"). They represent an important trend, because they are part of the movement toward paying for quality of patient care.[7]

These VBPs are important because they have aided in showing the way toward value. Their structure has provided an important foundation to build upon. In other words, they helped to make today's rapid changes possible.

Exhibit 27–1 Seven Federal Value-Based Programs

1. Hospital Value-Based Purchasing (HVBP)
2. Hospital Readmission Reduction (HRR)
3. Hospital Acquired Conditions (HAC)
4. Physician Value-Based Modifier (PVBM)
5. Skilled Nursing Facility Value-Based Program (SNFVBP)
6. Home Health Value-Based Program (HHVBP)
7. End-Stage Renal Disease (ESRD) Quality Initiative

Three Hospital Value-Based Programs

Three hospital programs are among the first value-based programs to be implemented by CMS. A brief description of each follows.

Hospital Value-Based Purchasing Program

This program provides incentive payments for acute care hospitals. The payment adjustments are based on quality of care, and are part of the Inpatient Prospective Payment System (IPPS). In other words, the hospital value-based purchasing (HVBP) program links payment to performance. The performance measures are adjusted (and typically increased) yearly. CMS has set a timeline for these adjustments that runs out to the year 2022.[8]

Hospital Readmission Reduction Program

The hospital readmission reduction (HRR) program provides incentive payments in order to reduce hospital readmissions, which are costly and may be unnecessary. Reductions may be accomplished in two ways: improving the coordination of transitions of care to other care settings and improving the quality of care provided.[9]

Hospital Acquired Conditions Program

This program works in reverse: It reduces payments instead of making incentive payments. In this case, those hospitals whose patients get the most hospital-acquired conditions are penalized. In other words, the hospitals that rank worst in hospital acquired conditions (HACs) are the ones that have their payments reduced.[10]

Four Other Value-Based Programs

These four programs cover multiple care settings, as described below.

Physician Value-Based Modifier Program

This program for physicians is also one of the original value-based programs to be implemented by CMS. The program payments began in 2015 and have been paid to ever-expanding groups of physicians over 2016 and 2017. The program expands to include other clinicians in 2018.

As the title implies, when an eligible claim is submitted, the payment is adjusted, or modified, based on particular quality and cost measures performance. In other words, when the modifier is applied to payment, it rewards both lower costs and higher quality performance. (Note that the Physician Value-Based Modifier (PVBM) Program is also known as the Value-Modifier [VM] Program.)[11]

Skilled Nursing Facility Value-Based Program

This program provides incentive payments to skilled nursing facilities (SNFs). The payments reward SNFs based on the quality of care provided. In other words, payment is received for quality of care, not quantity of care. At the time of this writing, the skilled nursing facility value-based program (SNFVBP) continues to develop. This development is expected to progress in stages.[12] However, the IMPACT Act is moving post-acute care facilities (PACs) toward standardization and interoperability. This legislation, which includes SNFs, may affect certain aspects of the SNF value-based program due to standardization efforts.

Home Health Value-Based Program

This program was first implemented on January 1, 2016, as a home health value-based program (HHVBP) model in nine states. Payment for those participating in the model is based on quality performance. In an interesting concept, the participating home health agencies (HHAs) will compete on value in order to receive quality performance incentive payments.

At the time of this writing, the HHVBP continues to develop. This development is expected to progress in stages.[13] However, as with SNFs, the HHA value-based program may be impacted by legislative efforts toward standardization and interoperability.

End-Stage Renal Disease Quality Initiative Program

The End-Stage Renal Disease (ESRD) Quality Initiative Program is a disease-specific program. It concerns outpatient dialysis or ESRD facilities , and it too was one of the original programs to be implemented by CMS. This program provides incentive payments for better quality of care, and it also reduces payments to those facilities that do not meet particular standards of performance. In other words, this program also links payment to performance.[14]

Value-Based Payments

The traditional method to pay for service delivery is by volume. Instead, CMS is now beginning to pay for value and quality. For example, CMS announced two related goals for Medicare fee-for-service payments, as follows.

Payment Goal One

"Thirty percent of Medicare payments are tied to quality or value through alternative payment models...by the end of 2016, and 50% [will be] by the end of 2018."[15] (The various types of alternative payment models are described elsewhere in this chapter.) According to CMS estimates, this aggressive 2016 timeline was actually exceeded.[16]

Payment Goal Two

Eighty-five percent of all traditional Medicare fee-for-service payments have been tied to quality or value by the end of 2016, and 90% will be by the end of 2018. This goal was accomplished through certain CMS programs, including the HVBP and the HRRP.[17] (These programs are also described elsewhere in this chapter.)

VALUE-BASED EDUCATION EFFORTS

The following examples illustrate just a few value-based education efforts. Note the digital impact of each, as all these examples are obtained online.

A Certificate in the Fundamentals of Value-Based Health Care

The Dartmouth Institute for Health Policy and Clinical Practice (TDI) offers the TDI Certificate in the Fundamentals of Value-Based Health Care. To obtain the certificate, students must take six sequential online courses that center upon understanding and navigating high-value patient-centered healthcare delivery. Value-based improvement is measured by achieving outcomes that are not only better, but are achieved with the same or lower costs. And that improvement should be "...both scientifically and ethically sound and sustainable."[18]

An Online Course That Earns Continuing Education Credit

The Center for Continuing Education at Cleveland Clinic provides online courses that earn continuing education credits for healthcare professionals. One topic provided is entitled, "Value-Based Health Care"; this particular online course is included in the Disease Management Clinical Decisions series and is in the form of an interactive case study.[19]

Education Directed to Patients and Their Families

The Patient and Family Health Education Center at Cleveland Clinic provides information on a variety of healthcare topics. One topic is "Value-Based Care." The patient-directed information includes defining value-based care and explaining how such care reduces costs.[20]

Governmental Education for Professionals

CMS provides healthcare professional education products through the Medicare Learning Network, or MLN.[21] The MLN offers a wide variety of topics, many as either electronic downloads or print versions. Some provide continuing education credits as well. At this point in time, value-based information is most commonly found within quality measurement and/or regulatory payment updates.

VALUE-BASED LEGISLATIVE REFORM

Legislation is moving toward even more value-based programs. These programs accomplish their aims through both reporting and payments.

How Value-Based Reporting and Payments Came About: The Legislative Background

The following summary of legislative progress helps you to see the step-by-step progress toward value-based reform.

Initial "Digitizing" Steps

The early efforts toward "digitizing" health care covered a period of several years. One of the more important developments during this time was requiring Medicare providers to submit their claims for payment electronically. We consider this the first real step toward "digitizing," as every Chief Financial Officer wants to get claims paid, and a the conversion to electronic claim forms was thus established throughout the country.

HITECH Legislative Funding

The Health Information Technology for Economic and Clinical Health (HITECH) Act was part of the American Recovery and Reinvestment Act that was signed into law on February 17, 2009. The HITECH Act promoted the adoption and use of health information technology (HIT) and electronic health records (EHRs) through payment incentives. CMS described these EHR Incentive Programs in a single sentence: "The Medicare and Medicaid EHR Incentive Programs provide incentive payments to eligible professionals, eligible hospitals and critical access hospitals (CAHs) as they adopt, implement, upgrade or demonstrate meaningful use of certified EHR technology."[22]

The HITECH Act's legislative funding provided approximately $17 billion in incentives for hospitals and physicians. This law will impact future healthcare information management for many years to come (up to 2021 in the case of one program).

Value-Based Legislative Reform: The MACRA Act

A further legislative reform to the Medicare payment structure is now in place through the Medicare Access and CHIP Reauthorization Act of 2015 (MACRA). This Act is briefly described below. Note that the Act ends a method of payment to physicians that has been in place since the beginning of the Medicare program in the 1960s. This is truly a reform.

More Value-Based Legislative Reform: The IMPACT Act

Yet another legislative reform is now in place through the Improving Medicare Post-Acute Care Transformation (IMPACT) Act of 2014. This Act is also briefly described below. Note that, for the first time, interoperability will be required between and among the four types of post-acute facilities. This is another true reform.

Quick Facts About Physicians and the MACRA Act, MIPS, and APMs

MACRA reforms Medicare payments to physicians and certain clinicians via the following:

- Repealing the Sustainable Growth Rate (SCR) method of payment
- Replacing the SGR method with a new payment framework that emphasizes "giving better care, not just more care"
- Combining existing quality reporting programs into the single new payment framework.[23]

For the first two years, the individuals affected by the MACRA Act include physicians, physician assistants, nurse practitioners, clinical nurse specialists, and certified registered nurse anesthetists. Groups that include these eligible professionals are also included. In a second phase (from the third year onward), the Secretary can add more eligible professionals such as social workers, certified audiologists, and others.

The MACRA reforms help CMS to move toward the value-based goal of paying for both value and for better care. Physicians and other eligible professionals (EPs) can choose one of two quality programs: either the Merit-Based Incentive Payment System (MIPS) or the Alternative Payment Models (APMs). Both MIPS and APMs will go into effect over a period from mid-2015 through 2021 and beyond.[24]

What Is MIPS?

This new value-based program combines certain parts of existing quality reporting programs. The programs involved include certain sections of the Physician Quality Reporting System (PQRS), the Value Modifier (VM; also known as the Value-based Payment Modifier), and the Medicare Electronic Health Record (EHR) incentive program. (These stand-alone programs will be sunsetted, or ended, when they are combined into the new value-based program.)

Physicians and other eligible professionals will be measured in four areas. These performance areas include quality, resource use, meaningful use of certified EHR technology, and clinical practice improvement. (The first three areas come from the existing quality reporting programs, but the clinical practice improvement area is new.)

The MIPS payment method includes an automatic base increase for the period 2015 through 2019, followed by an additional increase applied from 2026 onward. These EPs are also at risk for positive or negative performance adjustments to their payments beginning in 2019.

What Are APMs?

APMs provide new methods of payment from Medicare to physicians and other eligible professionals. The MACRA Act considers the following entities to be APMs that are generally eligible for incentive payments:

- CMS Innovation Center Models
- Shared Savings Program Tracks
- Certain statutorily required demonstrations[25]

Specific types of entities within these general categories are then set out annually in a rule published by CMS. These "Advanced APMs" are considered to be advanced because they accept financial risk along with rewards (the rewards being the incentive payments).

The APM payment methods include a lump-sum incentive payment for some participating providers for the period 2019 to 2024. In addition, beginning in 2026, some providers can receive higher annual payments. In the future we can expect increased transparency of such physician-focused payment models (PFPMs). We can also anticipate the development of additional PFPMs as time goes on.

Other Provisions of the Act

Other provisions of the Act are detailed elsewhere, as the additional provisions are beyond the scope of this particular chapter.

Meaningful Use Is Not Dead, But Is Evolving

Meaningful use still exists. At a healthcare conference in the spring of 2016, CMS acting Administrator, Andy Slavitt, said that "the meaningful use program, as it has existed, will now be effectively over and will be replaced with something better."[26] However, various media sources reported only that meaningful use was dead, which is incorrect.[27] What Slavitt meant was that meaningful use is being incorporated into the MACRA Act's programs. Thus, meaningful use still exists, but its role has evolved. To see more about how this change has come about, see Appendix 28-A.

Quick Facts About Post-Acute Care and the IMPACT Act

The IMPACT Act of 2014 requires that standardized patient assessment data be reported by four types of post-acute care facilities, including SNFs, HHAs, inpatient rehabilitation facilities (IRFs), and long-term care hospitals (LTCHs). Note that hospice, another type of post-acute care facility, is not included in these requirements.

Data Interoperability

The Act specifies that "certain data elements must be standardized and interoperable to allow for the exchange and use of data among these PAC and other providers."[28] This will facilitate coordinated care and will "improve the long-term outcomes of beneficiaries receiving post-acute services across different care settings."[29] (Standardized data ensure that wording is comparable for purposes of assessment and scoring. Interoperability makes transmitting data across different systems possible.)

Transparency and Public Reporting

Transparency and public reporting is another important element in the IMPACT Act. The Act stipulates that there must be public reporting of PAC provider performance on both value-based aspects: quality measures and resource use.[30]

Other Provisions of the Act

Other provisions of the Act are detailed elsewhere. However, note that the Act also provided funding for much greater specificity in the reporting of nurse staffing.

QUALITY MEASUREMENT: THE CONCEPT

As one of the two foundations of value-based care, quality must be able to be studied and quantified. (The other value-based foundation is cost.) Note that types of quality measures can vary, as discussed within this section. Also note that developing quality measures is not just the first step in the process, but is an ongoing project. We hope that, in the future, public/private alignment will become commonplace.

Quality Measures in the Private Sector

This section discusses measures use linked to payment in a large alternative payment model and quality measures as used by an accrediting organization.

The California-Based Integrated Healthcare Association

The integrated healthcare association (IHA), working with health plans and physician organizations, launched a statewide pay-for-performance initiative over 15 years ago. This alternative payment model is based upon four elements, including "a common set of measures and benchmarks, health plan incentive payments, public reporting and public recognition awards."[31]

The IHA Value-Based Pay-for-Performance (P4P) program measures quality, cost, and resource use. The program's common measure set is evidence based and includes four major elements:

- Clinical quality
- Patient experience
- Meaningful use of HIT
- Resource use and total cost of care

To put the size of this program into perspective, participation in the Value-Based P4P includes "10 health plans and 200 California physician organizations with 35,000 physicians caring for

9 million Californians enrolled in commercial health maintenance organization (HMO) and point of service (POS) products."[32]

The National Committee for Quality Assurance

The National Committee for Quality Assurance (NCQA) is a private 501(c)3 not-for-profit organization that accredits health plans and that provides annual statistics about the quality of care delivered by these plans. The Committee has developed quality standards and performance measures for an array of healthcare organizations.

According to the NCQA website:

- Health plans earning NCQA accreditation at the present time must address an array of more than 60 standards, and reports on their performance are required in over 40 areas.
- Health plans are accredited in every state, the District of Columbia and Puerto Rico.
- These plans cover 109 million Americans.
- That figure accounts for 70.5% of all Americans in health plans.[33]

Quality Measures in the Public Sector

Value and quality are often intertwined when discussing value-based efforts. Certain quality measures have already been established for specific providers. These measures must first be recorded by the provider and then transmitted as appropriate. Within the public sector, CMS has a number of such quality reporting programs in place as follows.

Quality Reporting Programs

Examples of CMS Quality Reporting Programs are listed below. Note that additional programs may be developed in the near future. It is also expected that existing programs will be revised and refined, also in the near future.

Existing programs at the time of this writing include the following:

- Hospital Inpatient Quality Reporting (HIQR) Program
- Hospital Outpatient Quality Reporting (HOQR) Program
- Physician Quality Reporting System (PQRS)
- Long-Term Care Hospital (LTCH) Quality Reporting Program (QRP)
- Inpatient Rehabilitation Facility (IRF) Quality Reporting Program (QRP)
- Home Health Quality Reporting Program (HHQRP)
- Hospice Quality Reporting Program (HQRP).[34]

We understand that upgrading efforts are ongoing for these reporting programs. Such upgrades include greater transparency and ease of access.

Challenges in Quality Measure Implementation

The staff at CMS has identified a number of challenges that may occur in quality measure implementation from their viewpoint. This useful list of challenges can be divided into three segments as follows:

Issues related to patients and providers
  Engaging patients in the measure development process
  Reducing provider burden

Issues related to shortening and streamlining processes
  Shortening the period for measure development
  Streamlining data acquisition for measure testing

Issues related to development
  Developing meaningful outcome measures
  Developing patient-reported outcome measures (PROMS) and appropriate use measures
  Developing measures that promote shared accountability across settings and providers[35]

Challenges for the Manager

We cannot deny that challenges to quality measure implementation exist. The manager must deal with a whole variety of management issues related to these measures. The manager faces problems and challenges in both the development and implementation of quality measures. By their very nature such measures are metrics, and metrics must involve digital changes. Examples of the problems involved for the manager include the following:

- Hardware issues
- Software issues
- Training
- Staff stability and related turnover
- Uniform reporting during digital changes

To succeed, managers involved in measure development and implementation need support from the highest levels within the organization. This support must include funding for both required digital infrastructure and related staffing.

VALUE-BASED PUBLIC REPORTING IN THE PRIVATE SECTOR

Sharing information about quality reporting programs with the public is another important method of supporting value-based efforts. In this section, we discuss three different types of value-based public reporting.

Public Reporting by Providers and Health Plans

Two types of reporting about value-based efforts are described below. There are, of course, a number of other existing examples.

Annual Reporting of Program Results

The California-based Integrated Healthcare Association (IHA), in association with the California Office of the Patient Advocate (OPA), publicly reports value-based pay-for-performance results each year. These reports allow comparison between and among various health plans and providers. The intent is to "allow health care purchasers and consumers to make informed decisions about providers based on value."[36] Other reporting efforts by this partnership include reports on total cost of care performance by physician organizations and the Medical Group Medicare Report Card for "medical groups caring for seniors and people with disabilities enrolled in Medicare Advantage health plans."[37] In addition, each year the IHA also recognizes top-performing and most-improved physician organizations. Another IHA public recognition effort is the Excellence in Healthcare Award.[38]

An Overview of Annual Facts and Statistics

This type of report is typically an overview. The website containing the overview then allows the viewer to go to specific information about items of interest, including value-based efforts for the particular year. For example, Cleveland Clinic publishes an annual year-end "Facts + Figures" report. The two-page report provides a snapshot of the organization. Included, for our purposes, besides Mission, Vision, and Values, is a section titled "Quality, Safety, Transparency." This section mentions Quality and Patient Safety accountability that oversees improvement in quality and safety, all data driven. It also mentions "relentless focus on monitoring, recording and reporting quality and safety data."[39]

Public Reporting of Quality and Value by Other Organizations

A variety of other organizations also provide public reporting of quality and associated value. They include, among others, the National Quality Forum, the National Committee for Quality Assurance, the Leapfrog Group for Patient Safety, the Informed Patient Institute, and the Commonwealth Fund.[40]

Public Reporting of Physician Credentials and Experience

Another type of public reporting that websites provide is background information on physician groups and on individual doctors. To experiment, we typed our own GP's name into Google and seven websites came up that contained his credentials and experience.

These sites provide a type of value-based information, in that they can readily tell you, the consumer, important facts about the healthcare professional. Most sites contain information about specialties, experience, and credentials. You can find whether the physician has any sanctions, malpractice suits, or board actions against him or her. The site may also provide the results of patient satisfaction surveys or reviews, and possibly a comparative rating.

VALUE-BASED PUBLIC REPORTING IN THE PUBLIC SECTOR

This type of public reporting provides another layer of value by disseminating value-based information to interested parties. Within this section, we describe both national and state reporting examples as follows.

National Reporting Examples

Value-based quality measurement can be readily linked to public reporting. You may be familiar with one of the CMS "Compare" websites that publishes these quality measures. A brief description of four "Compare" sites follows.

Hospital Compare

The Hospital Compare website contains information about quality of care for over 4,000 hospitals in the United States.[41] The site contains a profile of each hospital. Besides general facility information and certain other measures that are reported, the particular measure of interest to us is "Payment and Value of Care."[42] This value-based measure is in three parts: "Medicare spending per beneficiary," "Payment measures," and "Value of care." The "Value of care" part is a combination of payment measures and quality-of-care measures.[43]

Physician Compare

At the time of writing, group practices are present on the "Physician Compare" CMS website. There are plans to add individual physicians and other healthcare professionals in the future. Also note that the site only includes those who are enrolled in the Medicare program.[44] The site contains a profile of each physician, including specialties, board certification, medical school and residency, and other information.[45]

The particular item of interest to us concerns participation in quality activities. If the physician or group practice participates in one or more of four quality activities, there is a green check mark on the profile page. (The site is careful to say, however, that "participation alone does not mean quality care has been achieved. Showing a commitment to quality is the first step in achieving quality care.")[46]

Nursing Home Compare

According to CMS, the Nursing Home Compare website contains information about both quality of care and staffing for all 15,000-plus nursing homes in the United States that are Medicare and Medicaid participating.[47] The site provides a five-star quality rating that covers quality measures, staffing, and health inspections. Each of these three elements is given an individual rating, and the three ratings are then combined to create an overall rating. The star rating is on a scale of 1 to 5, with 1 being the lowest and 5 being the highest score.[48] (The site does point out that there can be variation among states as to the inspection process and as to Medicaid program differences. Thus, it is best to compare facilities within a single state.)[49]

Home Health Compare

The Home Health Compare website contains information about the quality of care that is provided by home health agencies throughout the United States that are Medicare certified.[50] The site contains a profile of each agency, including type of ownership and services offered. The particular items of interest to us include information about quality measures, plus a "quality of patient care star rating."[51] The star rating is on a scale of 1 to 5, with 1 being the lowest and 5 being the highest score. Scores are based upon how the performance of a particular home health agency compares to that of other agencies.[52]

A State Reporting Example

According to an article in *Health Affairs*, just about one-half of the states in the United States have created some type of public reporting program.[53] As you might suspect, the content of these programs varies state by state. We provide one example, as follows.

The Utah Department of Health provides a Public Health Outcome Measures Report (PHOM). The report includes 109 public health measures in an online format that is easy to use. In this case, the purpose of public reporting is to "promote an understanding of the health status of the Utah population."[54] These measures, or indicators, are taken from another of Utah's websites, "Indicator-Based Information System for Public Health (IBIS-PH)," which contains even more detail.

FINANCIAL OUTCOMES

This section discusses several types of value-based financial outcomes.

A Financial Outcome Example

Intermountain Health (IH) provides an example of documented positive financial outcomes as follows. Intermountain Health is a Utah-based not-for-profit health system with 22 hospitals and 185 clinics in the Intermountain Medical Group, along with health insurance plans from SelectHealth. (Although it is not relevant to the example, IH is a pioneer in the use of telemedicine.) Intermountain piloted an integration of mental health with primary care a number of years ago. Every primary care patient at the Intermountain Medical Group clinics receives this screening, whether or not they are members of Intermountain's health plan. This value-based coordinated care model has improved outcomes for patients. Furthermore, Intermountain's financial outcomes are positive. Specifically, while costs per member are $22 higher up front, per-member costs are $115 lower overall annually. The annual reduced cost is due to fewer emergency room visits and other care.[55]

An Overview of Financial Outcomes as a Value-Based Business Model

The *Harvard Business Review* has published an article entitled "Turning Value-Based Health Care into a Real Business Model."[56] The authors begin by saying the shift from volume-based health care to value-based health care is inevitable. (We agree with this view.) While they discuss benefits in patient care, they also point out that sometimes short-term financial losses may be part of this shift to a value-based approach. In some cases, of course, the short-term loss may be offset by a long-term gain. The Intermountain example above is one of those cases.

The authors conclude that organizations' short-term financial losses were strategic. The benefits of these value-based strategic decisions include, for example, risk-management experience. Risk management is an integral part of many pay-for-performance alternative payment models, and gaining such experience would be valuable. Relationship building is another strategic benefit. Collaboration and alignment with stakeholders and physicians takes time and becomes even more important in moving toward a population-health approach. There is also a competitive advantage. In other words, in this value-based business model, each organization will gain competitively in the long run. This is because it will have already embraced and adapted to a value-based financial approach (the business model) while other organizations who have not done so will be left behind.

Large Interactive Systems Require Investment Dollars

Because of their size, large healthcare systems need large electronic health record systems. It follows that these large electronic systems require a substantial investment. In this section, we discuss two examples of such investments, both of which can be considered value-based financial outcomes.

Duke University Health System's Investment

North Carolina–based Duke University Health System (Duke) includes three hospitals along with physician practices, home care, hospice care, and support services.[57] In July 2012, Duke began a multi-year information systems project to unify electronic medical records across the health system. The new technology was to be implemented in three phases, from mid-2012 to spring 2014.[58] The project stayed on schedule; as of spring 2014, the system was operational in all three hospitals and 223 outpatient facilities.[59]

The investment in this project was widely reported to be $500 million. However, when the Duke Chief Medical Information Officer discussed related financial issues in a newspaper interview, he acknowledged $500 million as the gross cost, but also said the net cost was estimated at approximately $300 million, as follows.

He explained that the $500 million figure represented total ownership costs over a seven-year period. This amount included, therefore, the cost to maintain and upgrade the system over seven years, in addition to the initial costs to acquire and begin to use the technology. He also explained that the $500 million was the gross investment figure. If you add up all the costs to maintain and to support the 135 applications that are being replaced, and if you then subtract that cost from the $500 million, you wind up with a net new investment that is "a little bit more than $300 million."[60] Finally, he also pointed out that the project should be eligible to receive tens of millions of dollars in federal funding" that would help to partially cover costs of the investment.[61]

Kaiser Permanente's Investment

California-based Kaiser Permanente (KP) is a non-profit integrated health plan that includes 38 hospitals and over 600 medical office buildings and other facilities that are located in eight states plus the District of Columbia. The plan serves almost 10 million people.[62]

Kaiser Permanente claims that HealthConnect, the plan's comprehensive electronic record, is "one of the largest private electronic health systems in the world."[63] It took 10 years to build and became fully operational in 2010.[64]

InfoWorld interviewed Philip Fasano, the Chief Information Officer of KP, about the plan's EHR systems. The interviewer asked how much it cost to build the system, to which Fasano replied, "about $4 billion, a substantial amount of money, but we have 9 million members [so it costs about $444 per member]."[65] (Note that the interview occurred three years prior to the time of this writing, so the member count is different.) The CIO went on to make another important point: that it is necessary to continuously invest in the system during its lifetime.

DIGITAL OUTCOMES

This section discusses value-based digital outcomes that are important for physicians and for large healthcare systems.

How Would Digital Outcomes Benefit a Physician's Practice?

Value-based alternative payment models rely upon an array of performance measures that are reported electronically. The electronic submissions represent the record of the provider's performance. Thus, appropriate data collection and submission represents the positive digital outcome that should result in payment advantages.

For example, physicians and other eligible professionals are in the midst of transition to value-based payment models due to MACRA. This transition relies heavily upon electronic submission of performance data, which provides certain benefits. Specifically, the physicians who use certified EHRs and/or qualified clinical data registries (QCDRs) should benefit in two ways:

- Reduce data collection and the associated reporting burden
- Support timely performance

Figure 27–1 illustrates these points.

What Are Value-Based Digital Outcome Examples in Large Healthcare Systems?

This section provides outcome examples for two large systems.

Duke University Health System

Duke University Health System's (Duke's) information system project cost has been discussed in the preceding investment section. In this section, we discuss the project's digital outcomes.

The information system project's purpose was to unify electronic medical records across the system. It accomplished this purpose. Value-based outcomes include medical record access that is both seamless and in real time. Medical information can now be exchanged across all care settings. As the Duke press release states, quality, safety, speed, and efficiency have all been improved with implementation of the new system. In addition, 130 old clinical information systems became obsolete and were eliminated when the new system went online.[66]

The patient experience has been improved via the system's new online tool, "Duke MyChart." The patient can, among other features, view and/or request appointments, view their medical reports, request prescription refills, and send messages to healthcare providers.[67]

Finally, the organization's commitment to the project is underscored by another statistic. Duke provided 173,000 hours of training to faculty and staff in order to ensure a smooth transition. And it worked, too; the press release says neither patient care nor patient billing was significantly disrupted during the implementation process of this value-based system.[68]

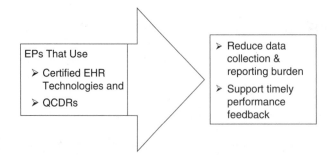

Figure 27–1 MACRA Electronic Specifications Provide Benefits.

Kaiser Permanente

The cost of KP's "HealthConnect" project has been discussed in the preceding investment section. In this section we discuss the digital outcomes for the entire KP online system. Note that KP covers the spectrum of care, as it is both a health plan (payer) and a provider of care. KP also has amassed a huge amount of electronic data that are being used for value-based purposes.

For example, HealthConnect is part of KP's online portal called "My Health Manager." This portal allows patients online access to such features as appointment scheduling, refills of prescriptions, messages to care providers, and so on. However, another valuable feature, called the online Patient Action Plan (oPAP), is also available. This web-based system concerns preventive care that is personalized for the individual patient in a health action plan. Researchers who studied the use of this patient-enabled health management tool found improved patient outcomes for preventive care.[69]

Clinicians also benefit from KP HealthConnect features. They have access to information about latest treatments and preventive care, and that access is already proving valuable. For example, in one pilot project, this access to information helped physicians to reduce coronary artery disease death by 76%.[70]

Another Outcome: Electronic Transmission Standards Must Be Updated and Maintained

Electronic transmission standards are important because they directly impact providers, health plans, and other stakeholders. These standards are coordinated with and are the beginning point for certified EHR technology. Both financial and digital outcomes depend upon such technology. Specific versions of the standards are acceptable for certified EHR technology at different points in time. As such, it is imperative that the related standards are updated and maintained at all times.

VALUE-BASED STRATEGIC PLANNING BY THE PRIVATE SECTOR

Leaders in the private sector already have their value-based strategic planning underway. We provide some examples of such planning within this section. Note that while there may be different approaches, the value-based aims are similar.

Recognizing That Value-Based Care Is a Long-Term Goal

The Cleveland Clinic has integrated the value-based concept throughout its organization, including research, education, and care delivery. Dr. Tony Cosgrove, President and CEO of Cleveland Clinic, has written in a blog that value-based health care is a "breakthrough that will change the face of medicine" and that " whether providers like it or not, healthcare is evolving from a proficiency-based art to a data-driven science."[71] Finally, one of the Cleveland Clinic's web pages summarizes the organization's strategic positioning: "[T]he ideal result is fewer readmissions, less frequent hospitalization and trips to the ER. Value-based care is a long-term goal."[72]

Taking a Patient-Centered View of Value

At the Mayo Clinic, it seems obvious that the Office of Value Creation must play an important role in value-based strategic planning. However, this Office does not operate within a silo. One of the "Quality at Mayo Clinic Update: How the Mayo Value Creation System Is Improving Patient Care" publications a few years ago makes this clear.

It says the organization, at that time, was working to define value, and the Office of Value Creation, the Value Program in the Center for the Science of Healthcare Delivery, Government Affairs, and Contracting were all working together toward this effort. Strategically speaking, "at this point, we are trying to take a patient-centered view of value at the levels of the care pyramid."[73] (And their concept at that point in time was a care "pyramid" consisting of complex care, intermediate care, and population health, with value definitions and detail for each level.) There is no doubt that this strategic approach has further evolved over time.

Focusing Upon Population Health as a Value-Based Strategy

Dartmouth-Hitchcock describes a focus upon population health that is strategic. This organization believes in the achievement of a sustainable health system. To quote one comment, "we believe the focus of organizations such as D-H should no longer be just on treating illness. We have an obligation to ensure health."[74]

Dartmouth-Hitchcock is a leader in value-based alternative-payment models that are risk based. This organization clearly believes that the incentives under such models will "move to keeping defined populations health as a way of controlling costs. Defined populations under new payment models are those 'attributed' to us because we are the entity responsible for their health and health care costs."[75]

VALUE-BASED STRATEGIC PLANNING BY THE PUBLIC SECTOR

A "national quality strategy" exists and this strategy guides planning throughout the U.S. Department of Health and Human Services (DHHS). The value-based and quality programs that are discussed within this chapter are an important part of CMS planning. Thus, because CMS is a part of DHHS, these value-based and quality issues are tied into national quality strategy as well. This section illustrates how CMS has fit its quality strategy goals into the national quality priorities.

National Quality Strategy

The National Quality Strategy (NQS) is led by the Agency for Healthcare Research and Quality (AHRQ) on behalf of the U.S. DHHS.[76] The NQS structure is summarized below.

Three Aims and Six Priorities

To summarize, the NQS is structured with three aims and six priorities. The three overarching aims are as follows:

- Better care
- Healthy people/healthy communities
- Affordable care[77]

Details about the six priorities for NQS are discussed in the following section, especially as to how they interrelate to the CMS quality strategy.

Nine Strategic Levers

The NQS also created nine "levers." Used in this sense, the term "levers" may be core business functions, resources, and/or actions, any of which may be activated in order to align to the quality strategy. These strategic alignment elements are as follows:

- Measurement and feedback
- Payment
- Health information technology
- Innovation and diffusion
- Public reporting
- Learning and technical assistance
- Certification, accreditation, and regulation
- Consumer incentives and benefit designs
- Workforce development

The strategic levers are also summarized in **Exhibit 27–2**.

The Agency has included a phrase for each lever, as follows, to better describe how the levers work should work. **Table 27–1** illustrates the appropriate phrase for each of the nine levers.[78]

Why Are the NQS Levers Important?

The levers are important because they show how all aspects of value-based and quality programs fit into the national strategic plan. We can recognize one or more of these nine levers in each of the private and public sector value-based efforts that are discussed within this chapter.

How Do CMS Quality Strategy and Goals Fit into the National Strategy?

CMS quality strategy coordinates with the national quality strategy's priorities. In other words, the CMS strategy fits into the national strategy because CMS has adopted the NQS priorities as the six CMS goals. A description of this sequence follows.

National Quality Strategy Priorities Are Converted into Domains

In order to implement these priorities, they are converted into domains. Six domains represent the priorities of the NQS. These domains, as described in the CMS Quality Strategy, are as follows:[79]

- Efficiency and Cost Reduction Domain
- Care Coordination Domain

Exhibit 27–2 Nine Strategic Levers

Nine levers that can be activated for strategic alignment:

1. Measurement & feedback
2. Payment
3. Health information technology
4. Innovation & diffusion
5. Public reporting
6. Learning & technical assistance
7. Certification, accreditation, & regulation
8. Consumer incentives & benefit designs
9. Workforce development

Table 27–1 How the Strategic Levers Should Work

The Lever	How It Should Work
Measurement and Feedback	Provide performance feedback to plans and providers to improve care
Payment	Reward and incentivize providers to deliver high-quality, patient-centered care
Health Information Technology	Improve communication, transparency, and efficiency for better coordinated health and health care
Innovation and Diffusion	Foster innovation in healthcare quality improvement and facilitate rapid adoption within and across organizations and communities
Public Reporting	Compare treatment results, costs, and patient experience for consumers
Learning and Technical Assistance	Foster learning environments that offer training, resources, tools, and guidance to help organizations achieve quality improvement goals
Certification, Accreditation, and Regulation	Adopt or adhere to approaches to meet safety and quality standards
Consumer Incentives and Benefit Designs	Help consumers adopt health behaviors and make informed decisions
Workforce Development	Investing in people to prepare the next generation of healthcare professionals and support lifelong learning for providers

Reproduced from The National Quality Strategy: Fact Sheet, AHRQ Publication No. 14-M006-EF, www.ahrq.gov/workingforquality/nqs/nqsfactsheet.htm

- Clinical Quality of Care Domain
- Safety Domain
- Person and Caregiver Centered Experience and Outcomes Domain
- Population and Community Health Domain

Detail for each of these domains is contained in **Table 27–2**.

Strategic Goals for Quality

This section discusses various national and agency aspects of strategic goals.

Linking National and CMS Strategies

To take this coordination a step further, CMS has adopted the domains just described as its "framework for measurement." This methodology is important because it links NQS strategy—and resulting domains—directly and efficiently to CMS strategic goals and their measurement. Thus, each National Quality Priority Domain as just described is linked to a specific CMS Quality Strategy Goal. In other words, six national domains equal six CMS goals. Details for each of these CMS goals are contained in **Table 27–3**.

Table 27–2 National Quality Strategy Priorities Are Converted to Domains

National Priority Domains	Details
Efficiency & Cost Reduction	Cost Efficiency Appropriateness
Care Coordination	Patient and family activation Infrastructure and processes for care coordination Impact of care coordination
Clinical Quality of Care	Care type (preventive, acute, post-acute, chronic) Conditions Subpopulations
Safety	All-cause harm HACs HAIs Unnecessary care Medication safety
Person and Caregiver Centered Experience and Outcomes	Patient experience Caregiver experience Preference and goal-oriented care
Population and Community Health	Health behaviors Access Physical and social environment Health status

Table 27–3 National Quality Strategy Domains Are Linked to CMS Quality Strategy Goals

National Priority Domains	CMS Goals
Efficiency & Cost Reduction	Make care affordable
Care Coordination	Promote effective communication & coordination of care
Clinical Quality of Care	Promote effective prevention & treatment of chronic disease
Safety	Make care safer by reducing harm caused while care is delivered
Person and Caregiver Centered Experience and Outcomes	Help patients & their families be involved as partners in their care
Population and Community Health	Work with communities to help people live healthily

More About CMS Strategic Quality Measure Development

This chapter provides an overview of NQS Priorities and Domains. The national priorities are converted into six national domains (see Table 27–2). This chapter also shows how these domains can then be linked to CMS goals (see Table 27–3). (Note that CMS goals are part of CMS's own quality strategy.) (Also note that Exhibits 27–1 and Table 27–1 in this chapter address another aspect of strategic planning. These two exhibits describe "levers" that can be activated to better achieve important strategic alignment.)

CONCLUSION: THE FUTURE

This section contains a brief look into the future.

Required Implementation Changes Still to Come

Future legislative and regulatory changes will certainly occur. Some are predictable at this time, while others are not. At the time of writing, for example, we cannot reasonably predict the direction that multiple value-based alternative payment models may take. Likewise, we cannot predict the outcome over the next few years of the current multiple challenges to other aspects of healthcare legislation.

Leadership: The Essential Ingredient

One thing is clear, however. If an organization is to meet its value-based goals, leadership support and encouragement is essential. This quote sums it up very well: "[T]he investment required is as much in leadership as in dollars."[80]

The "Glide Path"

In conclusion, we expect interpretations of the various value-based and health information technology strategic priorities, along with their supporting rules and regulations, to emerge over a considerable period of years. A formidable base of knowledge has been laid as a foundation for these directions. One official, who must have had an aviation background, was reported to have said we were now on the "glide path" to success in the area of health information technology, meaning that the sailing (or flying) would be smooth from now on. We hope he was correct.

INFORMATION CHECKPOINT

What is needed?	A descriptive document about value-based health care.
Where is it found?	In the planning office or in the financial division; possibly on the organization's website. (But be careful not to borrow proprietary information that belongs to the organization.)
How is it used?	Its use depends upon the item you have found. Potential uses include strategic planning or an analysis of potential financial impacts. Other uses could be for informational or educational purposes.

📖 **KEY TERMS**

Alternative Payment Model (APM)

Electronic Health Record (EHR)

Eligible Professional (EP)

IMPACT Act

MACRA

Meaningful Use (MU)

Merit-Based Incentive Payment System (MIPS)

Value-Based Program (VBP)

Value Modifier (VM)

OTHER ACRONYMS

ESRD-QIP: End-Stage Renal Disease Quality Initiative Program
HAC: Hospital Acquired Conditions Program
HIQRP: Hospital Inpatient Quality Reporting Program
HHQRP: Home Health Quality Reporting Program
HHVBP: Home Health Value-Based Program
HOQR: Hospital Outpatient Quality Reporting Program
HQRP: Hospice Quality Reporting Program
HRR: Hospital Readmission Reduction Program
HVBP: Hospital Value-Based Purchasing Program
IRF-QRP: Inpatient Rehabilitation Facility Quality Reporting Program
LTCH-QRP: Long-Term Care Hospital Quality Reporting Program
PQRS: Physician Quality Reporting System
PVBM: Physician Value-Based Modified Program
SNFVBP: Skilled Nursing Facility Value-Based Program

📋 **DISCUSSION QUESTIONS**

1. Using your organization as a point-of-reference, how would you define "value-based care"?
2. If senior management appointed you to chair a committee to adopt such a concept, whom would you include?
3. How would you describe a patient-centered view of value?
4. Identify the essential elements of a National Quality Strategy. Describe how they are interrelated.
5. Describe the recent key elements to legislative reform of the Medicare payment structure.
6. Why are value-based digital outcomes important for healthcare providers?

NOTES

1. Mayo Clinic, "Quality at Mayo Clinic: 2013 Update: How the Mayo Value Creation System Is Improving Patient Care," publication # MC6312-33rev0413, www.mayo.edu/pmts/mc6300-mc6399/mc6312-33.pdf, accessed April 14, 2016.

2. C. Weaver, "A Health-Care Model in Coal Country," *The Wall Street Journal*, September 27, 2015.

3. Cleveland Clinic, "Center for Value-Based Care Research," https://my.clevelandclinic .org/services/medicine-institute/research/Center-for-Value-Based-Care-Research, accessed April 14, 2016.

4. Brigham and Women's Hospital, "Patient-Centered Comparative Effectiveness Research Center," www.brighamandwomens.org/research/centers/pcerc/default.aspx, accessed April 14, 2016.

5. Dartmouth-Hitchcock, "Our Collaborations," www.dartmouth-hitchcock.org/about _dh/what_is_population_health.html, accessed April 14, 2016.

6. National Comprehensive Cancer Network, "About NCCN," www.nccn.org/about /default.aspx, accessed April 14, 2016.

7. Centers for Medicare and Medicaid Services [CMS], "CMS' Value-Based Programs," https://www.cms.gov/Medicare/Quality-Initiatives-Patient-Assessment-Instruments /Value-Based-Programs/Value-Based-Programs.html

8. CMS, "Hospital Value-Based Purchasing," last modified October 30, 2015, https://www .cms.gov/Medicare/Quality-Initiatives-Patient-Assessment-Instruments/hospital-value -based-purchasing/index.html?redirect=/Hospital-Value-Based-Purchasing/

9. CMS, "Readmissions Reduction Program (HRRP)," last modified April 18, 2016, https://www.cms.gov/medicare/medicare-fee-for-service-payment/acuteinpatientpps /readmissions-reduction-program.html

10. CMS, "Hospital-Acquired Condition (HAC) Reduction Program," www.cms.gov/Medicare /Quality-Initiatives-Patient-Assessment-Instruments/Value-Based-Programs/HAC /Hospital-Acquired-Conditions

11. CMS, "The Value Modifier (VM) Program," https://www.cms.gov/Medicare/Quality -Initiatives-Patient-Assessment-Instruments/Value-Based-Programs/VMP/Value -Modifier-VM-or-PVBM.html

12. CMS, "The Skilled Nursing Facility Value-Based Purchasing Program (SNFVBP)," https://www.cms.gov/Medicare/Quality-Initiatives-Patient-Assessment-Instruments /Value-Based-Programs/Other-VBPs/SNF-VBP.html

13. CMS, "The Home Health Value-Based Purchasing (HHVBP) Model," https://www .cms.gov/Medicare/Quality-Initiatives-Patient-Assessment-Instruments/Value-Based -Programs/Other-VBPs/HHVBP.html

14. CMS, "End-Stage Renal Disease (ESRD) Quality Incentive Program (QIP)," https:// www.cms.gov/Medicare/Quality-Initiatives-Patient-Assessment-Instruments/Value -Based-Programs/Other-VBPs/ESRD-QIP.html

15. CMS, "What Are the Value-Based Programs?" www.cms.gov/Medicare/Quality -Initiatives-Patient-Assessment-Instruments/Value-Based-Programs/MACRA-MIPS -and-APMs

16. U.S. Department of Health and Human Services, "HHS Reaches Goal of Tying 30 Percent of Medicare Payments to Quality Ahead of Schedule, March 2016, www.hhs.gov /about/news/2016/03/03/hhs-reaches-goal-tying-30-percent-medicare-payments-quality -ahead-schedule.html

17. Ibid.

18. The Dartmouth Institute, "The TDI Certificate in the Fundamentals of Value-Based Health Care," accessed April 14, 2016, www.tdiprofessionaleducation.org/tdi-certificate -program.html

19. Cleveland Clinic Center for Continuing Education, "Disease Management Clinical Decisions: Value-Based Health Care," www.clevelandclinicmeded.com/online/casebased/decisionmaking/value-based-care, accessed April 14, 2016.

20. Cleveland Clinic Patient and Family Health Education Center, "Diseases and Conditions: Value-Based Care," https://my.clevelandclinic.org/health/diseases_conditions/hic-value-based-care, accessed April 14, 2016.

21. MLN Homepage, Centers for Medicare and Medicaid Services, www.cms.gov/outreach-and-education/medicare-learning-network-min/mingeninfo/index.html, accessed September 17, 2016.

22. CMS, "EHR Incentive Programs: Getting Started," www.cms.gov/Regulations-and-Guidance/Legislation/EHRIncentivePrograms/Getting-Started.html

23. CMS, "What Are the Value-Based Programs?"

24. Ibid.

25. P.L. 114-10 (April 16, 2015) 129 STAT 121

26. B. Ahier, "Meaningful Use Isn't Quite Dead Yet," March 1, 2016, www.healthdata management.com/opinion/meaningful-use-isnt-quite-dead-yet

27. Ibid.

28. CMS, "IMPACT Act Spotlights and Announcements," last modified August 31, 2016, https://www.cms.gov/Medicare/Quality-Initiatives-Patient-Assessment-Instruments/Post-Acute-Care-Quality-Initiatives/IMPACT-Act-of-2014/Spotlights-and-Announcements-.html

29. Ibid.

30. P.L. 113-185 Sec. 2(g)(1) (October 6, 2014).

31. Integrated Healthcare Association, "Fact Sheet: Value Based Pay for Performance in California," September 2015, www.iha.org/sites/default/files/resources/vbp4-fact-sheet-final-20150925.pdf

32. Ibid.

33. National Committee for Quality Assurance, "About NCQA," www.ncqa.org/about-ncqa, accessed May 18, 2016.

34. 80 Federal Register (FR) 22067 (April 20, 2015).

35. Adapted from CMS, "CMS Quality Measure Development Plan (MDP)," December 18, 2015, page 8.

36. Integrated Healthcare Association, "Fact Sheet: Total Cost of Care," April 2015, www.iha.org/sites/default/files/resources/fact-sheet-total-cost-of-care-2015.pdf

37. Integrated Healthcare Association, "Results and Public Reporting," accessed May 9, 2016, www.iha.org/our-work/accountability/value-based-p4p/results-public-reporting

38. Integrated Healthcare Association, "Fact Sheet: Total Cost of Care."

39. Cleveland Clinic, "Facts + Figures: 2015 Year-End," updated March 16, 2016, https://newsroom.clevelandclinic.org/wp-content/uploads/sites/4/2016/4/16-CCC-332-Facts-and-Figures_04.01.2016.pdf

40. Health Affairs, "Health Policy Briefs: Public Reporting on Quality and Costs," March 8, 2012, www.healthaffairs.org/healthpolicybriefs/brief.php?brief_id=65

41. Medicare.gov, "What is Hospital Compare?" www.medicare.gov/hospitalcompare/About/What-Is-HOS.html, accessed May 10, 2016.

42. Medicare.gov, "What Information Can I Get About Hospitals?" www.medicare.gov/hospitalcompare/About/Hospital-Info.html, accessed May 10, 2016.

43. Ibid.

44. Medicare.gov, "About Physician Compare," www.medicare.gov/physiciancompare /staticpages/aboutphysiciancompare/about.html, accessed May 10, 2016.

45. Medicare.gov, "Information Available on Physician Compare," www.medicare.gov /physiciancompare/staticpages/aboutphysiciancompare/informationavailable, accessed May 10, 2016.

46. Medicare.gov, "About the Data," www.medicare.gov/physiciancompare/staticpages/data /aboutthedata.html, accessed May 10, 2016.

47. Medicare.gov, "What is Nursing Home Compare?" www.medicare.gov/nursinghomecompare /About/What-Is-NHC.html, accessed May 10, 2016.

48. Medicare.gov, "What are the 5-Star Quality Ratings?" www.medicare.gov/Nursing HomeCompare/About/Ratings.html, accessed May 10, 2016.

49. Medicare.gov, "Strengths and Limitations," www.medicare.gov/NursingHomeCompare /About/Strengths-and-Limitations.html, accessed May 10, 2016.

50. Medicare.gov, "What is Home Health Compare?" www.medicare.gov/homehealthcompare /About/What-Is-HHC.html, accessed May 10, 2016.

51. Medicare.gov, "What Information Can I Get About Home Health Agencies?" www.medicare .gov/HomeHealthCompare/About/What-Information-Is-Available.html, accessed May 10, 2016.

52. Medicare.gov, "Quality of Patient Care Star Ratings," www.medicare.gov /HomeHealthCompare/About/Patient-Care-Star-Ratings.html, accessed May 10, 2016.

53. Health Affairs, "Health Policy Briefs: Public Reporting on Quality and Costs," www.healthaffairs.org/healthpolicybriefs/brief.php?brief_id=65, accessed March 8, 2012.

54. Utah Department of Health, "Public Health Outcome Measures Report," April 2014, http://ibis.health.utah.gov/phom/Introduction.html

55. L. S. Kaiser and T. H. Lee, "Turning Value-Based Health Care into a Real Business Model," *Harvard Business Review,* October 8, 2015, https://hbr.org/2015/10/turning -value-based-health-care-into-a-real-business-model

56. Ibid.

57. Duke University Health System, "Duke Human Resources: About Duke University Health System," https://www.hr.duke.edu/jobs/duke_durham/duhs.php, accessed May 10, 2016.

58. Duke University Health System, "Duke Starts to Transfer to Digital Electronic Health Records," www.wral.com/lifestyles/goaskmom/blogpost/11364264/?comment_order =forward, accessed September 17, 2016.

59. Duke University Health System, "Duke Medicine Completes Implementation of Electronic Health Records Across All Outpatient Facilities and Duke University Hospital," http:// corporate.dukemedicine.org/news_and_publications/news_office/news/duke-medicine -completes-implementation-of-electronic-health-records-across-all-outpatient-facilities -and-duke-university-hospital/view, accessed May 18, 2016.

60. D. Ranii, "Duke Kicks Off Digital Health Records Plan," www.ecu.edu/cs-admin/news /clips/upload/071812.pdf, accessed September 17, 2016.

61. Ibid.

62. Kaiser Permanente, "Who We Are," www.kaiserpermanentejobs.org/who-we-are.aspx, accessed May 19, 2016.

63. Kaiser Permanente, "About Us: Connectivity," https://share.kaiserpermanente.org /total-health/connectivity/, accessed May 19, 2016.

64. InfoWorld, "How Kaiser Bet $4 Billion On Electronic Health Records—And Won," May 2, 2013, http://www.infoworld.com/article/2614353/ehr/how-kaiser-bet–4-billion-on -electronic-health-records—and-won.html

65. Ibid.

66. Duke University Health System, "Duke Medicine Completes Implementation."

67. Duke University Health System, "Duke's New Medical Records System Improves Patient Experience," http://corporate.dukemedicine.org/news_and_publications/news _office/news/duke-s-new-medical-records-system-improves-patient-abilities-and-access -to-providers, accessed May 19, 2016.

68. Duke University Health System, "Duke Medicine Completes Implementation."

69. Kaiser Permanente, "Patient Access to Online Health Action Plans Enhances Rate of Preventive Care," https://share.kaiserpermanente.org/article/patient-access-to-online -health-action-plans-enhances-rate-of-preventive-care/, accessed May 19, 2016.

70. Kaiser Permanente, "About Us: Connectivity."

71. Z. Budryk, "How Value-Based Care Will Change Healthcare," September 26, 2013, http://www.fiercehealthcare.com/healthcare/how-value-based-care-will-change -healthcare/

72. Cleveland Clinic, "Diseases and Conditions: Value-Based Care."

73. Mayo Clinic, "Quality at Mayo Clinic."

74. Dartmouth-Hitchcock, "What Is Population Health?" www.dartmouth-hitchcock.org /about_dh/what_is_population_health.html, accessed April 14, 2016.

75. Ibid.

76. U.S. Department of Health and Human Services, "The National Quality Strategy: Fact Sheet," last updated September 2014, www.ahrq.gov/workingforquality/nqs /nqsfactsheet.htm

77. Ibid.

78. Ibid.

79. 80 FR 68667 (November 5, 2015).

80. L. S. Kaiser and T. H. Lee, "Turning Value-Based Health Care into a Real Business Model."

CHAPTER

New Payment Methods and Measures: MIPS and APMs for Eligible Professionals

28

INTRODUCTION

This chapter explores how new payment methods and quality measures work for physicians and other eligible professionals. The chapter has several parts, as follows, and each part contributes to an understanding of the choices among MIPS, APMs, and the related measures that determine their payment. Chapter parts include the following:

- Overview of MACRA and the payment choices that must be made
- Choice #1 is for MIPS incentives: how this choice is structured, who is eligible for MIPS, and facts about payment and reporting
- Details of the MIPS scoring process and how the scores become payment adjustments for the individual practitioner
- Details about the MIPS performance categories, how the related quality measures are created, and their timelines
- Choice #2 is for APM incentives: how this choice is structured, the various APM models, and facts about payment and reporting
- Details about the Advanced APM participation requirements and scoring standards

In conclusion, two reference sections are included: one for the three incentive programs as they existed before MIPS and one for existing alternative payment models.

This chapter should be read in conjunction with the preceding chapter, "Understanding Value-Based Health Care and Its Financial and Digital Outcomes." While this chapter describes how MIPS and APMs work, the preceding chapter provides a view of the healthcare industry's overall

Progress Notes

After completing this chapter, you should be able to

1. Distinguish between the two pay-for-performance choices in the Quality Payment Program.
2. Recognize the three existing incentive programs that were combined into MIPS.
3. Identify the four MIPS performance categories.
4. Describe how the MIPS Composite Performance Score uses weighted averages.
5. Identify the Advanced APM "significant participation" requirements.
6. Understand the Scoring Standards for APMs.
7. Discuss the framework for MACRA Quality Measurement.

value-based effort, along with the legislative sequence that came before the MACRA requirements. (See the section entitled "Value-Based Legislative Reform" in the preceding chapter.)

LEGISLATIVE REFORM AND MACRA: AN OVERVIEW

This section provides an overview of legislative reform as it pertains to MACRA.

The Legislative Act

The Medicare Access and CHIP Reauthorization Act of 2015 (MACRA) was signed into law on April 16, 2015. The law is grouped into categories, and each category is identified by a title number and heading. This chapter concerns new pay-for-performance incentives (MIPS and APMs) for physicians and other eligible professionals, which is located under Title I.[1]

The Repeal of SGR

Repeal of the Sustainable Growth Rate, or SGR, is a true legislative reform. The short history of SGR that follows explains why reform was necessary.

The SGR was a formula used to calculate Medicare payments to physicians. Each year, the formula compared increases or decreases in physician spending to increases or decreases in the gross domestic product (GDP). If the GDP increase exceeded the increase in physician spending, then the physicians' base rate payment amount would increase. However, if the physicians' spending increase exceeded the increase in the GDP, then the physicians' base rate payment amount would decrease.

An abbreviated SGR timeline looks like this:

1997: The SGR formula came into existence.
2002: The formula results in a 4.8% cut in the Medicare base payment rate (a wake-up call).
2003: A law blocking the formula's cuts was passed.
2004–2005: Congress passes annual "fixes" that disregard the formula's cuts.
2006: Another law was passed that made the annual cuts cumulative.
2009–2010: Congress passes annual "fixes" that disregard the cumulative cuts.
2015: The SGR formula is repealed by law.[2]

The problem with cumulative annual cuts is the resulting excessive reduction in base payment rates. This meant, for example, if last year's blocked cut was 4% and this year's cut was 5%, then the pay cut would now amount to a cumulative total cut of 9%, and so on, year after year.

Basically, at this point the SGR formula was broken. It was not sustainable. And to repeal it and replace the long-standing SGR formula with an entirely different approach to physician payment, as MACRA does, is true legislative reform.

New Pay-for-Performance Incentives (MIPS and APMs)

MACRA provides new physician pay-for-performance incentives that replace the repealed SGR formula. There are two methods, or types, of participation. The first type of participation is in the new Merit-Based Incentive Payment System, or MIPS. The second type allows incentive payments when requirements are met to be a qualifying participant in an Advanced Alternative Payment Model (APM).[3] The two payment methods and their related performance measures and/or requirements are described in the following sections of this chapter.

Other Provisions of the Act

As previously explained, subjects covered by this law are grouped into categories, and each category is identified by a title number and heading. Four other categories, and titles, are included in the Act. Title II concerns "extenders"; in other words, a series of programs and other funding efforts receive an extension within this title. Title III concerns an extension, or reauthorization, of the Children's Health Insurance Program (CHIP). (You will notice that CHIP is in the title of the law.) Title IV concerns offsets; these include certain limitations, updates and adjustments. The final Title V is labelled as "miscellaneous" and covers an array of other various subjects.[4]

PAYMENT CHOICES: MIPS VERSUS APMs

MACRA provides for two value-based pay-for-performance initiatives: MIPS and APMs. The new name for this overall payment approach is the Quality Payment Program. In other words, the Quality Payment Program includes both MIPS and APM types of incentive payments. Because MACRA provides two choices for payment, eligible professionals must generally opt for one or the other of these choices. **Figure 28–1** illustrates the two choices. Note that the start date ("Year 1") for both MIPS and APM incentive payments is 2019.

MIPS INCENTIVES

This section describes the MIPS payment structure and those eligible professionals who may be included and/or excluded from this initiative.

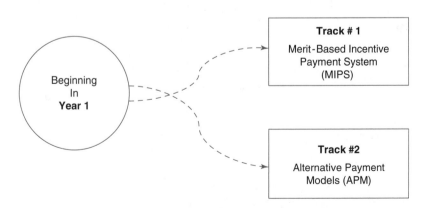

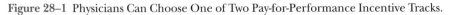

Figure 28–1 Physicians Can Choose One of Two Pay-for-Performance Incentive Tracks.

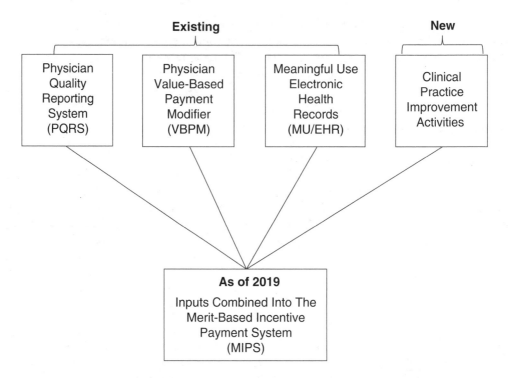

Figure 28–2 Four Pay-for-Performance Inputs Are Combined into MIPS.

MIPS Payment Structure

The MIPS payment structure consists of modified inputs from three existing programs, plus one new category. The three existing incentive programs whose modified measures are combined into MIPS inputs are described below. The fourth, new MIPS category is called Clinical Practice Improvement Activities. It is further described later in this chapter. **Figure 28–2** illustrates the four elements that provide inputs for the MIPS payment structure as of 2019.

Three Existing Incentive Programs Are Combined into MIPS

Many modified features of three existing incentive programs are combined into MIPS. They include the: Physician Quality Reporting System (PQRS) program, the Value Modifier program, and the Meaningful Use and Electronic Health Records Initiative.

These Three Programs End as Stand-Alones as MIPS Begins

At the time of this writing, payments will end in 2018 for these three programs. In other words, these programs became obsolete because the new Quality Payment Program (including both MIPS and APMs) takes over. **Figure 28–3** illustrates the changeover.

The payment penalties associated with the three existing incentive programs will also disappear as features of the programs are rolled into the MIPS payment structure. **Figure 28–4** illustrates the dissolution of such penalties.

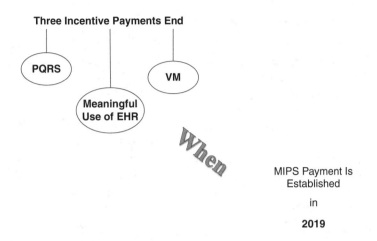

Figure 28–3 Three Incentive Program Payments End as MIPS Is Established in 2019.

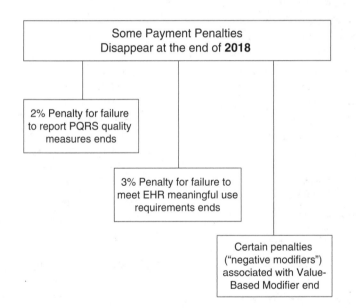

Figure 28–4 Some Payment Penalties Disappear at the End of 2018.

Eligible Professionals for MIPS

This section describes both eligible professionals included and excluded from MIPS as follows. Note that the Centers for Medicare and Medicaid Services (CMS) have chosen to use the term "eligible clinicians" instead of "eligible professionals." The description below uses the legislative term "eligible professionals."

Eligible Professionals Categories Subject to MIPS Will Increase

Five categories of eligible professionals (EPs) are subject to MIPS for the first two payment years. As of the third year, however, the Secretary has the right to add other types of eligible professionals, and eight more professional categories have been suggested for addition in the third year. **Exhibit 28–1** lists the five EPs types included in years one and two, plus the eight types that have been suggested beginning in year three.

Who May Be Excluded from MIPS?

As discussed previously, physicians and certain other eligible professionals have a choice between two payment methods; either MIPS or APMs. Therefore, certain eligible professionals who chose the APM methods may also be excluded from MIPS. In addition, some professionals will fall below the low-volume threshold and will be excluded. (The low-volume threshold is discussed in more detail in a following section of this chapter.) Finally, an eligible professional who is in the first year of participation in Medicare may be excluded from MIPS. **Exhibit 28–2** illustrates some reasons for exclusion.

HOW ARE MIPS PHYSICIANS AND OTHER ELIGIBLE PROFESSIONALS PAID?

This section summarizes performance scores and payment adjustments.

EPs Are Scored on Performance

Eligible professionals for MIPS are scored on performance. Their performance will be rated on a scale that ranges from maximum positive to neutral to maximum negative.

Summary of MIPS Payment Adjustments and Their Timelines

MIPS EPs receive an automatic base increase of 0.5% from 2015 through 2019. At the time

Exhibit 28–1 MIPS Eligible Professionals Inclusion Varies by Timeline

---

Definitely Included

For Years One & Two (2019 & 2020)*

- Physician
- Physician assistant
- Nurse practitioner
- Clinical nurse specialist
- Certified registered nurse anesthetist
- Groups that include such professionals

Possibly Included

From the third year onward (2021)*

- The Secretary can add other EPs such as:
- Physical therapists
- Occupational therapists
- Certified audiologists
- Clinical psychologists
- Speech-language pathologists
- Clinical social workers
- Nurse midwives
- Dietitians or nutrition professionals

*Timeline may change
SSA Section 1848 (g)(1)(c)(i)

Exhibit 28–2 Professionals Who May Be Excluded from MIPS

An eligible professional may be excluded from MIPS if he or she:

- Is a qualifying APM participant
- Is a partial-qualifying APM participant
- Is below the low-volume threshold for the performance period
- Is in the first year of Medicare participation

SSA Section 1848 (g)(1)(c)(ii)

MIPS Payment Adjustment Timelines							
MIPS	2015–2018*	2019	2020	2021	2022–2024	2025	2026 & Onward
(1) Automatic** Base Increase	0.5%	0.5%	0.0%	0.0%	0.0%	0.0%	0.25%
PLUS (2) Three Levels of Performance Adjustments at **RISK**							
Maximum Positive Adjustment***		+4%	+5%	+7%	+9%	+9%	
Neutral Adjustment		0.0%	0.0%	0.0%	0.0%	0.0%	
Maximum Negative Adjustment***		–4%	–5%	–7%	–9%	–9%	

*Note: PQRS, VM, and EHR remain in effect for the period 2015 to 2018.
**Automatic annual base conversion factor increase of 0.5% also in effect for period 2015–2018.
***Annual totals must be budget neutral.

Figure 28–5 MIPS Payment Adjustments and Timelines.
Modified from CMS, "Path to Value: The Medicare Access & CHIP Reauthorization Act of 2015," p. 9 and p. 18.

of this writing there is zero automatic base increase from 2020 through 2025, with a 0.25% increase applied from 2026 onward.

These EPs are then at risk for performance adjustments to their payments beginning in 2019. These payments are budget neutral. That means the total dollars paid out to successful providers will equal total dollars that reduce payments to unsuccessful providers. Thus, the budget neutral payments range from 4% maximum and minimum in 2019 increasingly upward to 9% maximum and minimum in 2025. The payment percentage amounts by year are illustrated in **Figure 28–5**.

MACRA also allows an extra bonus for exceptional performance. The bonus amount of $500 million dollars is exempt from budget neutrality and can be paid out over the first five years of the program. Participants become eligible for the bonus based on increases in their MIPS performance scores. (The scoring increase for exceptional performance is topped at an additional 10%.)[5]

MIPS COMPOSITE PERFORMANCE SCORE

This section provides an overview of the MIPS composite performance score.

Payment Adjustment Is Determined by Four Performance Categories Within the Composite Performance Score

The MIPS composite performance score (CPS) consists of four parts. Each part is a separate performance category within the composite score. (Note that some of their descriptive titles have changed, as indicated.)

- Quality
- Advancing Care Information (*a.k.a. Meaningful Use of Electronic Health Records*)
- Clinical Practice Improvement Activities
- Cost (*a.k.a. Resource Use*)

Each part (category) of the score is discussed in more detail in the following sections.

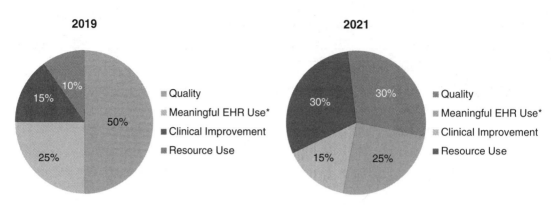

Figure 28–6 Weighted Averages for the MIPS Score Measures as Initially Proposed.
*As modified: now known as "Advancing Care Information"

The payment adjustment illustrated in Figure 28–5 begins with the clinician's (or group's) CPS. The CPS is a unified scoring system that converts measures and/or activities into points, allows partial credit, and provides advance information about what is needed for top-performance scoring.

MIPS Scoring Uses Weighted Averages

MIPS scoring uses weighted averages within the CPS that will change the performance categories weighting from year to year. **Figure 28–6** illustrates these changes. The figure shows how the distribution of weighted averages may shift from 2019 to 2021. In other words, the two years in this illustration show a different set of weighted averages among the four categories.

MIPS PERFORMANCE CATEGORIES

Each performance category is made up of a series of individual measures. The clinician chooses, within limits, which measures to report within each category. A brief summary about each category follows. The four categories are also illustrated in **Figure 28–7**.

Quality

This category contains streamlined measures from the PQRS and the Quality portion of the Value Modifier (VM) program. Required reporting for this category consists of six measures, rather than the nine measures previously required by PQRS. There is also more emphasis on outcome measurement. The Year 1 proposed weight of 50% subsequently became 60%.

As initially proposed, the eligible clinicians (EPs) or groups are allowed to choose the six measures that best reflect their practice. There are certain limitations to this choice. Of the six, one has to be either an outcome or a high-quality measure, and another has to be a crosscutting measure. (A crosscutting measure is one that can be applied across a number of providers and/or specialties; thus, these measures "cut across.") There is another available choice for specialists: they can choose a set of measures related to their particular specialty.[6]

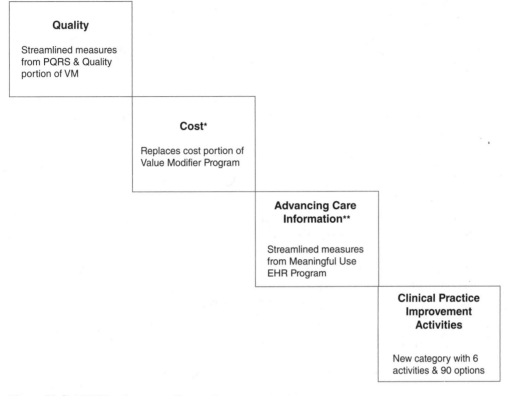

Quality

Streamlined measures from PQRS & Quality portion of VM

Cost*

Replaces cost portion of Value Modifier Program

Advancing Care Information**

Streamlined measures from Meaningful Use EHR Program

Clinical Practice Improvement Activities

New category with 6 activities & 90 options

Figure 28–7 MIPS Performance Categories.

*Cost a.k.a. Resource Use

**Advancing Care Information a.k.a. Meaningful Use

Advancing Care Information (also known as Meaningful Use of Electronic Health Records)

Meaningful use has gained a new name: Advancing Care Information (ACI). The ACI measures, originally derived from the Meaningful Use EHR program, have been modified and streamlined for use within MIPS. Quarterly reporting has been eliminated, as has the "all-or-nothing" threshold measurement of electronic health record (EHR) technology. Redundant measures and two objectives have been eliminated to reduce the reporting burden. The Year 1 weight is 25%.

For purposes of MIPS reporting, eligible clinicians or groups can choose measures that are most important within their practice. These customized choices will represent key measures of interoperability and information exchange. Flexible scoring has been implemented for all measures. The flexibility will help to promote care coordination. Thus better care coordination should result in better patient outcomes.[7]

Clinical Practice Improvement Activities (CPIA)

The new Clinical Practice Improvement performance category contains six types of activities proposed for Year 1:

- Expanded Practice Access
- Population Management

- Care Coordination
- Beneficiary Engagement
- Patient Safety and Practice Access
- Participation in an APM

The Year 1 weight is 15%.

The CMS proposed rule sets out measures of more than 90 activities within this category. Eligible clinicians or groups can choose six measures among these that best reflect goals for the practice. (At least one activity must be chosen in order to avoid a zero score.)[8]

Cost (also known as Resource Use)

The cost category will assess all the applicable resource use measures that are applicable to the particular clinician or group. This category replaces the cost portion of the Value Modifier program. Over 40 episode-specific measures have been added in order to address specialty concerns. Year 1 weight proposed at 10% subsequently became zero.

The eligible clinician or group does not have to report measures for this category. Instead, CMS performs the calculation. To do so, CMS will compare resource use across practices that involve similar care episodes and similar clinical condition groups.[9]

HOW MIPS SCORING WORKS

The clinician's (or group's) chosen measures, as reported, are accumulated into annual totals. The clinician's totals from each category's measures as reported are converted into points.

How Do Points Earned Become Percentage Scores?

The next step is for points earned to become percentage scores. You will recall that there are weighted averages within the composite performance score. Figure 28–6 illustrates these weights for both 2019, which is Year 1 for the Quality Payment Program and MIPS, and for 2021.

Accordingly, the Year 1 maximum score possible for each performance category will equal that category's weight within the overall score (the Composite Performance Score). The Year 1 maximum percentage scores are therefore proposed as follows:

Quality = 50%, subsequently changed to 60%.
Advancing Care Information = 25%
Clinical Practice Improvement Activities = 15%
Cost = 10%, subsequently changed to zero.

(Note that these percentages are as shown in Figure 28–6.)

Points are turned into percentage scores in this manner. First, the clinician earns points by reporting his or her chosen measures for the first three performance categories listed previously. (You will recall that the "Cost" category does not require the reporting of measures because it is calculated by CMS from claims and volume information.)

There are a certain number of points needed to reach the maximum score for each of the first three performance categories listed above. An example follows.

Table 28–1 MIPS Scoring by Performance Category: An Example

MIPS Performance Category	Maximum Possible Score (stated as a percentage)	Total Points Needed to Reach the Maximum Score
Quality	50	80 to 90*
Advancing Care Information (a.k.a. Meaningful Use)	25	100
Clinical Practice Improvement Activities	15	60
Cost (a.k.a. Resource Use)	10	CMS calculates average score of all resource measures that can be attributed

*Depending on group size.
Modified from CMS Quality Program Executive Summary Table 1, p. 10 (May 2016).

Quality = 80 to 90 points (depending on group size)
Advancing Care Information = 100 points
Clinical Practice Improvement Activities = 60 points

Table 28–1 illustrates the Year 1 proposed percentages and total points as just discussed.

Dr. Brown's Scores: An Example

The points earned by an individual (or a group) are mathematically converted into the relevant percentage. For example, Dr. Brown's practice earns all 60 points in the Clinical Practice Improvement Activities category, so that portion of his weighted composite performance score will be the full 15%. But due to office staff errors, some measures for the Advancing Care Information (a.k.a. Meaningful Use) category were not properly reported for part of the performance period. As a result, Dr. Brown's practice only earned 50 points, or one-half, of the 100 points that are needed in order to reach the maximum score. Therefore, his percentage score for this category will be 12.5%, or one-half of the 25% maximum possible score. (Refer to the left-hand column in Table 28–1 to further understand the maximum possible scores as expressed in percentages.) All told, Dr. Brown's four performance category percentage scores looked like this:

Quality = 37.5%
Advancing Care Information = 12.5%
Clinical Practice Improvement Activities = 15.0%
Cost = 8.0%

The four performance category composite scores would then be converted into a total composite score using the weighted averages as shown in Figure 28–6. How Dr. Brown's scores affect his payment adjustment is the subject of the next section.

How Do Scores Become Payment Adjustments?

This section discusses the overall process of computing scores and converting them into payment adjustments.

Measures Are Submitted During the Performance Period

First, the physician (or group) records and submits selected measures during the performance period. (We have already discussed how each practice can choose measures to report within the four performance categories. More detail about performance periods appears in a following section.) After all these data are collected, properly reported measures are analyzed and outcomes are calculated. The resulting computations are then converted into scores and the scores, in turn, are converted into payment adjustments. An overview of this process follows. (While the following section provides a general descriptive overview, the actual computations are quite sophisticated and are beyond the scope of this text.)

Five Steps from Measures to MIPS Payment Adjustment

This section provides a general overview of five steps that would generally convert submitted measures into MIPS payment adjustments. For purposes of our description, we will assume that Analyst Jane works for CMS and is going to perform all five steps. (This is not realistic, of course, as individual teams of analysts would be segmenting the process into individual team responsibilities.) We will also assume that Dr. Brown's individual composite score is the end result of this example.

Step 1: First, Analyst Jane and her team will analyze the submitted measures from all over the country. These represent measures for the Quality, Advancing Care Information, and Clinical Practice Improvement Activities performance categories as submitted during the performance period. The national analysis will, of course, include Dr. Brown's submitted measures for the performance period. (The team will also compute relevant benchmarks for comparative purposes.)

Step 2: Analyst Jane and her team will compute costs and certain other outcomes from CMS data sources. These calculated outcomes primarily represent the Resource Use (Cost) performance category. (Note that some of these computations may be based on the prior year's data rather than performance period data.)

Step 3: Analyst Jane and her team will have already standardized the data from the four performance categories and will have performed a series of statistical analyses. Now they compute the national means and medians. They divide the results of this analysis into quartiles. Using the quartile results, they apply standard deviation computations to divide their analysis into three national tiers. The three tiers are labelled as high, average, and low.

Step 4: Next, Analyst Jane does two things. First, she finds the individual physician or group's composite, or multiple-part, performance score. In our example, that would be Dr. Brown's composite performance score. Then, she assigns the doctor's score to one of the three national tiers. The doctor's score will thus fall into a high, average, or low tier.

Step 5: Now that Analyst Jane knows which tier Dr. Brown's score is in, she will compute the doctor's payment adjustment. (Her computation must also take budget neutrality into account.) This payment adjustment will have one of three possible outcomes: it will result in a positive, neutral, or negative payment adjustment for Dr. Brown.[10]

Figure 28–8 illustrates the five-step process just described. Note that this process would be repeated each time a performance period ends. (Note also that the exact process will probably be modified over time.)

At the time of this writing we understand that first, an eligible MIPS participant should be able to view preliminary results, and second, that there may be certain appeal rights established.

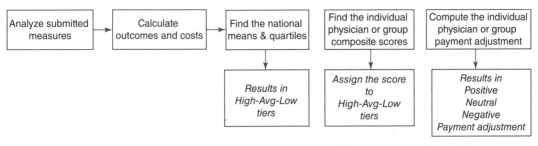

Figure 28–8 How MIPS Scoring Works: An Overview.

MIPS REQUIRED REPORTING AFFECTS PAYMENT

This section discusses required reporting and the related performance periods.

Required Reporting

Reporting on required measures is important because the reported measures directly impact future payment adjustment amounts. Complete reporting—that is, reporting on every measure that is has been previously selected—is necessary in order for the measures to be recognized when they are submitted. In other words, an incomplete set of measures may not be counted. Accuracy in recording is equally important, of course.

What Is a Performance Period?

A performance period is a designated time span that is used to capture data. The data that are captured measure how well that facility or professional or group is performing. At the time of this writing, for example, the MIPS program performance period covers a one-year period, and that period is a calendar year.[11]

How Does Performance Period Reporting Affect Payments?

This section discusses the reporting and scoring timeline along with feedback opportunities.

Timeline

The measures reported during a performance period are analyzed to help determine a payment adjustment that is based on quality and value performance. CMS has provided an example of the timeline for the first performance period under MIPS as follows.

The first MIPS performance period, for example, is calendar year 2017. CMS uses the following year (2018 in this example) for analysis and scoring of the data collected in the prior year. Then the next year (2019 in this example) is when the first MIPS payment adjustments are made. In other words, the performance period reporting made two years ago directly affects the payment adjustments received in a current year.[12]

Feedback

CMS is expected to provide feedback to the physicians and groups who are MIPS participants. At the time of this writing, the first feedback was anticipated in the middle of the performance period year. (This would give an opportunity for adjustments to the participant's reporting process.) The second feedback was then anticipated in the middle of the analysis-and-scoring year (the year in between the performance period and the payment-adjustment year).

Sunsetting Existing Programs

In discussing timelines, it is important to understand that previously existing incentive programs remain in existence for the period 2015 through 2018. During that four-year period, providers are still being paid under these programs. (The three programs include the PQRS, the Value-Modifier, and the Meaningful Use of EHR.)

DATA SUBMISSION

This section describes the allowable options proposed for submitting required data.

Individual Reporting

Individuals can choose among various options for data submission. The four performance categories differ somewhat in available options. These differences are described as follows.

Quality Performance Category Options

Data submission choices include submission through EHRs or through a Qualified Registry or Qualified Clinical Data Registry (QCDR). Claims submitted by providers are also part of quality data submission, as are administrative claims. ("Administrative claims" means CMS will perform any needed computations, and no special submission is required from the participant.)

Advancing Care Information (ACI) Performance Category Options

Submission choices for ACI include through EHRs, a Qualified Registry, or a QCDR. Attestation is another available choice for this category. Administrative claims are also part of the process, but, again, no special submission is required.

Clinical Practice Improvement Activities (CPIA) Options

Submission choices for CPIA also include through EHRs, a Qualified Registry, a QCDR, or through attestation. Once again, administrative claims are part of the process but no action is required on the part of the participant.

Resource Use (Cost) Performance Category Options

The Resource Use category entirely uses the administrative claims computation process, so no action at all is required by the participant.[13]

Group Reporting

Groups have a couple of additional options. In the case of the Quality Performance category, groups may also choose the CAHPS for MIPS Survey option. Groups of 25 or more may use the CMS Web Interface when submitting data for the Quality, ACI, and CPIA categories.[14]

Reporting by Intermediaries

CMS has proposed to allow certain intermediaries to submit performance category data on behalf of eligible clinicians. At the time of this writing, the allowable intermediaries include health information technology (HIT) vendors who obtain their data from the eligible clinicians' certified EHR technology, CMS-approved (certified) survey vendors, Qualified Registries and QCDRs.[15]

APM INCENTIVES—(CHOICE #2)

These alternative payment models, or APMs, represent innovations in how to compensate physicians and other eligible professionals.

Advanced APMs According to MACRA

MACRA considers the following to be Advanced APMs:

- CMS Innovation Center Models under section 1115A (other than a healthcare innovation award)
- The Shared Savings Program
- A demonstration under section 1866C
- Demonstrations required by Federal law

These APMs are considered "advanced" because the participants accept risks along with rewards (the rewards being the incentive payments). To be eligible for such payment, particular criteria about EHR usage and reporting of quality measures must be met.[16]

Eligible Advanced APMs Proposed for Year 1

CMS proposes specific criteria for Advanced APMs through rulemaking. These criteria fit within MACRA's description of entities as listed above. At the time of writing, the eligible Advanced APMs proposed for Year 1 are as follows:

- Comprehensive Primary Care Plus (CPC+)
- Medical Shares Savings Programs—Tracks 2 and 3
- Next Generation ACO Model
- Comprehensive End-Stage Renal Disease Care (CEC) Model
- Oncology Care Model

It is important to note that the Comprehensive End-Stage Renal Disease Care Model is a large dialysis organization arrangement. Likewise, the Oncology Care Model is a two-sided risk arrangement. **Figure 28–9** summarizes these models. It is also important to note that some changes to the types of Year 1 proposed models may occur before actual implementation.

The eligibility for Advanced APMs will be reviewed annually. Thus, while these models are proposed for Year 1, we are still at the beginning of this transition to value-based performance payment models. As such, we can expect a series of modifications, expansions, and revisions as time goes on. We can therefore expect that the choices among future multiple payment approaches will increase. We can also expect increased transparency through public reporting as these models develop and mature.[17]

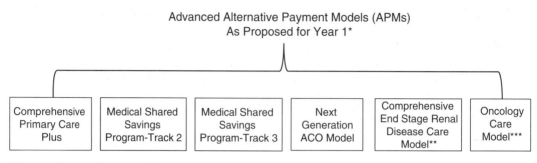

*Other models may subsequently be included.
**A large dialysis organization arrangement.
***A two-sided risk arrangement.

Figure 28–9 Advanced Alternative Payment Models (APMs) as Proposed for Year 1.

Other Payer Advanced APMs: An Upcoming Option

Another interesting option is expected to be in effect for payment in 2021. (If so, this means the relevant performance-reporting period may be two years prior, or 2019.) This proposed option is another type of APM, called Other Payer Advanced APMs. As the name suggests, data from payers other than Medicare could be taken into account when determining a provider's participation status. These other payers could be either private insurers or particular state Medicaid programs.

Participation requirements for these Other Payer Advanced APMs would be as follows:

- Use certified EHR technology.
- Provide payment based on quality measures that are comparable to measures in the MIPS quality performance category.
- Bear more than a nominal amount of risk for monetary losses (or be a particular comparable type of Medicaid Medical Home Model.)[18]

ELIGIBLE PROFESSIONALS WITHIN APMs

Eligible Professionals for APMs fall into one of two categories: Qualifying (QEPs or QPs) and Partial Qualifying (PQEPs). This distinction is important because APM payment adjustments and their related timelines vary between QEPs and PQEPs. Also, note that MACRA refers to Eligible Professionals. However, CMS proposes to use a different term within its rule making. The equivalent CMS term is "Eligible Clinicians."

Qualifying Eligible Professionals (a.k.a. Qualifying Eligible Clinicians) Defined

Qualifying eligible professionals (QEPs) meet all thresholds (as defined in the scoring section of this chapter) and are at risk. "At risk" means financially at risk. In other words, the eligible professional/clinician will bear some financial burden based on performance.

Partial Qualifying Eligible Professionals (a.k.a. Partial Qualifying Eligible Clinicians) Defined

Partial qualifying eligible professionals (PQEPs) meet slightly reduced thresholds and are at risk. They also bear some financial burden based on their performance.

The Pathway Toward Becoming a Qualifying APM Participant (QP)

It is important to understand that the EPs/ECs within an Advanced APM entity may *collectively* meet the necessary threshold for participation. In other words, everyone who is eligible within a particular Advanced APM may receive the same score and thus the same payment adjustment. This is a key distinction that can easily be overlooked or misunderstood. The sequence of progression, or pathway, for eligible clinicians toward becoming a Qualifying APM Participant (QP) is illustrated in **Figure 28–10**.[19]

Four Steps to Find if the Eligible Clinician Will Become a Qualifying APM Participant

CMS has published four steps that illustrate whether or not an eligible clinician within an Advanced APM will become a QP. (Remember that these clinicians will be collectively meeting the necessary thresholds.) The four steps are as follows:

1. QP determinations are made at the Advanced APM Entity level.
2. CMS calculates a Threshold Score for each Advanced APM Entity.
3. The Threshold Score for each method is compared to the corresponding QP threshold.
4. All the eligible clinicians in the Advanced APM Entity become QPs for the payment year.[20]

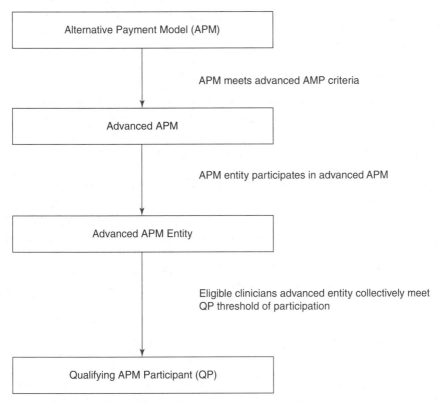

Figure 28–10 Qualifying APM Participant (QP) Pathway.
Modified from 81 Federal Register 28295 Figure B (May 9, 2016).

The result: If the threshold scores for the Advanced APM Entity are above the appropriate threshold, then all the eligible clinicians in the Advanced APM Entity will become QPs for that particular payment year. However, if the threshold scores for the Advanced APM Entity are below the corresponding QP threshold, then none of the eligible clinicians will become QPs for that payment year. In other words, the determination is all or nothing at the time of this writing.

It is also important to understand that the threshold scores are derived each year from a calendar year performance period. The performance period will be two years prior to the payment year, and is thus aligned with the MIPS performance period.[21]

HOW ARE ADVANCED APM EPs PAID?

This section discusses payment adjustments and timelines. Note that the following comments about payment refer to scoring thresholds. A description of such thresholds appears in the scoring section of this chapter.

Qualifying Eligible Professionals (QEPs) Payments

This section describes payment details for QEPs.

Incentive Payments 2019 Through 2024

If QEPs meet their thresholds, they receive an annual lump sum incentive payment of 5.0% from 2019 through 2024. These QEPs will also be excluded from MIPS adjustments. At the time of this writing, beginning in 2026, qualifying participants may receive higher fee schedule updates.[22] A timeline payment summary appears later in this section.

QEP Incentive Payment Base Period Versus QP Performance Period

It is important to understand the difference between base period and performance periods for Advanced APM Qualifying Professionals/Clinicians. The performance period will be two years prior to the payment year, as previously discussed, and is aligned with MIPS performance periods.

The incentive payment base period is for a different purpose. It is used to calculate how much the 5% incentive lump sum will be. To do so, the relevant payments for services are added up; then 5% of that figure equals the 5% incentive lump sum to be received. (The relevant payments to be added up are based on "the estimated aggregate payments for professional services furnished the year prior to the payment year...e.g. the 2019 APM Incentive Payment will be based on 2018 services."[23]

This cycle is repeated each year. For example, as CMS explains it, the first cycle would be as follows: 2017 = QP Performance Period; 2018 = Incentive Payment Base Period (to calculate the 5%); 2019 = Payment Year. Then the second cycle starts. It would be: 2018 = QP Performance Period; 2019 = Incentive Payment Base Period; 2020 = Payment Year. And the cycle would keep repeating for the duration of the 5% incentive payments.[24]

Partial Qualifying Eligible Professionals (PQEPs) Payments

This section describes payment details for PQEPs.

Some eligible professionals/clinicians may be participating in an Advanced APM that does not meet the standard threshold as previously described. Instead, this Advanced APM meets a slightly reduced threshold. Therefore, these eligible professionals/clinicians are considered to be Partial Qualifying Eligible Professionals/Clinicians, or PQEPs.

The PQEPs receive no lump sum incentive payment. They can either choose to participate in MIPS, or they can choose to opt out of MIPS. If they choose to participate in MIPS, they will receive favorable weights in the MIPS scoring. If they choose to opt out instead, they will be held harmless. In other words, they would receive no favorable payment adjustment, but neither would they be subject to a MIPS negative adjustment.[25]

Summary of APM Payment Adjustments and Their Timelines

In discussing timelines, it is important to understand that any previously existing payment methods remain in existence for the period 2015 through 2018. In other words, during that four-year period, providers are still being paid under these methods.

At the time of this writing, the APM payment adjustments are scheduled to commence in 2019. As previously discussed, these APM payment adjustments are based upon the results of reporting for a performance period two years prior to 2019. Thus, measures reported in 2017 represent the performance period for Year 1 (2019) APM incentive payments. **Table 28–2** summarizes both the payment information and the timelines as discussed.

What Is the "Intermediate Option" for Payment Adjustment Choices?

"Intermediate Option" is the term for flexibility of choice between the MIPS and APM tracks. First, as we have previously described, partially qualifying EPs can choose whether or not they want to receive the MIPS payment adjustment. Second, the APM/MIPS participants would get credit toward their score within the category of Clinical Practice Improvement Activities. CMS has proposed aligning MIPS standards and APM standards in order to "make it easy for clinicians to move between them."[26]

Table 28–2 APM Payment Adjustments and Timelines (as Proposed)

APMs Payment Adjustments	2015–2018*	2019	2020	2021	2022–2024	2025	2026 Onward
Qualifying EPs (QEPs; meet all thresholds and are at risk) Annual Lump Sum Payment		5.0%					Higher fee schedule updates starting in 2026
Partial Qualifying EPs (PQEPs; meet slightly reduced thresholds and are at risk)		No lump sum payment; can choose to participate in MIPS **OR** No lump sum paid; can opt out of MIPS and be held harmless					To be determined

*Note: PQRS, VM & EHR remain in effect for the period 2015 to 2018.
Modified from CMS, "Path to Value: The Medicare Access & CHIP Reauthorization Act of 2015," p. 18.

Table 28–3 Advanced APMs: Required Participation by Year (as Proposed)

Required participation through an Advanced APM*	Payment Years					
	2017	2018	2019	2020	2021	2022 & Later
Percentage of payments	25%	25%	50%	50%	75%	75%
OR						
Percentage of patients	20%	20%	35%	35%	50%	50%

*Requirements for percentage of significant participation, by year.
Modified from CMS Quality Payment Program Overview Fact Sheet Table 1, p. 5 (October 14, 2016).

HOW SIGNIFICANT PARTICIPATION WORKS

This section discusses Advanced APM participation requirements.

What Is Significant Participation in an Advanced APM?

Significant participation is expressed in terms of ever-increasing percentages. In other words, participation must be met in each applicable payment year in either of the following two ways: percentage of payments through an Advanced APM or percentage of patients through an Advanced APM.

At the time of this writing, participation percentages for APM payments range from 25% to 75% over a six-to-seven year period. Likewise, participation percentages for APM patients range from 20% to 50% over the same six-to-seven year period. **Table 28–3** illustrates the progression of these timelines.

Will These Requirements Change Over Time?

It is to be expected that specific requirements will be edited and perhaps modified as time goes on. In addition, "CMS will continue to modify models in coming years to help them qualify as Advanced APMs."[27]

ADVANCED APM PARTICIPATION STANDARDS

This section discusses participation standards that are applicable to Advanced APMs.

Participation Standards for Advanced APMs

The initial proposed standards for Advanced APMs include three particular areas, as follows.

Financial Risk

The financial risk standards involve the level of financial risk. If financial risk requirements are not met, then CMS could take action in several ways. Possible CMS actions include requiring repayment, withholding current payments due, or reducing future rates to equal the required repayment penalty. In other words, the APM would lose money. (Of course, if the APM exceeds the standards, it should gain, because it would receive incentive payments.) The proposed initial financial risk standards must be met in three ways, including total risk, marginal risk, and a minimum loss rate.

Comparable Measures

This standard requires that the APM measures be comparable to MIPS measures within the quality performance category. As you will recall, to be comparable the measures must always be valid and reliable. They must also be evidence-based and at least one of the measures must be an outcome measure (assuming there is an appropriate measure available).

Certified EHR Technology (as Proposed)

This standard requires that in the first year of the performance period, 50% of the APM clinicians must use certified EHR technology. And for the second year of the performance period 75 percent of the APM clinicians must use certified EHR technology.[28]

Required Reporting for the First Year

CMS has proposed that all EPs will be reporting through MIPS for the first year. This requirement is imposed because they want to determine whether the particular EP (or group) can actually meet the Advanced APM requirements.

Accurate and complete reporting of measures is always important. However, complete reporting is especially important when the provider is attempting to qualify for participation as an Advanced APM. Overall scoring standards for APMs are the subject of the following section.

SCORING STANDARD FOR APMs

The APM scoring standard implements uniformity across the various types of APMs. Goals include reducing reporting burdens while maintaining the goals and objectives of the individual APM entity. (Meeting the requirements for this standard can also be viewed as a necessary first step toward becoming an Advanced APM.)

Criteria for Eligibility

Eligibility criteria for APM entity scoring standards include the following:

- The APM participates in an agreement with CMS.
- The APM bases its payment incentives on performance, using quality and cost-utilization measures.
- The APM includes at least one eligible MIPS clinician on a CMS participation list.

(Note that the eligible clinician's name must be on an APM participation list by the end of the MIPS performance year. If not, the clinician has to report under standard MIPS methods instead.)[29]

Types of APM Entities That Qualify

At the time of this writing, the following types of APM entities qualified for the APM scoring standard:

- Comprehensive Primary Care Plus (CPC+)
- Medical Shares Savings Programs (all tracks)
- Next Generation ACO Model
- Comprehensive End-Stage Renal Disease Care (CEC) Model

- Oncology Care Model (OCM)
- All other APMs that meet the criteria for the scoring standard

The Standard Aggregates Scores

Under the standard, all MIPS scores for eligible clinicians are combined, or aggregated; weighted; and averaged to arrive at a single score at the level of the APM entity. This means that all the eligible clinicians within that APM will receive the exact same MIPS composite performance score. The standard has streamlined both reporting and scoring. Also, wherever possible, the scoring standard uses performance measures that are related to that APM.

Performance scores under the standard use the same performance categories as does MIPS. At the time of this writing, it appears that the Resource Use category will usually be not applicable and thus will not contribute to the score. The remaining three categories (Quality, ACI, and CPIA) will be weighted when computing the final composite score. However, the weights may vary according to the type of APM entity.

CREATING PHYSICIAN-FOCUSED PAYMENT MODELS (PFPMS)

This section focuses upon how more physician-focused payment models may be created.

Legislative Intent

The underlying legislative intent is to encourage the creation of physician-focused payment models (PFPMs) as per the following quotation. Alternative Payment Models "provide incentive payments for certain eligible professionals (EPs) who participate in APMs, by exempting EPs from the MIPS if they are qualifying APM participants, and by encouraging the creation of physician-focused payment models (PFPMs)."[30]

A New Committee

The overall phrase used to describe these models is "physician-focused payment models" or PFPMs. A new committee will have the responsibility for reviewing and assessing possible new models. Its title is the "Physician Focused Payment Model Technical Advisory Committee."[31]

BUILDING THE MEASUREMENT DEVELOPMENT PLAN FOR MIPS AND APMs: DEVELOPING NEW QUALITY MEASURES

Measuring quality and value are important for MIPS and APMs because quality and value are the foundation of the new payment system for EPs. Since MIPS measures are more fully developed than those of APMs, there are differences between MIPS and APMs as to their implementation timelines. MIPS measures are more developed and are ready for the first stages of implementation. APMs, on the other hand, are taking longer in the initial stages of development. Our focus on measuring quality and value centers upon MIPS for that reason.

What Is the Measure Development Plan (MDP)?

The Measure Development Plan (MDP) has been created in response to a MACRA requirement. The law requires that a draft plan for the development of quality measures be developed and posted on the CMS.gov website.[32] A final plan is then posted at a later date. The final plan is supposed to take comments regarding the draft plan into consideration. The plan's full title is "CMS Quality Measure Development Plan: Supporting the Transition to the Merit-based Incentive Payment System (MIPS) and Alternative Payment Models (APMs) (Draft)."[33] Introductory commentary states that the law provides

> both a mandate and an opportunity for the Centers for Medicare & Medicaid Services (CMS) to leverage quality measure development as a key driver to further the aims of the CMS Quality Strategy:
>
> * Better Care,
> * Smarter Spending, and
> * Healthier People.[34]

The purpose of the MDP is twofold: "to meet the requirements of the statute and serve as a strategic framework for the future of clinician quality measure development to support MIPS and APMs."[35]

Creating New Quality Measures for MIPS

New quality measures are an important part of the MIPS payment structure. The basic sequence for creating these new measures is as follows:

* First, start with existing measures. These are contained in the PQRS, in the VM program, and in the Meaningful Use (MU) requirements of the Medicare EHR Incentive Program.
* Next, align and harmonize these measures. In other words, the existing measures may be combined, expanded, and/or enhanced.
* Then add new measures. New measures will be needed to fill gaps. A process is in place to identify these "identified measure and performance gaps."[36] When adding the new measures, stakeholder comments may be considered. (Such comments may be gathered in response to a published Request for Information, or RFI.) In addition, measures that private payers are using may be considered.

New MIPS quality measures will result from this process. **Figure 28–11** illustrates the process just described. Note also that any quality measures developed for APMs must be comparable.

TIMELINES FOR DEVELOPING QUALITY MEASURES

This section discusses various measure development timelines.

Timelines Initially Set by MACRA

MACRA called for the initial draft Measure Development Plan (MDP) to be published as of January 1, 2016. A comment period followed. Then the final MDP was published in May 2016.

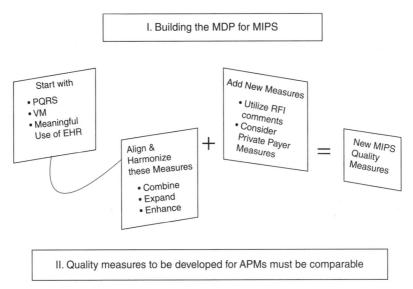

Figure 28–11 Building the MDP for MIPS and APMs: Creating New Quality Measures.

The Act further called for updates to the MDP to be published annually or otherwise as appropriate.[37] Thus we expect to see annual updates, as required, published on a regular annual schedule. Any updates that might be otherwise appropriate, of course, are unpredictable.

Procedural Timelines

CMS has another set of procedural timelines to comply with. A final rule about quality measure development will be published each year by CMS no later than the first of November.[38] Within the regulatory rule-making process, a Call for Measures will be published in the first half of each year. This allows stakeholders to submit their input. After the Call for Measures ends in June of each year, a proposed rule will most probably be published with a multi-month comment period. Only then will the final rule be ready to be published on the first of November.

A FRAMEWORK FOR MACRA QUALITY MEASUREMENT

This section discusses quality measurement concerning a framework for measurement along with related priorities and domains.

Required Priorities and Domains for Quality Measures Development

MACRA sets out specific requirements for development of quality measures as follows.

MACRA-Required Priorities for Types of Measures

The Measure Development Plan (MDP) required by MACRA has been described in a previous section of this chapter. MACRA further requires that the Measure Development Plan take four priorities into account when creating the quality measures. The four priorities are as follows:

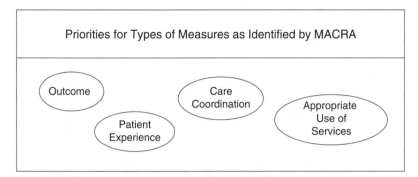

Figure 28–12 Four Priorities for Types of Quality Measures as Identified by MACRA.
Data from MACRA Section 102(1)(D)(4-16-15).

- Outcome measures (including patient reported outcome and functional status measures)
- Patient experience measures
- Care coordination measures
- Measures of appropriate use of services (including measures of over use)[39]

Figure 28–12 illustrates this requirement.

MACRA-Identified Quality Domains

MACRA also sets out specific quality domains for use in quality measure development. MACRA says "the term quality domains means at least the following domains" and five domains are then listed as follows.

- Clinical care
- Safety
- Care coordination
- Patient and caregiver experience
- Population health and prevention[40]
- An additional sixth quality domainis under consideration by CMS. It is: efficiency and reduction

(Note that this addition is permissible, as the legislative wording is "...at least the following....")
Figure 28–13 illustrates these requirements. The addition of an efficiency and reduction domain is especially logical, because it ties into the National Quality Strategy (NQS) domains. In other words, with this addition, these six domains mirror the six NQS domains that are the subject of the next section in this chapter.

A Framework for Quality Measurement

CMS has published a Framework for MACRA quality measurement that is linked to NQS domains. The framework is mapped to the six National Quality Strategy (NQS) domains as follows. Note that the details following each domain's title are a part of CMS's framework. (Note also that some domain titles vary slightly as they are expanded from the NQS titles as listed above.)

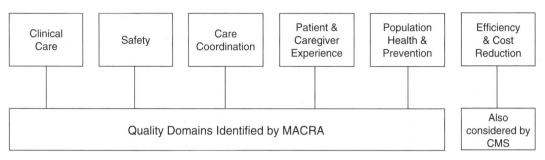

Figure 28–13 Six Quality Domains for Quality Measures Development.
Data from SSA Section 1848 (s)(1)(D).

Clinical Quality of Care

- Care type (preventive, acute, post-acute, chronic)
- Conditions
- Subpopulations

Safety

- All-cause harm
- Hospital-acquired conditions (HACs)
- Hospital-associated infections (HAIs)
- Unnecessary care
- Medication safety

Care Coordination

- Patient and family activation
- Infrastructure and processes for care coordination
- Impact of care coordination

Person- and Caregiver-Centered Experience and Outcomes

- Patient experience
- Caregiver experience
- Preference- and goal-oriented care

Population and Community Health

- Health behaviors
- Access
- Physical and social environment
- Health status

Efficiency and Cost Reduction

- Cost
- Efficiency
- Appropriateness[41]

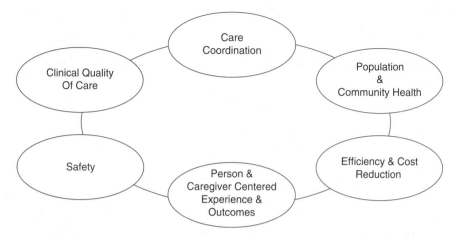

Figure 28–14 CMS Framework for Measurement Mapped to National Quality Strategy Domains. Modified from 80 FR 68668 (November 5, 2015).

We have illustrated this linkage in **Figure 28–14**. CMS has published two more comments concerning the framework:

- Measures should be patient-centered and outcome-oriented whenever possible.
- Measure concepts in each of the six domains that are common across providers and settings can form a core set of measures.[42]

Other Measure Development Considerations

Other measure development considerations include the following:

- Coordinate across various measure developers.
- Consider how clinical practice guidelines and best practices can be used in the measures.
- Use an evidence-based approach for certain measures where relevant.

It is also important to realize that measures will be reassessed and revised over time. We can therefore expect that more future efforts toward standardization and ease of use for all measures.

More About National Quality Strategy's Priorities and Domains

This chapter uses a four-part sequence to show how CMS develops quality measures. First, the Measure Development Plan for MIPS is described. (See Figure 28–11.) Second, the priorities for quality measures that are identified (and thus required) by MACRA are described. (See Figure 28–12.) Third, the quality domains that are identified (and thus required) by MACRA legislation are described. (See Figure 28–13.) And fourth, this chapter then shows how the CMS framework for measurement ties back into the six NQS domains. (See Figure 28–14.)

CONCLUSION: BENEFITS AND COSTS OF THE QUALITY PAYMENT PROGRAM

Implementing the Quality Payment Program results in both benefits and costs.

Benefits and Costs

One benefit of the new MIPS program is an increase in the attention to quality of care. The measures' metrics provide information that may be used for internal comparative performance purposes. Another benefit concerns the program feedback about cost of care. The cost of care as computed by CMS may provide financial information based on a national benchmark. Comparing this national baseline financial information to the provider's own costs, also as computed by CMS, may be especially valuable for future financial planning.

Costs of program participation include costs of new software plus potential hardware upgrades. Staff training is essential and is of course another cost. The potential time lag in cash flow at the point of implementation should also be recognized.

Public reporting can be considered either a benefit or a cost. This depends upon the organization's public image and the results that are posted within the public reporting venue.

Ingredients for Success

Success of this value-based program begins with proper measure choices and continues with measure development and implementation. Proper implementation first means the right choices. Another crucial element is sufficient training of a focused staff who understands the implications.

Success Also Depends Upon the Use of Qualified Electronic Transmission Standards

Success also depends upon complying with all digital requirements involving use of qualified electronic transmission standards. Funding must be made available for sufficient hardware and software, along with proper training of staff. Timely updates on software and staff training are essential. In addition, an electronic disaster plan should be in effect and up-to-date.

Organizational Implications

Leadership must be responsible for seeing that quality and financial incentives align properly. Such alignment could well result in a move away from so-called "silo," or vertical, departmental responsibilities. Assigning responsibilities differently (not departmentally) could potentially result in horizontal networks of responsibility that are organized around patient groups with similar needs.

Finally the organization's leadership must recognize that the digital age has arrived. It is here, and the inevitable change that it brings must be recognized and dealt with in order to achieve success.

THREE INCENTIVE PROGRAMS AS THEY EXISTED BEFORE MIPS: A REFERENCE

This information is provided to serve as a bridge between what came before MIPS and what has followed. It can be used for both comparative and reference purposes.

Physician Quality Reporting System (PQRS)

The Physician Quality Reporting System (PQRS) is a quality reporting program concerning covered professional services within the Medicare Part B Physician Fee Schedule (MPFS).[43] PQRS applies to both individual EPs and group practices and is intended to improve the quality of care provided to patients. CMS considered the following factors as the minimum when EPs are selecting measures for reporting. The minimum factors include:

- Clinical conditions usually treated
- Types of care typically provided (e.g., preventive, chronic, acute)
- Settings where care is usually delivered (e.g., office, emergency department [ED], surgical suite)
- Quality improvement goals for 2016
- Other quality reporting programs in use or being considered[44]

Practitioners can see, after the fact, how often they met a particular quality measure and thus can assess their overall quality performance.

Beginning in 2015, the program applied a negative payment adjustment to certain individual EPs and PQRS group practices. Those practitioners received negative payment adjustments because they did not satisfactorily report data on quality measures for the relevant performance period. Each year's results stand alone, so a negative adjustment in one year does not necessarily mean a negative result for the following year. In other words, reporting satisfactorily for the 2016 performance period year would avoid a negative payment adjustment in the 2018 PQRS program year. Finally, for those who might be wondering, PQRS originally had another name: It was previously known as the Physician Quality Reporting Initiative.

Value-Based Payment Modifier (Value Modifier)

The Value-Based Payment Modifier, or Value Modifier (VM), provides a budget-neutral payment adjustment to a physician (or group) based upon "the quality of care compared to the cost of care furnished to Medicare fee-for-service beneficiaries during a performance period."[45]

The VM uses a two-part composite score. The quality composite score is primarily calculated from submitted PQRS data. (The quality score also includes three outcome measures that are calculated by CMS from Medicare claims data.)[46] The cost composite score includes performance cost measures and is calculated by CMS by primarily using claims data. The cost measures, also calculated by CMS, include six performance cost measures.

The VM provides eligible practitioners with a positive, neutral, or negative payment adjustment. It is important to note that the VM adjustment is separate from the PQRS as described previously. However, the quality measures for the two programs have been aligned. The VM was phased in; it first applied to groups of 100 or more eligible professionals. By 2016, the VM was applicable to groups of 10 or more eligible professionals.[47]

Meaningful Use (MU) and the Electronic Health Records (EHR) Incentive Program

The EHR Incentive Programs were first implemented in 2011. The program was designed to encourage providers to "adopt, implement, upgrade and demonstrate meaningful use of certified EHR technology."[48] Medicare EHR incentive program payments to eligible professionals, eligible hospitals, and critical access hospitals have come to an end. Meaningful use, as defined above, was still required, however, and at the time of this writing negative payment adjustments have been imposed for non-use through 2018. (Note, however, that Medicaid incentive program payment adjustment continues until 2021.)

Meaningful use is determined by reporting upon certain objectives and measures. Within the Medicare program, implementation progresses in three stages: Stage 1, Stage 2 (now Modified Stage 2), and Stage 3. (The numerous Medicaid program variations are beyond the scope of this book.) At first, the Medicare EHR Incentive Program required choices among "core" and "menu" objectives and measures. However, as of 2016, the program has been streamlined. All providers are now required to attest to a single set of objectives and measures.[49] The streamlining also means that the number of objectives has been reduced.

Meaningful Use measures have been modified and incorporated into the new Quality Payment Program (MIPS and APMs), a Medicare program that is presently scheduled to commence payment in 2019. And MU has gained a new name within the Quality Payment Program. It becomes "Advancing Care Information" instead. For more details about the current status of Meaningful Use in its new Advancing Care Information form, see Appendix 28-A at the end of this chapter.

ALTERNATIVE PAYMENT MODELS: A REFERENCE

This information is provided to serve as a bridge between existing APM models and those models that qualify for incentive payments as Advanced APMs. In other words, these models were in operation before new Quality Payment Program criteria were set. We intend this information to be used for both comparative and reference purposes.

A brief description of various models follows. (A full discussion of such models is beyond the scope of this text.)

Accountable Care Organizations (ACOs)

The Medicare program offers various ACO programs, as follows.[50]

Medicare Shared Savings Program

Under this program, hospitals, eligible providers, and suppliers can come together in a Shared Savings Program ACO. The program was created to "facilitate coordination and cooperation among providers to improve the quality of care for Medicare Fee-For-Service (FFS) beneficiaries and reduce unnecessary costs."[51] The ACO that meets performance standards and lowers the growth in costs will be rewarded. Note also that data about the shared savings program ACOs is made public.[52]

Advance Payment ACO Model

This interesting model came about through input from stakeholders. There was concern that smaller ACO groups would not be able to pay for the necessary investment in infrastructure and staff. (This investment would be required in order to achieve the desired care coordination.) Therefore, this Advance Payment ACO model is intended to assist rural providers and physician-based groups by providing cash up front. This cash is not a grant or a gift; instead it is cash advanced from the shared savings that the ACO group is expected to earn.[53]

Furthermore, the advance payment design recognizes that there are both fixed start-up costs and variable start-up costs. For that reason, according to CMS, each of these ACOs will receive the following three types of advance payments. Note that two are upfront, one fixed and one variable, while the third payment is monthly. The ACO will receive:

- An upfront, fixed advance payment
- An upfront, variable advance payment that is based on beneficiary numbers
- A monthly variable advance amount that is based on the size of the ACO [54]

Pioneer ACO Model

This model is intended for a more sophisticated group of organization and providers who are experienced in care coordination. In other words, they do not have a learning curve. Two design elements are especially interesting in this model. First, these groups are expected to move more quickly from the shared savings plan into a population-based payment model. That expectation is due to their prior experience. While the model is flexible, generally speaking, participants in the initial two years are held to a higher level of both shared savings and risk than those participants in the "regular" shared savings plan.[55]

The second interesting element is that this model is supposed to work in cooperation with private payers. It does that by "aligning provider incentives, which will improve quality and health outcomes for patients across the ACO, and achieve cost savings for Medicare, employers and patients.[56] (Note that at the time of this writing, this model was closed to new applicants.)

Patient-Centered Medical Homes

The easy-to-use phrase "patient-centered medical homes" actually refers to a CMS demonstration project with a long title. The demonstration's formal name is "The Federally Qualified Health Center Advanced Primary Care Practice, or FQHC APCP. It has a three-year life, unless it is subsequently extended and/or expanded. As the title suggests, only federally qualified health centers (FQHCs) can participate, and there is a strict set of criteria, terms, and conditions. Once accepted into the demonstration, each FQHC receives a monthly management fee for each applicable eligible Medicare beneficiary. The fee is paid quarterly and payment is automatic.[57]

Four Bundled Payment Models

The Bundled Payments for Care Improvement (BPCI) Initiative presently covers four care models. Payment is linked, or bundled, for multiple services that occur during a patient's episode of care. Organizations agree to episode-of-care payments that include both performance and financial accountability.[58] A brief comment about each of the four care models follows.

For Model #1, the episode of care equals the inpatient stay in an acute care hospital. Payment to the hospital is discounted from the usual Inpatient Prospective Payment System and payment to physicians is made separately under the Medicare Physician Fee Schedule.

Model #2 takes a different approach, as its payment is retrospectively bundled. The episode of care includes the inpatient stay, plus the post-acute care, plus all related services for are bundled for a period of up to 90 days after discharge from the hospital. The retrospective bundled payment adjustment is made after comparison to the target price, and such payment adjustment can either be positive or negative.

Model #3 is also retrospectively bundled and the episode of care is designated, or triggered, by a hospital stay. However, unlike the previous model, in this case the episode of care concerns only post-acute care provided to the patient. Once again, the retrospective bundled payment adjustment is made after comparison to a target price, and such payment adjustment can either be positive or negative.

Model #4 differs from that of Model #1. In this case one bundled payment is made to the hospital. This payment covers all the episode-of-care services, including those of the physicians. The hospital then pays the physicians and other professionals, using part of the bundled payment that it has received for this episode of care. (For those who are wondering, to complete the entire cycle the physicians must send a "no-pay" claim form to Medicare that sets out what services they performed.)[59]

Other New APM Models

Other new APM models will be developed in the near future. At the time of this writing, CMS has recently issued a "RFI" or Request for Information that seeks input about possible new physician-focused payment models or PFPMs.[60]

INFORMATION CHECKPOINT

What is needed?	Some description of the MACRA legislation, the Quality Payment Program, and/or MIPS and APMs.
Where is it found?	A newsletter or a training announcement or a planning committee report.
How is it used?	The use depends upon the particular item. Typical uses would be for general information or for training or planning purposes.

KEY TERMS

Accountable Care Organizations (ACOs)

Alternative Payment Model (APM)

Bundled Payment

Composite Performance Score

Eligible Professional (EP) (a.k.a. Eligible Clinician)

MACRA

Meaningful Use (MU)

Measure Development Plan (MDP)

Merit-Based Incentive Payment System (MIPS)

Partial Qualifying Eligible
   Professional (PQEP)
Patient-Centered Medical
   Homes
Performance Period

Physician-Focused Payment
   Models (PFPMs)
Qualifying Eligible
   Professionals (QEPs)

Sustainable Growth Rate
   (SGR)
Value-Based Program

DISCUSSION QUESTIONS

1. Describe how the Merit-Based Incentive Payment System (MIPS) and the Advanced Alternative Payment Model (APM) are illustrative of "pay-for-performance."
2. Put on your physician's hat. How would you determine which of the two incentive payment programs to participate in?
3. How did the Sustainable Growth Rate (SGR) work, and why was it ultimately repealed?

NOTES

1. 80 Federal Register 59102 (October 1, 2015).
2. B. Wynne, "May the Era of Medicare's Doc Fix (1997–2015) Rest in Peace. Now What?" *Health Affairs Blog*, April 14, 2015, Healthaffairs.org/blog/2015/04/14/may-the-era-of-medicares-doc-fix-1997-2015-rest-in-peace-now-what; also M. A. Carey, "Congress Is Poised To Change Medicare Payment Policy. What Does That Mean For Patients And Doctors?" *Kaiser Health News*, January 16, 2014, Khn.org/news/congress-doc-fix-sustainable-growth-rate-sgr-legislation
3. Centers for Medicare and Medicaid Services (CMS), "Proposed Policy, Payment, and Quality Provisions Changes to the Medicare Physician Fee Schedule for Calendar Year 2016," July 8, 2015, www.cms.gov/newsroom/mediareleasedatabase/fact-sheets/2015-fact-sheets-items/2015-07-08.html
4. 80 FR 59102 (October 1, 2015).
5. CMS, "Fact Sheet: Quality Payment Program Executive Summary," p. 5, https://www.cms.gov/Medicare/Quality-Initiatives-Patient-Assessment-Instruments/Value-Based-Programs/MACRA-MIPS-and-APMs/NPRM-QPP-Fact-Sheet.pdf, accessed May 23, 2016.
6. CMS, "The Medicare Access and CHIP Reauthorization Act of 2015: Quality Payment Program," https://www.cms.gov/Medicare/Quality-Initiatives-Patient-Assessment-Instruments/Value-Based-Programs/MACRA-MIPS-and-APMs/Quality-Payment-Program/MACRA-NPRM-Slides.pdf, accessed June 6, 2016.
7. Ibid.
8. Ibid.
9. Ibid.
10. The computation steps overview as described was generalized from the composite score steps used to calculate the 2016 Value Modifier. CMS, "CMS Fact Sheet: Computation of the 2016 Value Modifier," September 2015, www.cms.gov/Medicare/Medicare-Fee-for-Service-Payment/PhysicianFeedbackProgram/downloads/2016-VM-Fact-Sheet.pdf

11. CMS, "Hospital Value-Based Purchasing," September 2015, www.cms.gov/Outreach-and-Education/Medicare-Learning-Network-MLN/MLNProducts/downloads/Hospital_VBPurchasing_Fact_Sheet_ICN907664.pdf

12. CMS, "MIPS: Advancing Care Information Performance Category," p. 41, www.cms.gov/Medicare/Quality-Initiatives-Patient-Assessment-Instruments/Value-Based-Programs/MACRA-MIPS-and-APSs/Advancing-Care-Information-Presentation.pdf, accessed June 7, 2016.

13. CMS, "MACRA: Quality Payment Program," pp. 39–40.

14. Ibid.

15. 81 FR 28280 (May 9, 2016).

16. P.L. 114-10-(April 16, 2015) 129 STAT.121.

17. MACRA, "Delivery System Reform, Medicare Payment Reform: What's the Quality Payment Program?" https://www.cms.gov/Medicare/Quality-Initiatives-Patient-Assessment-Instruments/Value-Based-Programs/MACRA-MIPS-and-APMs/MACRA-MIPS-and-APMs.html, accessed March 17, 2016.

18. 81 FR 28165 (May 9, 2016).

19. Ibid., 28295.

20. CMS, "MACRA: Quality Payment Program," pp. 63 and 68.

21. Ibid.

22. Ibid., pp. 70–71, and CMS. Qualifying Eligible Professionals (QEPs) Payments, www.cms.gov/Medicare/Quality-Initiatives-Patient-Assessment-Instruments/Value-Based-Programs/MACRA-MIPS-and-APMs, accessed March 17, 2016.

23. CMS, "MACRA: Quality Payment Program," pp. 70–71.

24. Ibid.

25. Ibid., p. 86.

26. CMS, "Fact Sheet: Quality Payment Program ES," p. 4.

27. Ibid., p. 3.

28. Ibid., p. 11.

29. CMS, "MACRA: Quality Payment Program," pp. 87–92.

30. 80 Federal Register (FR) 63485 (October 20, 2015).

31. P.L. 114-10 (April 16, 2015) 129 STAT. 115.

32. P.L. 114-10 Sec 102 (April 16, 2015).

33. CMS, "CMS Quality Measure Development Plan: Supporting the Transition to the Merit-based Incentive Payment System (MIPS) and Alternative Payment Models (APMs)." (Baltimore, MD: Author, 2015), https://www.cms.gov/Medicare/Quality-Initiatives-Patient-Assessment-Instruments/Value-Based-Programs/MACRA-MIPS-and-APMs/Final-MDP.pdf

34. Ibid., p. 3; also, CMS, "CMS Quality Strategy 2016," (Baltimore, MD: Author, 2015).

35. Ibid., p. 3.

36. Ibid., p. 4.

37. Sec 1848(s)(1)(A).

38. Ibid.

39. MACRA Sec.102(1)(D).

40. MACRA Sec. 102(1)(B).

41. 80 FR 68668 (November 5, 2015).

42. Ibid.

43. CMS, "Physician Quality Reporting System," last modified August 8, 2016, www.cms.gov /Medicare/Quality-Initiatives-Patient-Assessment-Instruments/PQRS

44. CMS, "Measures Codes," last modified August 31, 2016, www.cms.gov/medicare/quality -initiatives-patient-assessment-instruments/pqrs/measurescodes.html

45. CMS, "CMS Fact Sheet: Computation of the 2016 Value Modifier," September 2015, www .cms.gov/Medicare/Medicare-Fee-for-Service-Payment/PhysicianFeedbackProgram /downloads/2016-VM-Fact-Sheet.pdf

46. https://www.cms.gov/Medicare-Fee-for-Service-Payment/PhysicianFeedbackProgram /ValueBasedPaymentModifier.html

47. CMS, "Value-Based Payment Modifier," accessed January 20, 2016, www.cms.gov /Medicare/Medicare-Fee-for-Service-Payment/PhysicianFeedbackProgram /valuebasedpaymentmodifier.html

48. CMS, "Medicare and Medicaid EHR Incentive Program Basics," last modified January 12, 2016), https://www.cms.gov/regulations-and-guidance/legislation/ehrincentive programs/basics.html

49. CMS, "2016 Program Requirements," https://www.cms.gov/Regulations-and-Guid- ance/Legislation/EHRIncentivePrograms/2016ProgramRequirements.html, accessed June 9, 2016.

50. CMS, "Accountable Care Organizations (ACOs)," last modified January 6, 2015, www.cms .gov/Medicare/Medicare-Fee-for-Service-Payment/ACO/index.html

51. CMS, "Shared Savings Program," http://www.cms.gov/Medicare/Medicare-Fee-for-Ser- vice-Payment/sharedsavingsprogram/index.html?redirect=/SharedSavingsProgram, accessed September 19, 2016.

52. Ibid., pp. 1–2.

53. CMS, "Advance Payment ACO Model," pp. 1–2, last modified February 19, 2016, https:// innovation.cms.gov/initiatives/Advance-Payment-ACO-Model

54. Ibid., p. 2

55. CMS, "Pioneer ACO Model," https://innovation.cms.gov/initiatives/Pioneer-ACO- Model/, accessed April 6, 2016.

56. Ibid., p. 1

57. CMS, "Federally Qualified Health Center Advanced Primary Care Practice (FQHC APCP) Demonstration Fact Sheet," www.cms.gov/Medicare/Demonstration-Projects/ DemoProjectsEvalRpts/downloads/fqhc_fact_sheet.pdf, accessed April 6, 2016.

58. CMS, "Bundled Payments for Care Improvement (BPCI) Initiative: General Informa- tion," p. 1, https://innovation.cms.gov/initiatives/bundled-payments, accessed April 6, 2016.

59. Ibid., pp. 2–3.

60. CMS, MACRA RFI (CMS-3321-NC), http://www.innovation.cms.gov/Files/x/macra-faq .pdf, accessed June 30, 2016.

Meaningful Use: Modified and Streamlined with a New Name

28-A

HOW MEANINGFUL USE HAS EVOLVED

This section provides background information that leads to a better understanding of the current program.

Meaningful Use's New Name Applies to Physicians and Other Eligible Professionals

As we have learned, in the accompanying chapter, "Meaningful Use of Certified Electronic Health Records (EHRs)" has a new name. It is now known as Advancing Care Information (ACI). It is important to understand that the new name applies to usage by physicians and other eligible professionals.

ACI is now one component in the Merit-Based Incentive Payment System (MIPS). And MIPS is one of two methods contained in the overall Quality Payment Program. The legislation that created the new incentive program is known as the Medicare Access and CHIP Reauthorization Act of 2015 (MACRA). This Act applies to physicians and other eligible professionals. The accompanying chapter to this Appendix describes details of the Quality Payment Program, including both MIPS and Advanced Alternative Payment Methods (APMs). (For simplicity purposes, in the remainder of this Appendix, when we say "physicians," we actually mean "physicians and other eligible professionals.")

Physicians and Hospitals Have Different Meaningful Use Programs

Meaningful Use (MU) programs are in place for physicians and for hospitals. Separate incentive programs have been implemented for physicians and for hospitals. A very brief background summary follows.

Hospitals Retain the "Meaningful Use" Name for Now

The hospital Medicare program incentive payments spanned a four-year period. Then, beginning in fiscal year 2015, eligible hospitals that were not meaningful users of certified EHR technology became subject to payment adjustments.[1] In other words, negative payment adjustments (reductions) now apply if eligible hospitals are not meaningful users.

Do not be confused by different terminology. At the time of this writing, hospitals still use the term "meaningful use" (although it is possible that may change in the near future). At present, the new name "Advancing Care Information" only applies to the physician and other eligible professionals. However, the hospital's meaningful use program has also been streamlined. Its measures are undergoing an alignment process that is beyond the scope of this text.

Physicians Use the New ACI Name Upon Quality Payment Program Implementation

The original Medicare program incentive payments for physicians spanned a similar period. Then, beginning in calendar year 2015, eligible physicians who were not meaningful users of certified EHR technology also became subject to payment adjustments.[2] In other words, physicians were also subject to negative payment adjustments (reductions) if they were not meaningful users. They remained subject to these reductions until MACRA's Quality Payment Program (QPP) was implemented.

Meaningful Use had to Be Demonstrated Every Year

The Centers for Medicare and Medicaid Services (CMS) made it clear that meaningful use had to be demonstrated every year as follows. "EPs must demonstrate meaningful use every year in order to avoid Medicare payment adjustments. For example, an eligible professional that demonstrates meaningful use for the first time in 2013 will avoid the payment adjustment in calendar year (CY) 2015, but will need to demonstrate meaningful use again in 2014 in order to avoid the payment adjustment in CY 2016."[3]

Reporting Periods for MU Used to Vary by Type of Provider

The typical reporting period covers 12 months. However, the beginning month and the ending month will vary between two types of providers. (At the time of this writing, the difference still existed.) The physician and eligible professional reporting period is a CY. A CY runs like the calendar does, from January 1 to December 31. The hospital reporting period, on the other hand, is a fiscal year (FY). Specifically, it is the federal fiscal year. This reporting period runs from October 1 of one year to September 30 of the following year.

However, as of 2016, MU reporting for hospitals was also converted to a CY.[4] This change means comparison of like data is easier because the reporting periods match.

CHANGES TO ALLOWABLE MU STAGES

This section discusses allowable MU stages plus a modification of one stage.

MU Has Progressed Stage by Stage

This section provides background information about the stages of meaningful use.

Three Original Stages of Meaningful Use

The original meaningful use programs progressed in three stages:

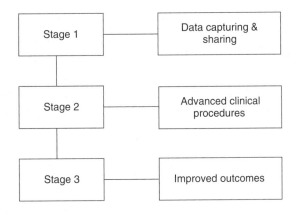

Figure 28-A–1 Three Initial Stages of Meaningful Use.
Courtesy of J.J. Baker and R.W. Baker, Dallas, Texas.

- Stage 1, which included data capture and sharing
- Stage 2, which included advanced clinical processes
- Stage 3, which included improved outcomes

Figure 28-A–1 illustrates this progression.

Stages Progressed Through a Rolling Implementation

The program allowed a rolling implementation. Under this concept, eligible providers had a choice as to what year they would enter the program. Note that while numerous other changes to MU have occurred, at the time of this writing providers may still choose which year to enter the program.

Stage 2 Was Modified

Meaningful use stages have been streamlined when preparing for use as ACI in the QPP. In another process, however, Stage 2 Meaningful Use previously underwent a series of changes to make MU more user-friendly. Therefore, the Stage 2 MU in use until QPP implementation has been termed Modified Stage 2.

Allowable Stages of Meaningful Use in the First Year

In 2015 or 2016, a provider demonstrating meaningful use for the first time was allowed to use Modified Stage 2. In 2017 or 2018, the provider demonstrating meaningful use for the first time was allowed to use either Modified Stage 2 or Stage 3. By 2018, everyone is scheduled to use Stage 3. In other words, only one single version of meaningful use (Stage 3) will be allowable.[5]

The end to multiple stages also ended the necessity for rolling implementation. These changes then allowed a smooth progression to the streamlined MU that became ACI within the QPP. **Table 28-A–1** illustrates allowable implementation by year from 2015 through 2019 and into the future.

Table 28-A–1 Meaningful Use Stages by First Year

First year demonstrating meaningful use	Stage of Meaningful Use				
	2015	2016	2017	2018	2019 & Future Years +
2015	Modified Stage 2	Modified Stage 2	Modified Stage 2 or Stage 3	Stage 3	Stage 3
2016	n/a	Modified Stage 2	Modified Stage 2 or Stage 3	Stage 3	Stage 3
2017	n/a	n/a	Modified Stage 2 or Stage 3	Stage 3	Stage 3
2018	n/a	n/a	n/a	Stage 3	Stage 3
2019 & Future Years 2019+	n/a	n/a	n/a	n/a	Stage 3

Modified from CMS "Table: Stage of Meaningful Use Criteria by First Year" EHR Incentive Programs (4-14-2016).

CHANGES TO MEANINGFUL USE REQUIREMENTS

Prior to ACI, new participation requirements were put into place for the period 2015 to 2017. Objectives and measures were simplified at the same time.

New Participation Requirements Began

New Medicare participation requirements were put into place for the period 2015 to 2017. The CMS focus for both Modified Stage 2 and Stage 3 was as follows:

- Advanced use of certified EHR technology to support health information exchange and interoperability
- Advanced quality measurement
- Maximized clinical effectiveness and efficiencies[6]

Objectives and Measures Were Simplified

For the period 2015 to 2017, all providers use one single set of objectives and measures. This change simplifies the original "core and menu" structure that was previously in effect. For this period, the number of objectives was also reduced. Hospital objectives were reduced to nine while eligible professional objectives were reduced to 10.7.

Some providers were also able to claim certain "alternate exclusions." One example of an alternate exclusion is as follows. A provider who was scheduled to be in either Stage 1 or Stage 2 in 2016 may be allowed to claim an alternate exclusion for certain Public Health Reporting measures. This exclusion may be allowable if it requires "acquisition of additional technologies that they did not previously have or did not previously intend to include in their activities for meaningful use."[8] In other words, alternate exclusions are short-term aids that help the transition of MU stage implementation.

CONCLUSION: ADVANCING CARE INFORMATION BECOMES THE NEW MEANINGFUL USE

This section clarifies certain aspects of the transition from MU to ACI.

The Methodology Still Uses Objectives and Measures

A number of changes have been made to MU as it became ACI. However, the basic measurement structure remains. This means objectives and measures are still in use within the new advancing care information.

Three Types of ACI Measures

Each ACI objective is accomplished by meeting a particular set of measures that belong to that specific objective. At the time of this writing, there are three types of such measures as described below.

System-Based Measures

System-based measures ask three questions, as follows:

- What function of our certified EHR technology system must be enabled?
- Do we meet the required threshold?
- Are we excluded from the measure?

Action-Based Measures

Action-based measures also ask three questions, as follows:

- What actions must we take?
- Do we meet the required threshold?
- Are we excluded from the measure?

Percentage-Based Measures

Percentage-based measures ask four questions, as follows:

- What makes up the denominator?
- What makes up the numerator?
- Do we meet the required threshold?
- Are we excluded from the measure?

Figure 28-A–2 further illustrates this concept.

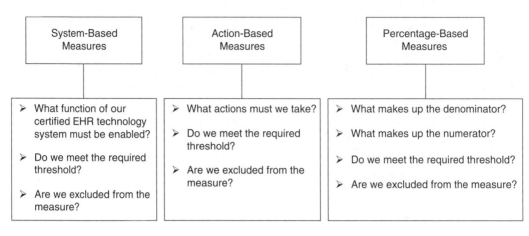

Figure 28-A–2 Three Types of Meaningful Use Measures.
Courtesy of J.J. Baker and R.W. Baker, Dallas, Texas.

Computing a Percentage-Based Measurement

ACI objectives may often use the percentage-based measures as described above. Therefore, managers need an understanding of how these measures are calculated. This section first discusses numerators and denominators, and then provides a six-step computation method.

Numerators and Denominators

To compute a percentage, you must first calculate a fraction, as illustrated in the six-step method that follows. A fraction has two parts: the numerator is the top number and the denominator is the bottom number. The line between the two parts signifies the division function. The denominator indicates the total number of parts available to be divided and the numerator indicates the number of parts of the denominator that are taken.

Why Is This Subject Important?

CMS has provided specifications for computing measures. Each specification for a percentage-based measure sets out what the composition of the denominator should be and what the composition of the numerator should be. Therefore, it is important to understand the consequences of selecting a denominator and the consequences of what the numerator will be. We understand that electronic software will actually perform the calculations, but managers should know how the method works in order to better understand the results produced for their organization.

A Six-Step Computation Method

It works this way:
Step 1: Determine your denominator.
Step 2: Determine your numerator.
Step 3: Calculate the fraction (including the decimal).
Step 4: Convert the fraction to a percentage.
Step 5: Refer to the threshold percentage that is set for this particular measure.
Step 6: Compare your percentage to the threshold percentage; it must meet the threshold in order to count. (That is, it must meet a minimum level.)

For additional detail about the six steps, see the Supplemental Materials section entitled "The Mechanics of Percentage Computation."

Exceptions

Be aware that certain exceptions exist for particular measures. These exceptions don't have to be included in the numerator or denominator, so they won't count against you.

Summary

In summary, the Advancing Care Information performance category has a mix of new and older items. The overall ACI concept is working toward a more user-friendly method.

ACRONYMS

ACI = Advancing Care Information
APM = Alternative Payment Model
CHIP = Children's Health Insurance Program
CY = Calendar Year
EHR = Electronic Health Record
FY = Fiscal Year
MACRA = Medicare Access and CHIP Reauthorization Act of 2015
MIPS = Merit-Based Incentive Payment System
MU = Meaningful Use
QPP = Quality Payment Program

NOTES

1. CMS, MLN #904626, p. 1.
2. ARRA Division B. Title IV Section 4101 (HITECH Act).
3. CMS, "Understanding 2018 Medicare Quality Program Payment Adjustments (v1.03/1/2016)," p. 3, March 2016, www.cms.gov/Medicare/Quality-Initiatives-Patient-Assessment-Instruments/PQRS/Downloads/Understand2018MedicarePayAdjs.pdf
4. CMS, "Medicare and Medicaid EHR Incentive Program Basics," last modified January 12, 2016, www.cms.gov/regulations-and-guidance/legislation/ehrincentiveprograms/basics.html
5. CMS, "Stage of Meaningful Use Criteria by First Year: EHR Incentive Programs," April 14, 2016.
6. CMS, "Medicare and Medicaid EHR Incentive Program Basics."
7. CMS, "2016 Program Requirements," www.cms.gov/Regulations-and-Guidance/Legislation/EHRIncentivePrograms/2016ProgramRequirements.html, accessed June 9, 2016.
8. Ibid.

Standardizing Measures and Payment in Post-Acute Care: New Requirements

THE IMPACT ACT: NEW DIRECTIONS FOR POST-ACUTE CARE

This section focuses upon provisions of the IMPACT Act legislation, along with legislative intent.

Legislative Provisions

The Improving Medicare Post-Acute Care Transformation (IMPACT) Act of 2014 was signed into law on October 6, 2014. Major provisions of the Act are discussed as follows.

Purposes of the IMPACT Act

The IMPACT Act describes five particular purposes for the legislation as follows:

- Enable comparable data and quality across post-acute care (PAC) settings
- Improve Medicare beneficiary outcomes
- Facilitate coordinated care by allowing provider access to longitudinal information
- Improve hospital discharge planning
- Provide data for research[1]

The purposes actually reach beyond the post-acute settings; see, for example, "Improve hospital discharge planning," and "Provide data for research," which implies future results of such research that may stretch into many years. **Exhibit 29–1** illustrates this aspect of the legislation.

Requirement of the IMPACT Act: Standardizing Measures

The Act requires the reporting of standardized patient assessment data and standardized quality measure data. The Act further requires that the standardized data be

Progress Notes

After completing this chapter, you should be able to

1. Identify five purposes of the IMPACT Act.
2. Identify four types of facilities affected by the IMPACT Act.
3. Understand three reasons for focusing attention on post-acute care (PAC) settings.
4. Understand the concept of a core set of measures within domains.
5. Describe standardized data.
6. Define interoperability.

Exhibit 29–1　Five IMPACT Act Purposes

> **Purposes of the IMPACT Act include**
>
> - Enable comparable data & quality across PAC settings
> - Improve Medicare beneficiary outcomes
> - Facilitate coordinated care by allowing provider access to longitudinal information
> - Improve hospital discharge planning
> - Provide data for research
>
> Modified from CMS, "The IMPACT Act of 2014 and Data Standardization," *MLN Connects*, p. 5 (October 21, 2015).

interoperable. Such standardized data enables electronic-related uniformity, exchangeability, and comparability across PAC settings. (See the section about standardized data and interoperability later in this chapter for further details.)

Standardized assessment data allows additional cross-setting outcomes. Such outcomes include the following:

- Quality care
- Improved outcomes
- Coordinated care
- Improved discharge planning[2]

Table 29–1 lists both electronic-related and other benefits.

Moving Toward Creating a Uniform PAC Payment System

The Act proposes a uniform payment system to be created across the four post-acute care settings listed below. At the time of this writing, the proposed system is termed a "Proposed Alternative Post-Acute Care Payment Model."

Other Provisions of the Act

Implementing verifiable and auditable data collection about staffing in skilled nursing facilities (SNFs) has been funded in the amount of $11 million. Facilities are required to "electronically submit...direct care staffing information, including information for agency and contract staff, based on payroll and other verifiable and auditable data in a uniform format," which may then be audited in order to verify staffing information.[3] (See the "Regulations" section in the preceding chapter entitled "Staffing: Methods, Operations and Regulations" for specific details.)

Among other provisions, hospice facilities are to be inspected every three years.[4] In addition, both hospitals and PAC providers are affected by regulations to be promulgated about the discharge planning process.[5]

Table 29–1　IMPACT Act Requirements

Electronic-Related	All Other
• Data element uniformity	• Quality care & improved outcomes
• Exchangeability of data	• Coordinated care
• Comparing data & quality across all PAC settings	• Improved discharge planning

Modified from CMS, "The IMPACT Act of 2014 and Data Standardization," *MLN Connects*, p. 4 (October 21, 2015).

Facilities Affected by the IMPACT Act

This legislation concerns four different care settings that provide care after acute care treatment (thus "post-" or "after-" acute care). The four care settings include the following:

- Skilled nursing facilities (SNFs)
- Home health agencies (HHAs)
- Inpatient rehabilitation facilities (IRFs)
- Long-term care hospitals (LTCHs)

Exhibit 29–2 illustrates the care settings that are impacted.

Exhibit 29–2 Facilities Affected by the IMPACT Act

Skilled Nursing Facilities (SNFs)	Home Health Agencies (HHAs)	Inpatient Rehabilitation Facilities (IRFs)	Long-Term Care Hospitals (LTCHs)

Physicians and other eligible professionals are not part of this legislation.

WHY FOCUS ATTENTION ON POST-ACUTE CARE?

The Centers for Medicare and Medicaid Services (CMS) point out three valid reasons for turning attention to these post-acute care facilities. The reasons, illustrated in **Exhibit 29–3** include the following:

- Escalating PAC costs
- PAC data standards and/or data interoperability are lacking
- Meeting the goal of setting payment rates by individual patient characteristics instead of by care setting[6]

Note also that physicians and other eligible professionals are not part of this legislation. Hospitals, however, are somewhat affected due to coordination of discharge planning requirements.

Control Escalating PAC Costs

The costs are substantial. As illustrated in **Table 29–2**, Medicare spending amounted to $58.9 billion in 2014 across the four types of facilities.[7] These costs are projected to continue to increase.

    (The authors will mention that fraud also plays some part in inflating these costs, particularly in HHAs, but chasing fraud is the responsibility of another division of CMS [Fraud & Abuse Enforcement for Program Integrity] and is well beyond the scope of this text.)

Set Data Standards and Ensure Digital Interoperability

Value-based programs need accountability in order to work, and that accountability results from recording standard measures. Setting uniform standards across all four care settings allows accountability. Ensuring that digital information can be transmitted across these settings (interoperability) is another key element of such standardization.

Exhibit 29–3 Three Reasons to Focus Attention on Post-Acute Care

- Escalating PAC costs
- PAC data standards and/or interoperability are lacking
- Goal of setting payment rates by individual patient characteristics instead of the care setting (i.e., alternative PAC payment model)

Modified from CMS, "The IMPACT Act of 2014 and Data Standardization," *MLN Connects*, p. 5 (October 21, 2015).

Table 29–2 Post-Acute Care Statistics

Provider	Facilities	Beneficiaries	Medicare Spending (in Billions)
Nursing Homes	15,000	1.7 Million	$28.7
Home Health Agencies (HHAs)	12,311	3.4 Million	18.0
Inpatient Rehabilitation Facilities (IRFs)	1,166	373K	6.7
Long-Term Care Hospitals (LTCHs)	420	124K	5.5

Modified from: www.cms.gov/Medicare/Quality-Initiatives-Patient-Assessment-Instruments.html

Create an Alternative Post-Acute Care Payment Model

Setting payment rates by individual patient characteristics is an important goal. This goal can be accomplished by creating an alternative post-acute care payment model that reaches across the four care settings. As Table 29–2 illustrates, almost 29,000 facilities and almost 5.6 million beneficiaries could be affected by creating such a "cross-setting model."

A NEW ALTERNATIVE PAYMENT MODEL FOR FOUR CARE SETTINGS

This section discusses three aspects of the new PAC alternative payment model.

The New Alternative Model Would Combine Four Care Settings into One Payment

The new Alternative Post-Acute Care Payment Model proposes to primarily do two things. First, the model would establish a universal PAC payment system. In other words, payment across the four care settings would be unified. Second, the model would eliminate the present payment methods for the four care settings, because these methods would all be replaced by the new unified model.

Exhibit 29–4 illustrates the primary features of the new method. To summarize, the alternative model would set payment rates in accordance with characteristics of individual patients, instead of in accordance with the type of care setting.

Exhibit 29–4 Proposed Alternative PAC Payment Model

- Establish a unified PAC payment system
- Set payment rates according to characteristics of individuals
- Eliminate present payment tied to PAC care setting

Why the New Payment Model Is Possible

The new model is possible because each of the four affected care settings has some type of patient assessment instrument: SNFs use the Minimum Data Set (MDS), HHAs use the Outcome and Assessment Information Set (OASIS), IRFs use the IRF-Patient Assessment Instrument (PAI), and LTCHs use the Continuity Assessment Record and Evaluation (CARE). Therefore, if major information exists in some form on each type of assessment, then standardizing the data makes the new

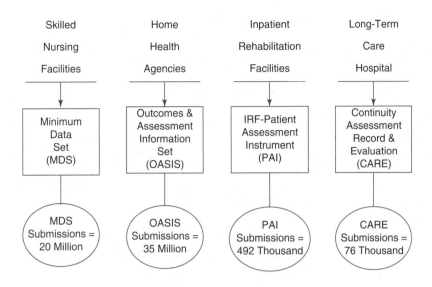

Figure 29–1 Post-Acute Care (PAC) Assessment Instrument Submissions.
Data from www.cms.gov/Medicare/Quality-Initiatives-Patient-Assessment-Instruments.html

model possible. This is because, of course, standardization then allows "cross-setting" across the four care settings.

The SNFs and HHAs have by far the most assessment instrument annual submissions. At the time of this writing, 2014 information reported 35 million OASIS (HHA) submissions and 20 million MDS (SNF) submissions. The combined 55 million submissions from these two care settings far overshadow numbers from the remaining two care settings. Their combined total of 568,000 (492,000 PAI [IRF] and 76,000 CARE [LTCH] amounted to just about one percent of the 55 million from the combined SNFs and HHAs.[8] **Figure 29–1** illustrates this information.

First Steps: Implementing Uniform Measures in Three Phases

This PAC reform depends upon uniform measures across four care settings. Phase I covers specifications of applicable measures, followed by data collection and analysis of the uniform measures. In Phase II, providers among the four care settings receive confidential feedback. The feedback reveals how they have performed on the uniform measures they reported. In Phase III, public reporting is implemented. This reporting makes performance by provider open information to the public. (Note also that providers may receive preview reports before their information is made public.) **Figure 29–2** illustrates these phases.[9]

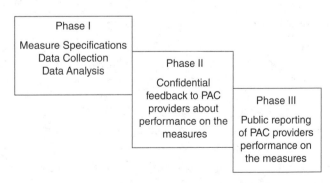

Figure 29–2 PAC Measurement Implementation Phases.

STANDARDIZED DATA AND INTEROPERABILITY: THE KEYS TO PAC REFORM

This section discusses standardization and interoperability.

Why Does the IMPACT Act Require Standardized Data?

Legislative reform has now introduced "cross-setting" to post-acute care. At the time of this writing, each type of post-acute facility has its own set of assessment information. (The SNFs have the MDS, the HHAs have OASIS, and so on.) This "silo" of electronic data does not, and typically cannot, cross over into a different type of facility. In "cross-setting," those information barriers are eliminated. Information can readily flow back and forth throughout the four types of post-acute facilities—the government term for this easy flow is "interoperability."

The cross-setting concept runs throughout the IMPACT Act as described within this chapter. In other words, standardized data enables electronic-related uniformity, exchangeability, and comparability across the various post-acute care settings. (See the section about standardized data and interoperability later in this chapter for further details.)

Table 29–1 previously listed three electronic-related elements that are enabled by standardizing assessment data. They include the following: Data element uniformity; exchangeability of data; comparing data and quality across all PAC settings. Note that all these requirements are possible because of today's digital technology status in health care. The adoption of electronic health records (EHR) nationwide was the key that allows today's improvements to recording and submitting electronic data.

What Is Standardized Data?

This section defines standardized data and provides two examples.

Standardized Data Defined

To standardize is to make uniform. In this case, standardized data are data that are both uniform and comparable. For example, each of the four types of PAC facilities has some type of assessment instrument that they are already using. Certain data elements from each of these assessment instruments have been selected to be standardized. These uniformly reported items will then be precisely comparable across each type of facility.

One Example

The example used in one CMS training session was "eating." All four instruments had some type of "eating" assessment item, but the wording was different for each.[10] Standardized data would make sure that the wording (and intent of the assessment) is the same for each.

Another Example

"Mobility" is another example used in the training session. Of all 17 mobility items listed, 8, or just over half, were present on the instruments for SNFs, IRFs, and LTCHs.[11] Even though individual wording may be different from assessment to assessment, the opportunity for standardization is present.

What Is Interoperability?

This section defines and discusses the concept of interoperability.

Interoperability Defined

In this case, interoperability means the ability to operate or, actually, to transmit across the data systems used by the various types of PAC facilities. Thus certain elements of a skilled nursing home's data should be in a standard format that is comparable to the standard format for those elements that rest in, say, a home health agency.

The Key to Achieving Outcomes

The IMPACT Act requires that such data be interoperable because we need for such data to be transmitted back and forth across the various care settings. This interoperability, along with standardization, are the keys to achieving the anticipated outcomes.

STANDARDIZING ASSESSMENT AND MEASURE DOMAINS FOR PAC PROVIDERS

This section discusses various aspects of measurement criteria.

Background

The CMS has evolved a framework for measurement that serves as a basic structure for measurement criteria. The criteria within this framework can be applied to measurements required within the IMPACT Act legislation, as follows.

Types of measures utilized for the PAC reform should have two basic characteristics: all adopted measures should be patient-centered and outcome-oriented.[12] Note that an outcome-oriented measure should be used whenever possible. Therefore, not every measure will or can be measuring outcomes as such.

The Concept: A Core Set of Measures

The CMS measurement framework hinges upon domains. Certain domains can be commonly identified across the four PAC settings and their respective providers. Thus it is possible to create a core set of measures framed within these domains. This point is especially important because it is a basic concept that underlies the PAC reform approach.

Note that the IMPACT Act specifically identifies assessment and measure domains that are required under this law. Therefore, it is especially important to recognize them and their underlying concept. **Figure 29–3** illustrates both measure types discussed above along with the "core set" concept. A discussion of required domains for both assessments and measures follows.

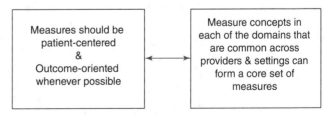

Figure 29–3 Two Structural Elements in the CMS Framework for Measurement.

Adapted from 80 FR 68668 (November 5, 2015).

Exhibit 29–5 Five PAC Standardized
Assessment Domains

- Functional status
- Cognitive function & mental status
- Special services, treatments & interventions
- Medical conditions & comorbidities
- Impairments

Modified from CMS, "IMPACT Act of 2014 and Data Standardization," *MLN Connects,* pp. 33–37 (October 21, 2015).

Assessment Domains That Must Be Standardized

The IMPACT Act specifies five assessment domains that must be standardized. They include the following:

- Functional status
- Cognitive function and mental status
- Special services, treatments, and interventions
- Medical conditions and comorbidities
- Impairments[13]

Note that additional domains may be added, but these five are the original basic requirements. **Exhibit 29–5** illustrates this information.

Measure Domains That Must Be Standardized

The IMPACT Act also specifies eight measure domains that must be standardized. These eight domains can be divided into three groups, generally based on intent behind the information to be gained. Refer to **Exhibit 29–6** to find descriptive phrases for each domain.

Exhibit 29–6 Eight PAC Standardized
Measure Domains

---

1. Functional status, cognitive function, & changes in function & cognitive function
2. Skin integrity & changes in skin integrity
3. Medication reconciliation
4. Incidence of major falls
5. Transfer of health information & care preferences when an individual transitions
6. Resource use measures, including estimated Medicare spending per beneficiary
7. Discharge to community
8. All-condition risk-adjusted potentially preventable hospital readmission rates

Modified from CMS, "IMPACT Act of 2014 and Data Standardization," *MLN Connects,* pp. 33–37 (October 21, 2015).

The first and largest group of measure domains consists of patient care information. These general types of care information are as follows:

- Various functional status and cognitive function measures for the individual patient
- Skin integrity, etc., typically centering upon pressure ulcers and/or their prevention
- Reconciliation of the patient's various medications
- Number of major falls the patient has experienced

The second group of measure domains consists of information about a patient moving between care settings and/or being discharged from care, including:

- Information transfer and care preferences as an individual patient moves from one care setting to another
- Information about the individual patient being discharged from any care setting (i.e., "into the community")
- Information about hospital readmission rates (in particular, readmissions that may be preventable)[14]

The final "group" is actually a single item that represents measures about resource use. Resource use is typically a value-based measure. As such, the grouping is expected to utilize estimated Medicare spending per beneficiary. Certain methodology adjustments for resource use may be aligned as necessary, including spending per beneficiary and time period(s), plus geographic and other relevant adjustments.[15]

The reporting of these quality measures is to occur "through the use of a PAC assessment instrument." Therefore, the relevant assessment instruments are to be modified "as necessary" to enable their use for such reporting.[16]

ELECTRONIC REPORTING TIMELINES FOR PAC PROVIDERS

This section discusses timeline requirements.

Time Required for Measure Development

CMS estimates that developing these quality measures will take six months to two years. The development process includes public and stakeholder input along with guidance from the Measure Applications Partnership (MAP).[17] It is therefore possible that some timelines may be revised. (The Measure Application Partnership is a multi-stakeholder partnership that guides the selection of performance measures for federal health programs.)[18]

PAC Provider Timelines

At the time of this writing, certain standardized assessment domains will be implemented for SNF, IRF, and LTCH providers as of October 1, 2018, and for HHAs as of January 1, 2019. There is variation among the four providers as to the specific domain items they must initially report as of these dates. (For more information about these domains, see the section entitled "Standardizing Assessment and Measure Domains for PAC Providers," discussed previously.)

It is important to understand that SNF and LTCH providers should already have begun reporting certain quality and resource use measures two years earlier as part of their new value-based programs. Thus the SNF and LTCH providers may simply be adding new measures as required on October 1, 2018. This contrasts with IRF providers, who will be reporting their required measures for the first time as of October 1, 2018, and with HHA providers, who will be reporting their required measures for the first time as of January 1, 2019.

Payment Penalty for SNFs

Beginning in fiscal year 2018, SNF payment rates may be reduced if applicable data is not submitted. The payment rate reduction amounts to two percentage points.[19]

PAC Action Requirements

The most important action requirements for PAC providers are submission dates. According to CMS, "providers must submit standardized assessment data through PAC assessment instruments under applicable reporting provisions. The data must be submitted with respect to admission and discharge for each patient, or more frequently as required."[20]

Exhibit 29– 7 Action Requirements for PAC Providers

- Submit patient-specific standardized assessment data
- Submit through the appropriate assessment instrument (MDS, etc.)
- Begin to use standardized data no later than:

  October 1, 2018, SNF, IRF, LTCH
  January 1, 2019, HHA

Modified from CMS, "IMPACT Act of 2014 and Data Standardization," *MLN Connects*, p. 33 (October 21, 2015)

Also, at the time of this writing, IMPACT-required measures must begin to be submitted no later than October 1, 2018 for SNF, IRF, and LTCH providers. IMPACT-required measures for HHAs must begin to be submitted no later than January 1, 2019.[21] These dates are illustrated in **Exhibit 29–7**.

PUBLIC REPORTING: IMPACT ACT REQUIREMENTS

The IMPACT Act requires public reporting of PAC provider performance, including both quality measures and resource use measures.

Timeline for Public Reporting of Quality Measures

Note that public reporting includes not only reporting the measures themselves, but also includes the provider who is associated with those measures. The relevant data and information are to be made publicly available no later than two years after the measure's application date.[22]

Opportunity to Review

The Act stipulates that providers have the opportunity to review data and information that is to be made public. Thus the provider has the opportunity to both review and to submit corrections prior to any public reporting of the data.[23]

Required Improvements to the 5-Star Rating System

CMS has implemented certain improvements to the *Nursing Home Compare* website's 5-Star Rating System. This federal website provides information about every nursing home that participates in Medicare and/or Medicaid. *Nursing Home Compare* rates facilities using the 5-Star Rating System. Each facility is rated on a five-point scale for each of three domains (health survey, nurse staffing, and quality measures), plus a composite scale that combines the ratings for the three domains.[24]

Several revisions are directly tied to the Act, such as using payroll-based staffing reports and providing additional quality measures. A related improvement is a revised scoring methodology for the 5-Star Rating System that will take advantage of the data and information received from the payroll-based reporting and additional new quality measures.[25]

Two additional improvements are as follows. First, CMS and states have implemented focused survey inspections nationwide in order to verify staffing and quality measure information. Second, CMS has strengthened the requirements that states must maintain a user-friendly website and complete nursing home inspections in a timely manner so the current survey information can be included in the 5-Star Rating System.[26]

IMPACT ACT BENEFITS AND COSTS: A SUMMARY

This section discusses the Act's benefits, costs, and challenges.

Benefits

The IMPACT Act's benefits center upon requirements for quality improvement and a focus upon future payment reform. Quality improvement benefits include the following:

- Facilitate coordinated care among PACs
- Achieve improved outcomes
- Allow overall quality comparisons
- Allow "patient-centeredness"

Payment reform is anticipated through the creation of one or more Alternative Post-Acute Care Payment models. This type of model is based upon the individual patient's care and outcomes instead of the facility-based payment system now in place. Thus this quality- and value-based type of payment system has the potential to become a significant benefit for post-acute care.

Costs

PAC providers will encounter transitional costs, including the following:

- Required changes to hardware and software
- Related staff training
- Potential disruption of cash flow
- Planning costs for leadership

Most of the required changes are phased in over time, so certain implementation costs may also be phased in instead of occurring all at once.

Challenges

The Act's requirements face a challenge in implementing interoperability. A couple of years ago, the Office of the National Coordinator for Health Information Technology (ONC) made its annual report to Congress and noted that national interoperability had increased, but widespread interoperability remained a challenge.

The challenge included unchanged provider practice patterns and a lack of standardization among EHRs.[27] We believe the IMPACT Act's requirements address both of these challenges as related to post-acute care providers.

MEETING STRATEGIC GOALS

This section briefly discusses goals and their underlying strategy.

Background

The CMS goals for quality strategy are to support the three aims of National Quality Strategy (NQS). These three aims can be summarized as "better health; better healthcare; lower costs."[28]

The three NQS aims are converted into six NQS priorities. CMS, in turn, has adopted these priorities as strategic goals for quality. (The CMS goals appear below.)

The CMS Quality Strategy Goals

As described above, CMS has adopted a (slightly revised) version of the NQS priorities as its quality strategy goals. The CMS goals appear as follows. (The NQS domain phrase for each follows in parentheses.)[29]

- Promote effective communication and coordination of care (Care Coordination)
- Promote effective prevention and treatment (Clinical Quality of Care)
- Make care affordable (Efficiency and Cost Reduction)
- Strengthen person and family engagement (Person- and Caregiver-Centered Experience and Outcomes)
- Make care safer (Safety)
- Work with communities to promote best practices of healthy living (Population/Community Health)[30]

More about goals and the National Quality Strategy can be found in the chapter entitled "Understanding Value-Based Health Care and Its Financial and Digital Outcomes."

Other Initiatives: Toward a Common Goal

Certain other initiatives are working toward the common goal of quality- and value-based patient care. For example, HHA regulations have been modernized "for the first time since 1989, with a focus on patient-centered, well-coordinated care."[31] Modernized improvements include requirements for a data-driven quality assessment, along with a performance improvement (QAPI) program.

The Road Map to Interoperability

The ONC is "the principal federal entity charged with coordination of nationwide efforts to implement and use the most advanced health information technology and the electronic exchange of health information."[32] It has created a 10-year Road Map to Interoperability that outlines goals for both governance and certification standards. It calls for consistency at federal, state, and private levels—an "unprecedented collaboration."[33] If such widespread interoperability can be accomplished, then technology could seamlessly support patients' health. The IMPACT Act is an important step toward that goal of seamless digital technology.

CONCLUSION: INNOVATION IN THE DIGITAL AGE

This section discusses the process of innovation, leadership and the future.

Innovation Defined

Innovation may be defined as "the introduction of something new; a new idea, method, or device," while "to innovate" is defined as "to effect a change in; to make changes."[34] In light of this, the scope of reforms proposed for PAC settings, along with the digital conversions involved, would certainly qualify as innovations.

How do leaders of an organization approach an innovative project? E. M. Rogers, a communication and innovation researcher, comments upon reaction to an innovation as follows:

> An innovation presents an individual or an organization with a new alternative or alternatives, with new means of solving problems. But the probabilities of the new alternatives being superior to previous practice are not exactly known by the individual problem solvers. Thus, they are motivated to seek further information about the innovation to cope with the uncertainty that it creates.[35]

We visualize this type of information-seeking information approach as a sequential decision process, as discussed in the following section.

The Process of Leadership Decisions Affects Innovation

Leadership decisions are often made in a series of stages. **Figure 29–4** illustrates three decision stages that may lead to adoption, for example, of a particular approach to PAC reform digital choices. The three-stage decision process includes the following:

1. Gathers information: This stage seeks enough information to attain knowledge.
2. Forms an opinion: This stage uses the knowledge gained to reach an understanding that leads to forming an opinion.
3. Makes a decision: This stage uses the opinion that has been formed to make a decision.

The last stage, "Makes a decision," should result in one of two outcomes: The decision will either be positive (Yes: will adopt and implement) or negative (No: will not adopt). (There could be a third possible outcome on that last stage. R. W. once briefly worked with a boss who would never say "yes" or "no"; instead, his decision would be "Take no action either way.") We should also note that a negative decision might not always be final, as it might be reversed at a later date.

Bringing About Innovation

How can a manager help to bring about an innovative concept such as the legislative reforms that are the subject of this chapter? He or she can help first to understand and then to diffuse.

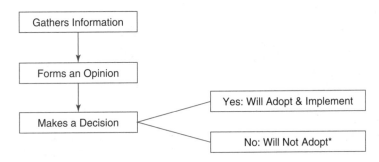

*Negative decisions may not be final.

Figure 29–4 Process Flow: Leadership Decision Stages.

Understanding the Required Framework

You as a manager can gather information and use it to understand the required framework. If requested, you can also actually assist in gathering information to provide to your upper-level management.

Diffusing the Information

You as a manager can also help to establish understanding about the innovative concept throughout your part of the organization. This could be by specific assignment or through informal information sharing. In either case, you would be assisting by helping to diffuse the information through individuals who need to know.

Management and the Impact of Leadership Changes

Two types of change in leadership may well impact the strategy and progress of healthcare technology management.

Leadership Change Within a Healthcare Organization

It seems obvious to say that leadership change within a healthcare organization may well result in a change in strategic direction. Still, this is often the case. Consequently, certain resources and/or initiatives may now receive more support, while some other resources and/or initiatives may have their funds and staffing cut, or even eliminated. It is important for a manger to be aware of this possibility, and be ready to defend his/her projects with current, well-organized information.

Leadership Change Within Legislative Bodies

Leadership change within legislative bodies can have a similar impact on projects in progress. This is especially true when it comes to funding, both current and future.

THE FUTURE: CHANGE IS INEVITABLE

The rate of change has accelerated in the digital age of health care. The IMPACT Act's reform legislation resonates across these four provider settings and beyond. It sets an interoperable quality- and vision-based vision of reform. While change is inevitable, it seems these PAC provider changes are in step with future patient-centered goals.

INFORMATION CHECKPOINT

What is needed?	Information about the new requirements affecting post-acute care facilities.
Where is it found?	Newsletters, blogs, or training materials
How is it used?	In general, to better inform healthcare providers. If your organization is a SNF, HHA, IRF, or LTCH, to educate staff about these required changes that are in progress.

KEY TERMS

Cross-Setting
Electronic Health Record (EHR)
Interoperability
IMPACT Act
Post-Acute Care (PAC)
Standardized Data
Value-Based Program

OTHER ACRONYMS

CARE = Continuity Assessment Record and Instrument
HHA = Home Health Agency
IRF = Inpatient Rehabilitation Facility
LTCH = Long-Term Care Hospital
MDS = Minimum Data Set
MAP = Measure Applications Partnership
NQS = National Quality Strategy
OASIS = Outcome and Assessment Information Set
ONC = Office of the National Coordinator for Health Information Technology
PAI = Patient Assessment Instrument
QAPI = Quality Assurance Performance Improvement
SNF = Skilled Nursing Facility

DISCUSSION QUESTIONS

1. Are you familiar with a post-acute care facility?
2. If so, how do you think these legislative requirements have affected that facility?
3. Do you think the requirements to standardize data and achieve interoperability are a good idea?

NOTES

1. P. L. 113-185 Sec. 2(a); also Centers for Medicare and Medicaid Services (CMS), "The IMPACT Act of 2014 and Data Standardization," *MLN Connects* (October 21, 2015), p. 5.
2. "The IMPACT Act of 2014 and Data Standardization," p. 4.
3. 80 Federal Register 46462 (August 4, 2015).
4. P. L. 113-185 Sec. 3(a)(1-2).
5. SSA Title XVIII Sec. 1899B (i)(1-3).
6. "The IMPACT Act of 2014 and Data Standardization," p. 5.

7. Ibid., p. 6.
8. Ibid., p. 6.
9. Sec. 1899B (e)(1)(A-C).
10. "The IMPACT Act of 2014 and Data Standardization," p. 10.
11. Ibid.
12. 80 FR 68668 (November 5, 2015).
13. Sec. 1899B (b)(1)(B).
14. Sec. 1899B (c)(1)(A-E).
15. Sec. 1899B (d)(2)(A-C).
16. Sec. 1899B (c)(2)(A).
17. "The IMPACT Act of 2014 and Data Standardization," p. 37.
18. National Quality Forum, "Measure Applications Partnership," www.qualityforum.org /setting_priorities/partnership/measure_applications_partnership.aspx
19. Sec. 1888 (e)(6)(A)(i).
20. "The IMPACT Act of 2014 and Data Standardization," p. 33.
21. Ibid.
22. Sec. 1899B (g)(1-4).
23. Ibid.
24. CMS, "Fact Sheet: Nursing Home Compare Five-Star Quality Rating System," www.cms .gov/medicare/provider-enrollment-and-certification/certificationandcomplianc /downloads/consumerfactsheet.pdf, accessed July 8, 2016.
25. CMS.gov, "CMS Announces Two Medicare Quality Improvement Initiatives," October 6, 2014, www.cms.gov/Newsroom/MediaReleaseDatabase/Press-releases/2014 -items/2014-10-06.html
26. Ibid.
27. D. Bowman, "ONC Interoperability Road Map Draft," p. 2, October 14, 2014, www .fiercehealthit.com/story/onc-interoperabiliity-road-map-draft-outlines-governance -certification-stand/2014-10-14
28. "The IMPACT Act of 2014 and Data Standardization," p. 18.
29. 80 FR 68668 (November 5, 2015).
30. "The IMPACT Act of 2014 and Data Standardization," p. 19.
31. "CMS Announces Two Medicare Quality Improvement Initiatives," p. 2.
32. HealthIT.gov, "Newsroom: About ONC," www.healthit.gov/newsroom/about-onc, accessed July 7, 2016.
33. "ONC Interoperability Road Map Draft," p. 1.
34. *Merriam Webster's Collegiate Dictionary,* 10th ed., s.v. "Innovation."
35. E. M. Rogers, *Diffusion of Innovations,* 4th ed., (New York: The Free Press, 1995), xvii.

ICD-10 Implementation Continues: Finance and Strategic Challenges for the Manager

© LFor/Shutterstock

ICD-10 E-RECORDS OVERVIEW AND IMPACT

This chapter provides an ICD-10 overview and describes the ICD-10 electronic records impact.

OVERVIEW OF THE ICD-10 CODING SYSTEM

The International Classification of Diseases, 10th Revision (ICD-10) is designed to "promote international comparability in the processing classification and presentation of mortality statistics."[1] The ICD is the international standard diagnostic classification for all general epidemiological issues, many health management purposes, and clinical use.[2]

This classification system has been developed by collaboration among the World Health Organization (WHO) and 10 international centers. Other countries that have already adopted ICD-10 include Australia, Canada, France, Germany, and the United Kingdom.[3]

ICD-10-CM AND ICD-10-PCS CODES

The National Center for Health Statistics (NCHS) is 1 of the 10 international centers collaborating with the WHO in the development and revisions of the ICD. The NCHS is an agency within the Centers for Disease Control and Prevention (CDC). As such, NCHS is the federal agency that is responsible for use of the ICD-10 in the United States.

WHO owns the ICD-10 copyright and has "authorized the development of an adaptation of ICD-10 for use in the United States for U.S. government purposes."[4] The NCHS, under the CDC, has developed a clinical modification of

Progress Notes

After completing this chapter, you should be able to

1. Understand the six benefits of transitioning to ICD-10.
2. Understand why the change to ICD-10 codes is a technology problem.
3. Identify the three types of ICD-10 implementation costs.
4. Understand how KPIs are used.
5. Describe ICD-10 KPIs' essential indicators.
6. Understand why situational analysis is particularly appropriate for electronic records implementation such as ICD-10.
7. Identify the four components of a SWOT analysis.

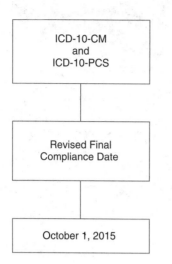

Figure 30–1 ICD-10 Revised Final Compliance Date.

the ICD-10, termed "ICD-10-CM." The ICD-10-CM replaces the ICD-9-CM. The ICD-10-CM diagnosis classification system has been developed for use in all types of healthcare treatment settings in the United States.[5]

Meanwhile, the Centers for Medicare and Medicaid Services (CMS) has developed a procedure classification system, termed the "ICD-10-PCS." The ICD-10-PCS is for use in inpatient hospital settings only within the United States.[6] (Note this difference: ICD-10-CM is for use in all types of healthcare treatment settings, while ICD-10-PCS is for use in inpatient hospital settings only.)

Final Revised ICD-10 Compliance Date

CMS has extended the deadline for ICD-10 compliance by one year. Thus the compliance date for ICD-10-CM and ICD-10-PCS is now October 1, 2015, instead of October 1, 2014, as reflected in **Figure 30–1**. CMS officials believe this extension "…will give covered entities the additional time needed to synchronize system and business process preparation and changeover to the updated medical data code sets."[7]

Providers and Suppliers Impacted by the ICD-10 Transition

The change from ICD-9 to ICD-10 has a ripple effect that impacts nearly every corner of the healthcare industry in the United States. The companies and organizations impacted by the ICD-10 transition include inpatient providers, outpatient providers, and an array of other support services and suppliers.

Figure 30–2 illustrates the entities that are affected by the ICD-10 transition. Inpatient providers impacted include both hospitals and nursing facilities. Outpatient providers include, at a minimum, physician offices, outpatient care centers, medical diagnostic and imaging services, home health services, other ambulatory care services, and durable medical equipment providers. Support services and suppliers include health insurance carriers and third-party administrators, along with the vendors who provide computer system design and related services.[8] Note that pharmacies (both chain and independent pharmacies) are substantially impacted by the required electronic transaction standards updates for pharmacies, while ICD-10 adoption is generally more of a peripheral issue for pharmacies.

E-RECORD STANDARDS AND THE ICD-10 TRANSITION

This section discusses Version 5010 of electronic record standards and provides an example of standards use.

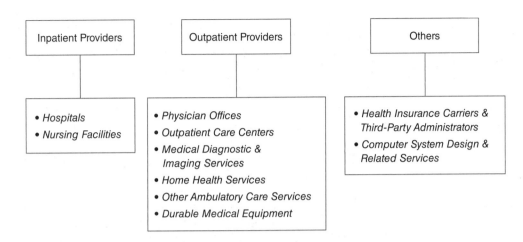

Figure 30–2 Inpatient and Outpatient Providers and Suppliers Impacted by the ICD-10 Transition.
Reproduced from 74 Federal Register 3357 (January 16, 2009).

Version 5010 of Standards and the ICD-10 Transition

Version 5010 of electronic transmission standards includes infrastructure changes that were necessary in order to prepare for the adoption of ICD-10 codes. A whole array of sequential rules and regulations has evolved over the last two decades to create these electronic transaction standards and to require their adoption—a full description of such rules and regulations is well beyond the scope of this text.[9]

Example of Standards Use

However, two particular items are of interest to us in the context of the ICD-10 transition:

1. It was necessary to update many electronic transaction standards in order to accommodate the new ICD-10 codes. The groups, or sets, of codes (termed "standard medical data code sets")[10] to be used in those electronic transactions also had to be updated. (Note that at the time of this writing, the current standard to be adopted is Version 5010, although new versions will inevitably be introduced in the near future.)[11]
2. When the Centers for Medicare and Medicaid Services (CMS) staff compute transition costs, they divide some of these costs between the updating of transaction standards such as Version 5010 (which they argue would have to occur anyway) versus the cost of adopting and implementing the ICD-10 codes. We will be referring to this cost-splitting in a later discussion of implementation costs.

ICD-10 BENEFITS AND COSTS

The ICD-10 transition process will require management decisions that take both costs and benefits into account. A brief summary follows.

Benefits

Management will need to account for what their own organization will realize in conversion savings as benefits. CMS identified six benefits of transitioning to ICD-10:

- More accurate payments for new procedures
- Fewer rejected claims
- Fewer improper claims
- Improved disease management
- Better understanding of health conditions and healthcare outcomes
- Harmonization of disease monitoring and reporting worldwide[12]

In regard to recognition of other benefits, see our comment about cost-splitting in a previous paragraph, as the same concept applies to splitting benefits. Thus, the systems conversion to Version 5010 also recognizes three types of benefits, including operational savings (better standards), cost savings (increase in electronic claims transactions), and operational savings (increase in use of auxiliary transactions).[13]

Managers should also decide what potential governmental financial assistance might be available to their own organization. The ICD-10 conversion is, of course, part (but not all) of this adoption process. It is therefore logical for management to consider part of the financial incentives offered as relating to this system conversion when analyzing benefits. The ARRA legislation described in previous chapters provides financial incentives for the timely adoption of electronic health records.

Costs

Management must make decisions about major costs incurred in the ICD-10 transition, including direct adoption costs and cash flow disruption costs. Some costs will be one-time costs, while other costs will become recurring costs, and this factor must also be considered in the decision-making process.[14]

Three Types of ICD-10 Adoption Costs

CMS acknowledges that transition costs from ICD-9-CM to ICD-10 code sets are unavoidable and are incurred in addition to the Version 5010 standards conversion costs.[15] Three recognized types of ICD-10 adoption costs include the following:

1. System changes
2. Training costs
3. Productivity losses

CMS believes that large providers and institutions will most likely need to make system changes and software upgrades. However, CMS also believes small providers may only need software upgrades.[16] This belief is based upon findings that the majority of small providers have simplistic systems.[17]

Details about training costs and productivity losses are addressed within this chapter. As a final note, also see our comment about cost-splitting in a prior paragraph. Thus, systems conversion to Version 5010 recognizes two similar types of cost: system implementation costs and transition costs.[18]

Cash Flow Disruption Costs

Code set transition has a learning curve for all users. Thus it is to be expected that a greater proportion of claims will be rejected during this learning curve. Rejected claims lead to cash flow disruption, and should be taken into account when decisions are made about implementation costs and benefits.

If certain contracts contain stipulations as to ICD-9 codes, these contracts may have to be renegotiated. The much greater specificity of the ICD-10 codes may make such renegotiation necessary in certain cases, and cash flow from contracts may be disrupted in the interim.

ICD-10 IMPLEMENTATION: SYSTEMS AFFECTED AND TECHNOLOGY ISSUES

ICD-10 implementation affects numerous computerized systems and creates complex technology issues, as discussed in the following sections.

Systems and Applications Affected by the ICD-10 Change

The ICD-10 technology changes that we will discuss in the following section impact a broad variety of systems and applications. It is important for the manager to fully understand the breadth and depth of change that is required by the technological transition from ICD-9 to ICD-10. **Figure 30–3** illustrates the types of systems and applications that must change.

Twenty-five different examples of various systems and applications are contained in Figure 30–3, divided into three categories as follows:

1. Necessary revisions to vendor software and systems
2. Systems used to model or calculate that are impacted
3. Specifications that will need to be revised[19]

Necessary Revisions to Vendor Software and Systems for Transition from ICD-9 to ICD-10 include:

Ambulatory systems
Billing systems
Patient accounting systems
Physician office systems
Practice management systems
Quality measurement systems

Emergency department software
Contract management programs
Reimbursement modeling programs

Financial functions such as:
    Code assignment
    Medical records abstraction
    Claims submission
    Other financial functions

Systems used to model or calculate are also impacted by the use of ICD-10 code sets:

Acuity systems
Decision support systems and content
Patient care systems
Patient risk systems
Staffing needs systems
Selection criteria within electronic medical
    records
Presentation of clinical content for support of
    plans of care

Specifications that will need to be revised for ICD-10 use include specifications for:

Data file extracts
Reporting programs and external interfaces
Analytic software that performs business analysis
Analytic software that provides decision support
    analytics for financial and clinical management
Business rules guided by patient condition or
    procedure

Figure 30–3 Systems and Applications Affected by the ICD-10 Change.

Reproduced from 74 Federal Register 3357 (January 16, 2009).

UNDERSTAND TECHNOLOGY ISSUES AND PROBLEMS

Examining the details of ICD-10 code set changes will help you more fully understand the technological problems that management will face in this transition. The scope of change is illustrated in the next three exhibits.

Comparison of ICD-9-CM and ICD-10-CM Diagnosis Codes

There were approximately 13,000 ICD-9-CM diagnosis codes; now ICD-10-CM has approximately 68,000 diagnosis codes, more than a 500% increase. ICD-9-CM diagnosis codes had three to five characters in length, while ICD-10-CM's characters are three to seven characters in length. This generally means input fields have to be lengthened in order to accommodate seven characters. In addition, ICD-9-CM's first digit may be alpha (E or V) or numeric, and digits two to five are numeric, while ICD-10-CM's first digit is alpha, digits two and three are numeric, and digits four to seven are either alpha or numeric. This change means reprogramming will be required for many applications. **Exhibit 30–1** sets

Exhibit 30–1 Comparison of ICD-9-CM and ICD-10-CM Diagnosis Codes

ICD-9-CM Diagnosis Codes	ICD-10-CM Diagnosis Codes
3–5 characters in length	3–7 characters in length
Approximately 13,000 codes	Approximately 68,000 available codes
First digit may be alpha (E or V) or numeric; digits 2–5 are numeric	Digit 1 is alpha; digits 2 and 3 are numeric; digits 4–7 are alpha or numeric
Limited space for adding new codes	Flexible for adding new codes
Lacks detail	Very specific
Lacks laterality	Has laterality
Difficult to analyze data due to nonspecific codes	Specificity improves coding accuracy and richness of data for analysis
Codes are nonspecific and do not adequately define diagnoses needed for medical research	Detail improves the accuracy of data used for medical research
Does not support interoperability because it is not used by other countries	Supports interoperability and the exchange of health data between other countries and the United States

Reproduced from 73 Federal Register 49803 (August 22, 2008).

out a comparison of ICD-9-CM versus ICD-10-CM diagnosis codes. The exhibit includes six benefits of the new code set in addition to the three differentials previously discussed in this paragraph.[20]

Comparison of ICD-9-CM and ICD-10-PCS Procedure Codes

There were approximately 3,000 ICD-9-CM procedure codes; now ICD-10-PCS has approximately 87,000 available procedure codes, or 29 times as many available codes. ICD-9-CM procedure codes had three to four numbers in length, while ICD-10-CPS's characters are alpha-numeric and seven characters in length. This generally means input fields have to be lengthened in order to accommodate seven characters and possibly reprogrammed to accept alpha characters. **Exhibit 30–2** sets out a comparison of ICD-9-CM versus ICD-10-PCS procedure codes. The exhibit includes seven benefits of the new code set in addition to the two differentials previously discussed in this paragraph.[21]

Exhibit 30–2 Comparison of ICD-9-CM and ICD-10-PCS Procedure Codes

ICD-9-CM Procedure Codes	ICD-10-PCS Procedure Codes
3–4 numbers in length	7 alpha-numeric characters in length
Approximately 3,000 codes	Approximately 87,000 available codes
Based upon outdated technology	Reflects current usage of medical terminology and devices
Limited space for adding new codes	Flexible for adding new codes
Lacks detail	Very specific
Lacks laterality	Has laterality
Generic terms for body parts	Detailed descriptions for body parts
Lacks description of methodology and approach for procedures	Provides detailed descriptions of methodology and approach for procedures
Limits DRG assignment	Allows DRG definitions to better recognize new technologies and devices
Lacks precision to adequately define procedures	Precisely defines procedures with detail regarding body part, approach, any device used, and qualifying information

Reproduced from 73 Federal Register 49803 (August 22, 2008).

AN EXAMPLE: COMPARISON OF OLD AND NEW ANGIOPLASTY CODES

Exhibit 30–3 sets out one example of the proliferation of codes. In the ICD-9-CM, angioplasty had one code (39.50). In the ICD-10-PCS, angioplasty has 1,170 codes.[22] *The Wall Street Journal* even used this example in a headline: "Why We Need 1,170 Angioplasty Codes."[23] (The original 1,170 codes have subsequently been reduced to 874, as shown in Exhibit 30–3.)

ICD-10 IMPLEMENTATION: TRAINING AND LOST PRODUCTIVITY COSTS

This section describes training and lost productivity costs for the ICD-10 transition. Also see this chapter's Appendix, entitled "ICD-10 Conversion Costs for a Midwestern Community Hospital."

WHO GETS TRAINED ON ICD-10?

CMS identified three types of individuals who would require varying levels of training on ICD-10. These included coders, code users, and physicians.

Coders

It is vital that coders receive adequate training on the ICD-10 coding changes. CMS, therefore, estimated training costs for both full-time and part-time coders. In producing cost estimates,

Exhibit 30–3 Comparison of Old and New Angioplasty Codes

Old Code:

ICD-9-CM
Angioplasty
1 code (39.50)

New Code:

ICD-10-PCS
Angioplasty Codes
854 codes

Specifying body part, approach, and device, including:

> 047K04Z Dilation of right femoral artery with drug-eluting intraluminal device, open approach
> 047K0DZ Dilation of right femoral artery with intraluminal device, open approach
> 047K0ZZ Dilation of right femoral artery, open approach
> 047K34Z Dilation of right femoral artery with drug-eluting intraluminal device, percutaneous approach
> 047K3DZ Dilation of right femoral artery with intraluminal device, percutaneous approach

Reproduced from CMS. "ICD-10-CM/PCS: The Next Generation of Coding," ICN #901044 (June 2015).

CMS assumed that full-time coders were primarily dedicated to hospital inpatient coding and that part-time coders worked in outpatient ambulatory settings. The difference is based on the job setting for a reason. CMS further assumed that all coders will need to learn ICD-10-CM, while the coders who work in the hospital inpatient job setting will also need to learn ICD-10-PCS.[24]

Code Users

CMS refers to the American Health Information Management Association (AHIMA) definition of code users as "anyone who needs to have some level of understanding of the coding system, because they review coded data, rely on reports that contain coded data, etc., but are not people who actually assign codes."[25] These users can be people who are outside of healthcare facilities: individuals such as researchers, consultants, or auditors, for example. Or these users might actually be inside the healthcare facility but are not coders. Such facility users might include upper-level management, business office and accounting personnel, clinicians and clinical departments, or corporate compliance personnel.[26]

Physicians

CMS believed that the majority of physicians did not work with codes and thus would not need training. The initial assumption was that only 1 in 10 physicians would require such knowledge. (CMS also believed that physicians would probably obtain the needed training through continuing professional education courses that they would attend anyway.)[27]

COSTS OF TRAINING

ICD-10 training costs were estimated for each category described above: coders, code users, and physicians.

Coder Training Costs

CMS initially assumed the following:

1. There were 50,000 full-time hospital coders that would need 40 hours of training per coder on ICD-10-CM and ICD-10-PCS. The 40 hours of training was estimated to cost $2,750, including lost work time of $2,200, plus $550 for the expenses of training, for a total of $2,750 per coder.
2. Training of full-time coders would start the year before ICD-10 implementation. It was further assumed that 15% of training costs would be expended in this initial year, 75% would be expended in the year of implementation, and the remaining 10% would be expended in the year after implementation.
3. There were approximately 179,000 part-time coders who would require training only on ICD-10-CM (and not on ICD-10-PCS). The part-time coders' training expense would amount to $110 for the expenses of training, plus $440 for lost work time, for a total of $550.[28]

Code Users Training Costs

CMS estimated there were approximately 250,000 code users, of which 150,000 would work directly with codes. Each code user was estimated to need eight hours of training at $31.50 per hour or approximately $250 apiece.[29]

Physician Training Costs

CMS estimated there were approximately 1.5 million physicians in the United States, of which 1 in 10 would require training. Each physician was estimated to need four hours of training at $137 per hour or approximately $548 apiece.[30]

COSTS OF LOST PRODUCTIVITY

CMS used a productivity loss definition as follows: "The cost resulting from a slow-down in coding bills and claims because of the need to learn the new coding systems."[31] Thus, the productivity loss slowdown reflects the extra staff hours that are needed to code the same number of claims per hour as prior to the ICD-10 conversion. (For instance, Jane normally codes x claims per hour; during the first month learning the new system, she slows down to xx claims per hour.)

CMS estimated that inpatient coders would incur productivity losses for the first six months after ICD-10 implementation; they further estimated that productivity would increase (and losses thus decrease) month by month over the initial six-month period until by the end of six months, productivity has returned to its former level. It was estimated that inpatient coders would take an extra 1.7 minutes per inpatient claim in the first month. At $50 per hour, 1.7 minutes equates to $1.41 per claim.[32] ($50.00 per hour divided by 60 minutes equals $0.8333 per minute times 1.7 minutes equals $1.41 per claim.)

CMS assumed the same six-month productivity loss period for outpatient coders. CMS further assumed that outpatient claims require much less time to code. In fact, the initial assumption was that outpatient claims would take one-hundredth of the time for a hospital inpatient claim. Thus, one-hundredth of the inpatient 1.7 minute productivity loss equals 0.017 minutes. At the same $50 per hour, one-hundredth of the $1.41 inpatient loss equals 0.014 per claim, or about 1.5 cents.[33] (To compute one-hundredth of $1.41, move the decimal to the left two places. Thus $1.41 becomes $0.014.) The reasoning for this small amount of coding time per claim is that physician offices "may use preprinted forms or touch-screens that require virtually no time to code."[34]

INTRODUCTION: ABOUT ICD-10 KEY PERFORMANCE INDICATORS

This section defines Key Performance Indicators (KPIs) for ICD-10 transition and maintenance.

What Are ICD-10 Key Performance Indicators (KPIs)?

As the name suggests, these indicators reveal problems regarding ICD-10 implementation and maintenance. The problems may affect productivity and/or cash flow.[35]

How Are ICD-10 KPIs Used?

The ICD-10 KPIs are typically used for two purposes. The KPIs will track your progress in transitioning, maintaining, and updating ICD-10 within your organization. KPIs will also provide opportunities for improvement. Typical improvements include system revisions and/or enhancements, plus specialized staff training to improve productivity lapses.[36]

KEY PERFORMANCE INDICATORS TO ASSESS ICD-10 PROGRESS

The following KPIs are grouped into six categories. The first two categories contain "essential indicators" that any organization should be able to generate.[37]

Four Essential Indicators About Claims

These four indicators should be available to you as they should be tracked by all healthcare organizations as key information regarding claim submission and payment:

Days to Final Bill: The number of days from time of service until the provider generates and submits claims.

Days to Payment: The number of days from the time the claim is submitted until the provider is paid.

Claims Acceptance/Rejection Rates: The percentage of claims that are accepted or rejected during payer "front-end" edits. Front-end edits are those a payer performs before the claim is entered into the payer's adjudication system.

Claims Denial Rate: The percentage of claims accepted into the payer's adjudication system that are denied.

Two Essential Indicators About Payment and Reimbursement Rates

These KPIs can give a picture of both payment amounts received per service and the rate of reimbursement against amounts billed.

Payment Amounts: Payment amounts that your organization receives for specific services, especially high-volume and resource-intensive services.

Reimbursement Rate: Cents on the dollar that your organization receives on claims versus the amount billed on those claims.

Four Coder Productivity Indicators

Productivity is measured by various methods as follows:

Coder Productivity: The number of medical records coded per hour. This indicator should be reviewed separately for each coder.

Volume of Coder Questions: The number of records that coders returned to clinicians with requests for more documentation needed in order to support proper code selection. Again, reviewing this indicator separately for each coder may reveal whether a problem exists with the individual coder or with the particular professional or department generating the source records.

Requests for Additional Information: The number of requests from payers asking for additional information required to process claims. Reviewing this indicator separately by payer may highlight specific coding issues.

Daily Charges/Claims: The number of charges or claims submitted per day. This is a pure productivity indicator for the department.

Three Internal Error Indicators

These indicators concern the individuals or departments that generate the initial information that coders use:

Incomplete or Missing Charges: The number of incomplete or missing charges, analyzed either by the week or the month. Again, separate reviews of particular departments will highlight problems to be solved.

Incomplete or Missing Diagnosis Codes: The number of incomplete or missing ICD-10 diagnosis codes on orders. If ICD-10 implementation is running smoothly, this indicator should almost be zero. Problems, on the other hand, could either be with individuals generating the information or possibly with the software they may be using.

Use of Unspecified Codes: The volume and frequency of unspecified code use. The use of unspecified codes may be perceived as a timesaving maneuver, but it should be tracked and corrected. Unspecified codes cause revenue losses.

Four External Error Indicators

These indicators concern actions by entities outside your own organization:

Clearinghouse Edits: This indicator can be approached in two ways. First, obtain and review the number and content of edits that are required by clearinghouses. Second, obtain and review the number of claims either accepted or rejected by clearinghouses.

Payer Edits: The number and reason for edits required by payers.

Return to Provider (RTP)/Fiscal Intermediary Shared System (FISS) Volumes: The number of rejections in the RTP/FISS volumes.

Medical Necessity Pass Rate: The rate of acceptance (or rejection) of claims with medical necessity content.

A Positive Usage Indicator

This indicator reveals best practices within the coding field:

Use of ICD-10 Codes on Prior Authorizations and Referrals: The number of orders and referrals that include ICD-10 codes.

USING KPIs TO TRACK ICD-10 IMPLEMENTATION PROGRESS

The first step in assessing ICD-10 implementation is to choose the particular KPIs that you intend to use. You may choose from the KPIs listed in **Exhibit 30–4**. Your next steps are as follows.[38]

Exhibit 30–4 Checklist for Assessing ICD-10 Progress: Key Performance Indicators

- Number of days to final bill
- Number of days to payment
- Claims acceptance/rejection rates
- Claims denial rate
- Payment amounts
- Reimbursement rate
- Coder productivity
- Volume of coder questions
- Payer requests for additional information
- Daily charges/claims
- Incomplete or missing charges
- Incomplete or missing diagnosis codes
- Use of unspecified codes
- Clearinghouse edits
- Payer edits
- RTP/FISS volumes
- Medical necessity pass rate
- Use of ICD-10 codes on prior authorizations & referrals

Modified from CMS, "ICD-10: Next Steps for Providers—Assessment & Maintenance Toolkit."

Establish Baselines

It is necessary to establish baselines, or points of comparison, for each of your chosen indicators.

These baselines should be pre-implementation—that is, from a period shortly before your organization implemented ICD-10 codes. If so, you will be able to compare pre- and post-implementation results for your assessment purposes.

Track Your Chosen Indicators

To properly assess KPIs, it is desirable to track your chosen indicators on a periodic pre-set schedule. The schedule should be reasonable as to the timing of assessment dates. For example, should assessments occur on a monthly, quarterly, or semi-annual basis?

Compare Against Baselines

Comparison of pre–ICD-10 implementation versus post–ICD-10 implementation is a most useful process. However, early transition results compared to later transition results are also helpful. In that case, you might find significant improvement in some areas and virtually no improvement in other areas.

Review Results

Some revisions may be desirable after tracking has been in place for several cycles. You may find that you are able to break results into smaller segments for more detailed results. For example, you may decide to keep separate track of authorization denials versus coding denials. Detail about reviewing such results appears in the following section.

REVIEWING KPI RESULTS

This section discusses the review of performance indicator results. Sometimes such reviews are called "troubleshooting," which is a good term to describe this process.

Review "Essential Indicator" Results for Claims and Payment

Taken together, the four essential indicators about claims and the two essential indicators about payment and reimbursement provide a snapshot of your ICD-10 implementation progress. When these six performance indicators from your baseline pre-implementation are compared to results post-implementation, problem areas that require action will be highlighted.

It is also good practice to compare indicators such as "Days to Final Bill" and "Days to Payment" against national or regional standards. If your organization is part of a multi-facility system, it is also a good practice to compare facility-specific results within the system.

Review Coder Productivity and Internal Error Indicator Results

The four coder productivity indicators allow an overview of the internal department or division responsible for coding. If your organization uses an outside billing service, then the important indicator would be "Requests for Additional Information." The outside billing service's requests for more information would be coming back to somewhere in your organization and would indicate an existing problem.

The three internal error indicators relate to places and people within the organization other than coders. If a claim has incomplete or missing charges and/or diagnosis codes, then the coders obviously cannot complete the claim and submit it for payment. In other words, the problem exists elsewhere. Segmenting this review by departments would assist in highlighting the problem area(s).

Review External Error Indicator Results

Claims are sent back by either payers or clearinghouses for further edits. These indicator results may be a people issue or a computer system issue. In either case, the result is unpaid claims and the reasons need to be addressed.

Other claims may be rejected. The results for this indicator have financial impact regarding cash flow. Segmenting the review by department is a good method to explore the reasons for such rejections.

Allow For Feedback

Try to provide a formal system for feedback regarding performance indicator results. One proven method is to create one single "issues list" that resides in one single location. Responsibility for providing the related feedback must then be formally designated.

CREATING ACTION PLANS TO DEAL WITH PROBLEMS

The KPIs are likely to reveal a series of different problems that will vary in their severity. Thus it makes sense to create a set of action plans that are designed to deal with this variety.

What Is an Action Plan?

An action plan consists of a series of steps (actions) that are intended to bring about change of some sort. Each step should be able to answer the following questions:

- What actions or changes will occur?
- Who will carry out these actions or changes?
- When will they take place, and for how long?
- What resources (such as funding and staff) are needed to carry out the actions or changes?
- How will information regarding the actions or changes be communicated (who should know what)?[39]

What Makes a Good Action Plan?

To be successful, your action plan needs to be complete, clear, and current. "Complete" means that the plan lists all the relevant action steps required to accomplish desired actions or changes. "Clear" means that the plan clearly answers the "who, when, what, and communication"questions. "Current" concerns whether the plan actually contains current work.[40] In other words, has the plan anticipated and addressed recently emerging issues, or is it already behind the times by the time it is released?

BUILDING SPECIFIC ACTION PLANS TO CORRECT DEFICIENCIES

This section outlines a selection of issues that could become part of specific action plans. The issues are divided between internal and external matters as follows.[41]

Internal Coding and Systems Action Plan Issues

Action plans typically point toward solutions. Different KPIs are designed to measure performance in different areas that impact productivity, payment, and cash flow. The following issues all require some type of solution.

Isolate Internal Coding Problems

- What codes are causing the most difficulty? What is the particular difficulty, and where within the organization does it originate?
- Who selects diagnosis codes, and who makes sure the codes adhere to guidelines (clinicians, billers, certified coders, others)?
- Would chart audits support selection of a particular ICD-10 code?
- When KPIs expose coding productivity issues, who specifically is responsible for seeing to supplemental training and subsequent tracking to assess any improvements? If such improvements are not forthcoming, what is the next step?

Isolate Internal Systems Problems

- Are certain system deficiencies regarding the ICD-9/ICD-10 transition not yet corrected?
- Are adjustments for annual ICD-10 updates not yet in place and are overdue?
- Have all systems implemented all available upgrades?
- Are there departmental "silo" issues (i.e., do IT [informational technology] supervisors and coding supervisors ever communicate)?

External Coding and Payer Action Plan Issues

Action plans provide structure while working to resolve issues with your payers and your external systems vendors. Producing the relevant data from your KPI process will serve to reinforce the concerns that you are expressing.

Isolate External Coding and Payer Problems

- Is code selection driven by vendor templates? If so, is this acceptable? Can it be changed? If not, why not? Who is responsible for finding out?
- Is the external systems vendor slow to install coding updates to your system? If so, who is responsible for pressuring the vendor to comply? What is the plan if such efforts fail?
- If KPIs expose a consistent claims edit and/or rejection problem with a particular payer, who is specifically responsible for addressing/solving issues with this payer? Under what time frame?
- If KPIs expose consistently slow payments from a particular payer, who is responsible for researching and resolving the issue? If such efforts fail, what is the next step?

Isolate External Systems Problems

- If KPIs expose productivity problems due to an outside systems vendor, is that vendor responsive to your organization's problems? If not, why not?
- Do contractual obligations with the system vendor hinder making changes? Is there a reasonable solution? Who is responsible for negotiating such a solution?
- Does the outside systems vendor provide experienced professionals to work with your staff, or is your organization a training ground for all the vendor's new employees? Is this a problem significant enough to justify inclusion in an action plan?

Untangling Internal Versus External Performance Problems: An Example

It is sometimes difficult to determine whether the root cause of a performance problem is within or outside the organization. An example follows.

This example centers upon the KPI for claims acceptance/rejection rates. For instance, certain problem areas can be isolated by computing the number of days in your accounts receivable for each payer. Problem areas can best be revealed by tracking the age of claims for each payer in 30-day intervals. Thus, how many of payer #1's claims are 0–30 days old? What about 31–60 days old? Or 61–90 days old? Or, even worse, 91–120 or 121-plus days old? What about payer #2? And so on.

In our experience, receiving payment for claims that are older than 90 days is questionable; these old claims should be red flags in your assessment. If you break down your aging assessment by payer, the culprits' red flags should be very evident. It may be that these old claims sitting in your accounts receivable are claims rejected by your payer. On the one hand, does this payer have an extraordinary number of rejected claims, and if so, why? On the other hand, within the internal department, who is responsible for responding to rejected claims by revising and refiling? (Or has the date for doing so on many of the old claims already passed you by?)

Another possibility is that the old claims residing in your accounts receivable are actually denied claims. Again, does the payer have an extraordinary number of denied claims, and if so, why? Or, within the internal departments, who is responsible for pursuing secondary payers? Why haven't they been doing so? Or are the claims so old that payment from anyone is not viable? If so, they should be written off the books as bad debts.

Understanding the Lines of Authority

As in the preceding example, it is helpful to clearly understand the lines of authority concerned with your issues. In other words, what department, office, division, or individual is in charge of the procedures that you are attempting to revise? What is the chance that this department, office, division, or individual will cooperate? It is likely that some member of the task force or one of your supervisors should be able to help define the applicable lines of authority that are relevant.

ICD-10 IMPLEMENTATION: SITUATIONAL ANALYSIS

System implementation on this scale requires multiple planning cycles. Recommendations for implementation planning that include situational analysis are described as follows.

IMPLEMENTATION PLANNING RECOMMENDATIONS

CMS recommends that healthcare organizations plan for implementation of ICD-10-CM/PCS by developing a three-step organizational plan that includes the following:

- Step 1: Situational Analysis
- Step 2: Strategic Implementation/Organizing
- Step 3: Planning for Strategic Control[42]

Figure 30–4 illustrates these steps. We believe that development of a timeline and a map of individual responsibilities should also be an important part of this planning process, as follows:

1. Situational Analysis: Situational analysis is defined and discussed in the following section.
2. Strategic Implementation and Organizing: The strategic implementation and organizing planning step includes acquiring the resources to implement the plan and evaluating the financial impact of the plan. In actual fact, these two steps should be reversed, as the scope of the financial impact should be considered before resources are acquired.
3. Planning for Strategic Control: Developing objectives should, of course, be the first step in planning for strategic control. The remaining planning recommendations are action steps. They include planning measurement tools, evaluation strategies, and actions to implement.[43]

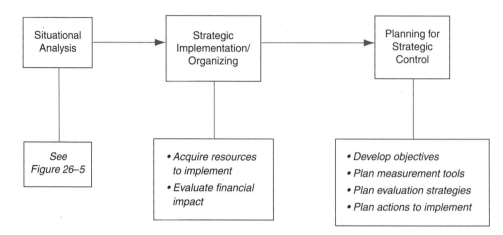

Figure 30–4 System Implementation Planning Recommendations.
Adapted from the Centers for Medicare and Medicaid Services, "ICD-10 Clinical Modification/Procedure Coding System." ICN #901044 (October 2008).

SITUATIONAL ANALYSIS RECOMMENDATIONS

This section provides background plus recommendations for an ICD-10 situational analysis.

Background

You will recall that situational analysis does two things. It reviews the organization's internal operations for strengths and weaknesses and it explores the organization's external environment for opportunities and threats. Thus it is called "SWOT," for strengths-weaknesses-opportunities-threats.

Situational analysis is particularly appropriate for the analysis of electronic records systems implementation such as ICD-10 because such implementation requires the collaboration of multiple knowledge areas. A meeting of the minds can better occur with the discipline that a situational analysis can impose. As we have previously said, it is a powerful tool when properly applied.

CMS Recommendations for ICD-10 Adoption

CMS recommends six steps for an ICD-10 adoption situational analysis. We believe the six steps should be divided into two parts. The first part contains strategic steps that must be addressed at the beginning of the project. The second part of the analysis contains developmental steps that we believe can only be properly accomplished after the strategic steps have been completed. (That said, however, we must also acknowledge that sometimes immovable deadlines and/or lack of sufficient planning resources do not allow the ideal two-part process.) **Figure 30–5** illustrates the CMS situational analysis recommendations for ICD-10 adoption.

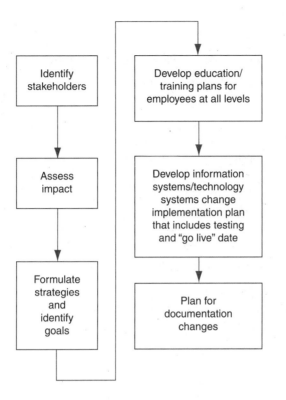

Figure 30–5 Situational Analysis Recommendations.

Adapted from the Centers for Medicare and Medicaid Services. "ICD-10 Clinical Modification/Procedure Coding System." ICN #901044 (October 2008).

Strategic Steps

The strategic steps that CMS recommends include three steps, as follows:

1. Stakeholders: Step 1 is to identify stakeholders. This traditional first step is an important beginning point for the analysis. The array of stakeholders will vary depending upon the size and nature of the healthcare organization. Payers should always be one of the stakeholders. Regulatory agencies may also be recognized as stakeholders.
2. Impacts: Step 2 involves assessing the impact of the ICD-10 transition. Impacts on all aspects of the organization should be recognized. As with stakeholders, the transition's impact will also vary significantly depending upon the size and type of healthcare organization.
3. Strategies and Goals: Step 3 involves formulating strategies and identifying goals. The larger the organization the more likely there will be competing strategies and goals. Compromises may have to be negotiated. Tight deadlines and/or lack of planning resources may work to shortchange this component of the situational analysis.[44]

Developmental Steps

The developmental steps that CMS recommends also include three steps, discussed as follows. Note that different knowledge areas are required for these different steps.

1. Training Plans: Training plans must be developed for employees at all levels. The cost of training for ICD-10-CM/PCS implementation is discussed and illustrated earlier in this chapter.
2. Systems Change Implementation Plan: Information systems and/or technology systems "change implementation plans" must be developed. These plans must include timelines and individual responsibilities. The timelines should leave sufficient time for testing. (Insufficient testing time is a common pitfall.) A "go live" date is another important part of this plan. If hardware and/or software vendors are involved in a facility's implementation plan, all timelines and the final "go live" date must also be coordinated closely with the vendor.
3. Documentation Change Plan: The documentation change plan will hopefully cover all areas of the organization where documents exist that will reflect ICD-10-CM/PCS changes. A document inventory is the ideal beginning point for a documentation change plan. The inventory allows for a full and complete change plan, but lack of resources often means completing the full document inventory is not possible.[45]

COMMENCING AN INFORMATION TECHNOLOGY SWOT MATRIX FOR ICD-10

This section discusses building a situational analysis matrix. The example used involves ICD-10 adoption as the project under consideration and information technology as the division or department involved in the project.

Background

Building a SWOT matrix can be an important strategic process. Each of the four components of a SWOT (strengths, weaknesses, opportunities, and threats) was discussed in a previous chapter about strategic planning. The SWOT analysis matrix containing all four components was also presented in that chapter. You will recall that the "Strengths" and "Weaknesses" sectors of the matrix were labeled "Internal," while the "Opportunities" and "Threats" sectors were labeled "External." We will use this format in the following section.

Building the Matrix

As to the internal components, the SWOT team or task force needs to evaluate resources and thus identify those that should belong in the strengths and weaknesses sectors of the SWOT matrix. For example, for an IT analysis such as the ICD-10 adoption issue, the team might enter "Financial Resources" as a main heading and "Capital Resources Available" as one of the Financial Resources subheadings in the strengths and weaknesses categories.

The team might also enter "Information Technology" as a main heading. Because this is an IT project, some of the subheadings in the strengths and weaknesses categories might include the following:

- IT Hardware Resources
- IT Software Resources
- IT Storage Capacity
- IT Staffing Capacity
- IT Staffing Knowledge Levels

Understand that the SWOT matrix is built as these resources are evaluated. As to the external components, the SWOT team or task force would likewise evaluate the external opportunities

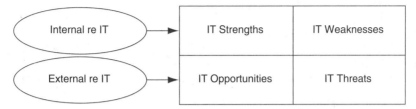

Figure 30–6 Basic Information Technology SWOT Analysis Format.

and threats as a parallel exercise. In an IT analysis such as the ICD-10 adoption issue, the team might logically enter the government's incentive payment as an external opportunity (potential dollars received) and an external threat (compliance requirements to be met).

The basic SWOT matrix in its present stage is illustrated in **Figure 30–6**. For further information about building a situational analysis, see the SWOT Worksheets and related Question Guides that appear as an Appendix to the Strategic Planning chapter.

SUMMARY

The four-part SWOT matrix is built as the key internal resources, both strengths and weaknesses, are evaluated, and the key external opportunities and threats are identified and evaluated. We can tie the CMS recommendations in the preceding section to the process of building a SWOT matrix as follows. Identifying stakeholders and commencing to assess impacts of the ICD-10 adoption are considered part of building the SWOT matrix. Formulating strategies and identifying goals would most likely come after building the initial matrix, because these actions would be influenced and should naturally carry forward from the evaluations performed as part of the SWOT matrix-building process. Finally, the remaining three developmental steps, each of which involves creating a plan, should all come as final steps in the situational analysis process.

As we have previously mentioned, there are a variety of approaches to performing a situational analysis, and this brief discussion features only the single approach as recommended by CMS. The important point is this: no matter what approach is utilized, a situational analysis is an important planning tool.

INFORMATION CHECKPOINT

What is needed?	An ICD-10 newsletter or course announcement or an ICD-10 training manual.
Where is it found?	Within your place of work or posted on the website of an industry trade organization.
How is it used?	It is used for the purpose of ICD-10 training.

KEY TERMS

Code Users
ICD-10 Codes
Key Performance Indicator (KPI)

Situational Analysis
SWOT Analysis
Version 5010 of Standards

DISCUSSION QUESTIONS

1. Do you believe your place of work (the organization) has been affected by the ICD-10 transition? If so, how has your organization been affected? If not, why not?
2. Has your own area of work been involved in the transition to ICD-10? If so, are you aware of how your organization managed the transition? (Through task force, planning committees, etc.)
3. Do you think using KPIs is a good idea? Does your organization use these types of indicators? If so, please describe.

NOTES

1. *National Center for Health Statistics, International Classification of Diseases, Tenth Revision* (ICD-10), www.cdc.gov/nchs/about/major/dvs/icd10des.htm
2. World Health Organization, Classifications, www.who.int/classifications/icd/en/
3. Centers for Medicare and Medicaid Services (CMS), "ICD-10 Clinical Modification /Procedure Coding System Fact Sheet." www.cms.hhs.gov/MLNProducts/downloads /ICD-10factsheet2008.pdf
4. National Center for Health Statistics (NCHS), About the *International Classification of Diseases, Tenth Revision, Clinical Modification* (ICD-10-CM), www.cdc.gov/nchs/icd /icd10cm.htm
5. CMS, "ICD-10-CM-PCS Fact Sheet."
6. Ibid.
7. 77 Federal Register (FR) 54665 (September 5, 2012).
8. 74 Federal Register (FR) 3357 (January 16, 2009).
9. CMS, "New Health Care Electronic Transactions Standards Versions 5010, D.0, and 3.0," Medicare Learning Network Fact Sheet ICN #903192 (January 2010).
10. 74 Federal Register (FR) 3328 (January 16, 2009).
11. 73 Federal Register (FR) 49745 (August 22, 2008).
12. 73 Federal Register (FR) 49821 (August 22, 2008).
13. Ibid., 49769.
14. Ibid., 49811.
15. Ibid., 49813.
16. Ibid., 49818.
17. Ibid., 49829.
18. Ibid., 49769.
19. 74 Federal Register (FR) 3348-9 (January 16, 2009).
20. 73 Federal Register (FR) 49803 (August 22, 2008).
21. Ibid.
22. CMS, "ICD-10-CM-PCS Fact Sheet."
23. J. Zhang, "Why We Need 1,170 Angioplasty Codes," *Wall Street Journal*, November 11, 2008.
24. 73 Federal Register (FR) 49814-5 (August 22, 2008).

25. Ibid., 49815-6.

26. Ibid., 49815.

27. Ibid., 49816.

28. Ibid., 49815.

29. Ibid., 49816 and 74 Federal Register (FR) 3346-7 (January 16, 2009).

30. Ibid., 49816.

31. M. Libicki and I. Brahmakulam, *The Costs and Benefits of Moving to the ICD-10 Code Sets* (Santa Monica, CA: RAND Corporation, 2004), 10, http://www.rand.org/pubs /technical_reports/2004/RAND_TR132.pdf

32. 73 Federal Register (FR) 49816 (August 22, 2008) and 74 Federal Register (FR) 3346-7 (January 16, 2009).

33. 73 Federal Register (FR) 49817 (August 22, 2008).

34. Ibid., 49816-7.

35. CMS, "ICD-10 KPIs at a Glance," March 9, 2016, www.cms.gov/Medicare/Coding/ICD10 /Downloads/ICD10KPIs20160309.pdf

36. CMS, "ICD-10 Next Steps for Providers: Assessment & Maintenance Toolkit," February 26, 2016, https://www.cms.gov/Medicare/Coding/ICD10/Downloads/ICD10NextStepsTool kit20160226.pdf

37. Certain KPI information within this section may be modified and/or condensed from "ICD-10 Next Steps...Assessment & Maintenance Toolkit."

38. Ibid.

39. Work Group for Community Health and Development at the University of Kansas, "Developing an Action Plan," http://ctb.ku.edu/table-of-contents/structure/strategic -planning/develop-action-plans/main, accessed July 14, 2016.

40. Ibid.

41. Some concepts within this section may be modified and/or condensed from "ICD-10 Next Steps."

42. CMS, "ICD-10-CM-PCS Fact Sheet."

43. Ibid.

44. Ibid.

45. Ibid.

ICD-10 Conversion Costs for a Midwestern Community Hospital

AUTHORS' NOTE

This CMS example illustrates the computation of hospital training costs and productivity loss costs and estimates a cost for system changes and upgrades in order to arrive at a total hospital ICD-10 conversion cost. We have numbered the paragraphs for easy reference. (And FYI, when the scenario below says "we" it means CMS, not the authors.)

INTRODUCTION

To further illustrate the computation of hospital ICD-10 conversion costs, CMS staff developed a scenario for a typical community hospital in the Midwest.[1] The material presented in the appendix was published in the proposed rule as an example of costs that might be incurred by a hospital. The data were drawn from the American Hospital Directory, available at www.AHD .com. While based on an actual hospital in a Midwestern state, the data have been altered to make calculations simpler.

THE SCENARIO

1. The hospital has 100 beds, 4,000 discharges annually, and gross revenues of $200 million. Using the factors presented in the impact analysis, we estimated training costs (including the cost of the actual training as well as lost time away from the job), productivity loss for the first six months resulting from becoming familiar with the diagnostic and procedure codes, and the cost of system changes.
2. For our scenario, we assumed that the hospital employs three full-time coders who will require eight hours of training at $500 per coder for $1,500 ($500 times 3). While they are in training, the hospital will have to substitute other staff, either by hiring temporary coders if possible, or by shifting staff. The estimated cost at $50 per hour is $1,200 (8 hours times 3 staff times $50 per hour).
3. In estimating the productivity loss, we are only looking at the initial six months after implementation. Therefore, we divided the annual number of discharges of 4,000 by 2 to equal 2,000. We assume that three-quarters of the discharges are surgical, giving us 1,500 discharges requiring use of PCS codes. Dividing this by six months yields an average monthly discharge rate of 250.

4. We performed a similar calculation for outpatient claims. Of the 13,000 outpatient claims, the monthly average is 1,083 (we do not distinguish between medical and surgical outpatient claims).

5. Applying the 1.7 extra minutes per discharge, we estimated it would take an extra 425 minutes (1.7 times 250) to code the discharges in the first month. At $50 per hour, the cost per minute is $0.83 ($50 divided by 60 minutes) and the cost per claim is $1.41 ($0.83 times 1.7). For the first month, the productivity loss for inpatient coding is $353 ($1.41 times 250). Assuming for simplicity's sake that the resumption of productivity over the six-month period would increase in a straight line, we divide the $353 by six to come up with $59. We reduce the productivity loss by this amount each month through the sixth month. The total loss for the six-month period is $1,233.

6. We apply the same method to determine the outpatient productivity loss. Based on our assumption that outpatient claims will require one-hundredth of the time for hospital inpatient claims, when applying the 0.17 extra minutes per claim, we estimate it would take an extra 18.41 minutes (0.017 times 1,083) to code the discharges in the first month. At $50 per hour, the cost per minute is $0.83 ($50 divided by 60 minutes) and the cost per claim is $0.14 ($0.83 times 0.017). For the first month, the productivity loss for outpatient coding is $15.28 ($0.014 times 1,083). Assuming for simplicity sake that the resumption of productivity over the six-month period would increase in a straight line, we divide the $15.28 by six, coming up with $2.55. We reduce the productivity loss by this amount each month through the sixth month. Thus the total loss for the first six months will equal $53.

7. In estimating the cost of system changes and software upgrades, we deliberately chose a value that we think overstates the cost. We assumed that the hospital will have to spend $300,000 on its data infrastructure to accommodate the new codes. Summing the training costs, productivity losses, and system upgrades, we estimate the total cost to the hospital will equal approximately $303,990. Finally, in order to determine the percentage of the hospital's revenue that would be diverted to funding the conversion to the ICD-10, we compared the estimated cost associated with the conversion to ICD-10 to the total hospital revenue of $200 million. The costs amount to 0.15% of the hospital's annual revenues.

8. We note that although the impact in our scenario of 0.15% is significantly larger than the estimated impact of 0.03% for inpatient facilities (set out in the rule), it is still significantly below the threshold the Department considers a significant economic impact. We are of the opinion that, for most providers and suppliers, payers, and computer firms involved in facilitating the transition, the costs will be relatively small.

NOTE

1. 73 Federal Register 49830 (August 22, 2008).

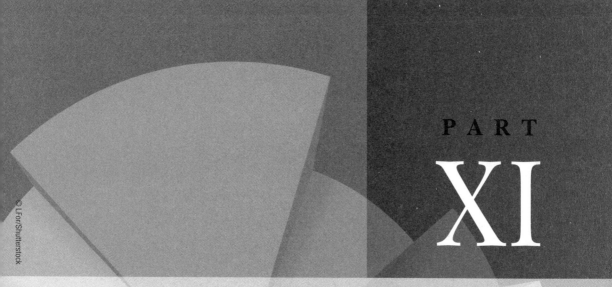

PART

XI

Case Studies

Case Study: The Doctor's Dilemma

THE OFFER: "SELL YOUR PRACTICE TO US"

This case study explores a doctor's dilemma: Should he sell his practice? Dr. John Matthews, a cardiac surgeon, has been approached by the administrator of Clinton Memorial Hospital to ascertain his level of interest in selling his practice. Dr. Matthews has admitting privileges at the hospital. He has been reading about the Feds' speeding up plans for value-based payments, wherein half of provider payments in five years will be linked to quality of care. In essence, the intent according to DHHS (U.S. Department of Health & Human Services) officials is to cut down on the volume of unnecessary procedures while improving patient outcomes.

Dr. Matthews understands that a complex time lies ahead. As the shift from volume to value gains momentum, both Clinton Memorial and his own practice will need to move quickly to understand the likely trajectory in their markets, to identify their desired role, and to make the significant structural and operational changes needed to succeed in the changing business model.

SEEKING TO UNDERSTAND HEALTHCARE FINANCE REFORM

While still considering the hospital's entreaty, Dr. Matthews feels that he needs to learn more about these concepts that constitute healthcare finance reform. At hospital medical staff meetings, accountable care organizations (ACOs) and bundled payments are frequently on the agenda. In general, Dr. Matthews has been able to ascertain that providers are wary of jumping head first into risk-sharing payment models, or risk contracting based on quality and cost.

Dr. Patrick Conway, Chief Medical Officer for the Centers for Medicare and Medicaid Services (CMS), said that through its Medicare Shared Savings Program (MSSP), 50% of all fee-for-service payments to providers will be tied to quality incentives (hitting quality metrics) through alternative payment models—particularly ACOs and bundled payments, which are also expected to slow the growth of healthcare costs. As the name implies, MSSP providers share in the savings through a percentage of funds that goes back to the ACO.

ACOs are provider groups that accept responsibility for the cost and quality of care delivered to a specific population of patients cared for by the groups' clinicians. Under these risk- and value-based payment models that reward achieving cost and outcomes of care, provider organizations have incentives to keep people well.[1] The organizations also provide data to be used in assessing their performance on cost and quality criteria.[2]

A bundled payment is a single payment to providers and/or healthcare facilities for all services to treat a given condition or provide a given treatment. Payments are made to the providers on the basis of expected costs for clinically defined episodes that may involve several practitioner types, settings of care, and services or procedures over time. When designed to improve value, bundled payments should include clear quality metrics focused on desired clinical outcomes that providers must achieve to maximize their payment.[3] These payments are perhaps even more key to reforming healthcare finance because they address specific issues of care and quality directly and could be more quickly adopted than ACOs.

RESEARCHING ACQUISITION VIEWPOINTS AND INDUSTRY TRENDS

Having achieved a better understanding of contemporary healthcare finance, Dr. Matthews turned his attention back to the acquisition question. Interestingly, Clinton Memorial's inquiry comes amidst a trend that, at first, found the acquisition rate of hospitals acquiring medical groups slowing in the past few years, with the apex having already occurred in 2011.[4]

A Negative View

The budgets of many of these same hospitals that once prioritized physician practice acquisitions are now in the red, causing administrators to rethink their practice acquisition strategies. A 2013 report from the Medical Group Management Association calculated a median loss for employing a physician to be $176,463.[5] This has led analysts such as Moody's to predict a pullback on physician practice acquisitions as costs continue to outpace revenue. In fact, Moody's identified physician employment as one of the largest expenses impacting hospitals' margin pressure.

Hospitals acquire physician practices in order to expand their networks, which they hope will in turn boost their revenues. However, in doing so, they also incur the costs associated with physician/employee salaries, benefits, office space, and necessary upgrades to IT infrastructures.

A Positive View

The above notwithstanding, the emerging macro view suggests something quite different. Provider mergers and acquisitions in the first three quarters of 2014 were up a robust 13.4% over the same period in 2013 according to Modern Healthcare's Merger and Acquisition Report.[6] This suggests that mergers, acquisitions, and partnerships will continue apace as healthcare reform reshapes the industry.

In fact, an outsize example of this trend is Baylor Healthcare System's recent merger with Scott & White Healthcare, a move that resulted in Texas's largest nonprofit healthcare provider. The merger produced a system that includes 48 hospitals, more than 40,000 employees, and more than $9 billion in assets.[7]

Another Industry Trend

Moreover, consolidation in the health industry is also occurring among insurers, with Anthem poised to acquire rival Cigna, and Aetna and Humana agreeing to a $37 billion marriage.[8] It should be noted, however, that regulators are not standing by idly.

The Federal Trade Commission is planning to block a merger between two large Illinois hospital groups, Advocate Health Care and North-Shore University Health System. Should the merger be approved, it would create a 16-hospital system that would dominate the North Shore area of Chicago.[9]

CONSIDERING OTHER PHYSICIANS' REACTIONS

Dr. Matthews also wants to know what other physicians think about practice acquisitions. He approaches the question from two directions, as follows.

What Others Who Sold May Have Believed

Amidst these complex trends, Dr. Matthews knows that many physicians who choose to sell their practices to a hospital or hospital system believe that doing so will allow them to spend more time with their patients. While it may appear that they have more regular hours and thus encounter fewer administrative hassles, they also end up feeling less productive because they lose the ability to have final say on their schedules. Instead, hospital administrators become the individuals in charge of setting doctors' office and on-call hours.

How Colleagues of His Who Sold Have Reacted

At this juncture, Dr. Matthews deemed it wise to call recently acquired physician colleagues to monitor how they reacted to the transition. He also knows there is a need for evidence-based management and business practice information that help physicians to better understand the business aspects of their practice.

WHAT WILL DR. MATTHEWS DECIDE?

We cannot predict the doctor's decision, because we do not have enough information about his practice's situation. But we can pose a question: Are doctors happier now, or are cost-cutting measures causing them to miss the autonomy of being a private-practice owner? And one thing is clear: Healthcare organizations must do better in incorporating change management and cultural integration into their merger and acquisition strategy.

NOTES

1. S. M. Shortell, "Creating Accountable Communities for Health," *H&HN: American Hospital Association*, July 2015.
2. S. M. Shortell, L. P. Casalino, and E. S. Fisher, "How the Centers for Medicare and Medicaid Innovation Should Test Accountable Care Organizations," *Health Affairs*, 29, no. 7 (2010): 1293–1298.
3. S. Delbanco, "The Payment Reform Landscape: Bundled Payment," *Health Affairs Blog*, July 2, 2014.
4. D. Doyle, "Why the Hospital Buying Spree May Be Coming to an End," Physician's Practice, March 29, 2014, www.physicianspractice.com

5. Medical Group Management Association, "MGMA Data Drive Cost and Revenue 2013," www.mgma.com, 2013.
6. B. Kutscher, "Expect More Not-for-Profit Hospital Mergers and Acquisitions," October 21, 2014, www.modernhealthcare.com/article/2014102/NEWS/31029964
7. G. Jacobson, "Baylor Health Care System, Scott & White Complete Their Merger," *Dallas Morning News*, Section D-1, March 2, 2016.
8. M. McArdle, "Supersizing the Health Industry," *The Week*, August 7, 2015.
9. R. Abelson, "Regulators Tamp Down on Mergers of Hospital," *New York Times*, December 19, 2015.

Case Study: Strategic Financial Planning in Long-Term Care

Neil R. Dworkin, PhD

BACKGROUND

John Maxwell, CEO of Seabury Nursing Center, a not-for-profit long-term care organization located in suburban Connecticut, had just emerged from a board of directors meeting. He was contemplating the instructions he had received from the board's executive committee to assess the financial feasibility of adding a home care program to the Center's array of services.

Seabury's current services consist of two levels of inpatient care, chronic care, and subacute units, and a senior citizens' apartment complex financed in part by the Federal Department of Housing and Urban Development. In keeping with its mission, Seabury has a reputation of providing personalized, high-quality, and compassionate care across all levels of its continuum.

The CEO and his executive team agreed to meet the following week to plan the next steps.

FRAMEWORK OF THE BOARD'S MANDATE

At its last retreat, the board made clear that, reimbursement and payment systems notwithstanding, Seabury must establish realistic and achievable financial plans that are consistent with their strategic plans. Accordingly, three points relative to integrating strategic planning and financial planning should hold sway:

1. Both are the primary responsibility of the board
2. Strategic planning should precede financial planning
3. The board should play an active role in the financial planning process

Ultimately, every important investment decision involves three general principles:

1. Does it make sense financially?
2. Does it make sense operationally?
3. Does it make sense politically?

The board's interest in a possible home initiative was guided by these stipulations, particularly as they relate to Seabury's growth rate in assets and profitability objectives. As a result of the financial downturn, the organization is experiencing declining inpatient volumes, a deteriorating payer mix, and a higher cost of capital, all of which have the potential to weaken its liquidity position.

Taking the strategic service line path to a home care program would be less capital intensive and should appeal broadly to the significant baby boomer population residing in its service area, whose preference would undoubtedly be to be treated in their homes.

INDUSTRY PROFILE

When John Maxwell convened his executive team the following week, he had already decided to present an overview of the home health industry as gleaned by Seabury's Planning Department. He prefaced his comments by drawing on recent research by the federal Agency for Healthcare Research and Quality that detailed why home health care in the 21st century is different from that which has existed in the past. He cited four reasons:

1. We're living longer and more of us want to "age in place" with dignity.
2. We have more chronic, complex conditions.
3. We're leaving the hospital earlier and thus need more intensive care.
4. Sophisticated medical technology has moved into our homes. Devices that were used only in medical offices are now in our living rooms and bedrooms. For example, home caregivers regularly manage dialysis treatments, infuse strong medications via central lines, and use computer-based equipment to monitor the health of loved ones.[1]

The CEO presented a profile of national home care data as compiled by the National Association for Home Care and Hospice as follows:

- Approximately 12 million people in the United States require some form of home health care.
- More than 33,000 home healthcare providers exist today.
- Almost two-thirds (63.8%) of home healthcare recipients are women.
- More than two-thirds (69.1%) of home healthcare recipients are over age 65.
- Conditions requiring home health care most frequently include diabetes, heart failure, chronic ulcer of the skin, osteoarthritis, and hypertension.
- Medicare is the largest single payer of home care services. In 2009, Medicare spending was approximately 41% of the total home healthcare and hospice expenditure.[2]

According to the U.S. Census Bureau, he continued, in 2010 Connecticut's population was 3,574,097 of which 14.4% were age 65 or older.[3] A Visiting Nurse Association (VNA) analysis of revenue by payer source in the state indicated that 60% of revenue was derived from Medicare.[4]

FEASIBILITY DETERMINATION

The CEO went on to explain that the feasibility determination would be based on initially setting the home care program's capacity at 50 clients because that was the minimum required for Certificate-of-Need (CON) approval in Connecticut. He distributed a model developed by healthcare finance expert William O. Cleverly (**Figure 32–1**), which presents the *logic* behind the integration of strategic and financial planning.

In essence, he said, financial planning is influenced by the definition of programs and services in consort with the mission and goals. The next step entails financial feasibility of the

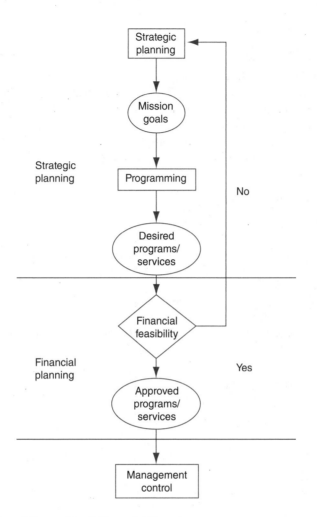

Figure 32–1 Integration of Strategic and Financial Planning.
Reproduced from W. O. Cleverley, *Essentials of Health Care Finance,* 7th ed. (Sudbury, MA: Jones & Bartlett), 289.

proposed homecare program. Among the components that should be considered in determining financial feasibility are the following:

- The configuration and cost of staff
- The prevailing Medicare and Medicaid reimbursement rates
- A projection of visit frequency by provider category based on the most prevalent clinical conditions
- The physical location of the program and its attendant costs (e.g., rent, new construction)
- A projection of cash flows

Direct care staff associated with the home care program includes:

- Medical Social Worker (MSW)
- Physical Therapist (PT)
- Home Health Aide (HHA)

- Registered Nurse (RN)
- Registered Dietitian (RD)

Maxwell indicated that it would be useful to create a scenario depicting a home health visit abstract incorporating prevailing Medicare and Medicaid reimbursement rates for a 70-year-old male with heart failure and no comorbidities in order to gain traction and project potential cash flow. As previously noted, heart failure is a condition frequently requiring home health-care services. Productivity in the home is typically based on the average number of visits per day by provider category. The visit scenario is depicted in **Table 32–1**.

Table 32–1 A Home Health Visit Scenario

Services	Visit Frequency	Payer	Rate	Rate x 4.2*	Medicare Cost	Medicaid Cost
Nursing (RN)	2x/month, every other week	Mc	$ 166.83	$ 700.69	$ 700.69	
Medical Social Worker (MSW)	Visits wkly for 4 wks	MA	$ 119.51	$ 501.94		$ 501.94
Physical Therapist (PT)	3x wkly for 2 wks	Mc	$ 103.22	$ 433.52	$ 433.52	
Home Health Aide (HHA)	Visits 4hrs MWF wkly for 60 days	Mc	$ 25.00	$ 1,260.00	$ 1,260.00	
Registered Dietitian (RD)	3x wkly for 1 wk	MA	$ 103.16			$ 309.48

Mc = Medicare

MA = Medicaid

*4.2 = The state's formula for the #wks/per month

Total monthly Medicaid budget = $826.95

Total monthly Medicare budget = $2,394.21

Once the board decides to move ahead with the home care program and it is approved by the state, implementation and ongoing operations becomes a management control issue (see the Cleverly model in Figure 32–1). The CEO refers to a proposed table of organization as illustrated in **Figure 32–2**.

Given the paucity of other home care programs in its service area, Maxwell knows that Seabury is likely to be accorded a green light.

As he and his team reflect on this, the looming question will be where will the clients come from? He knows that likely referral sources will include Seabury's subacute inpatient population and residents from its senior citizens' apartment complex who are "aging in place." Other likely sources will be recently discharged patients from the region's two community hospitals, both bereft of home care programs. A premium will be placed on effective case management, and direct marketing to the community will also be necessary.

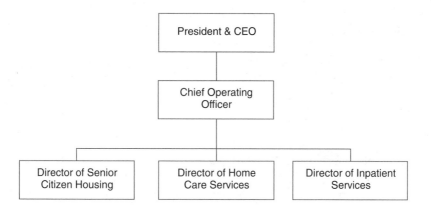

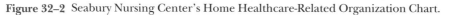

Figure 32–2 Seabury Nursing Center's Home Healthcare-Related Organization Chart.

NOTES

1. U.S. Department of Health and Human Services, "Human Factors Challenges in Home Health Care," *Research Activities*, no. 376 (December 2011).
2. National Association for Home Care and Hospice, *Basic Statistics about Home Care* (Updated 2010).
3. Department of Commerce, U.S. Census Bureau, *2010 Demographic Profile.*
4. Visiting Nurse Association, *VNA Healthcare Annual Report* (Hartford, CT: Hartford Healthcare, 2012).

Case Study: Metropolis Health System

BACKGROUND

1. The Hospital System

Metropolis Health System (MHS) offers comprehensive healthcare services. It is a mid-size taxing district hospital. Although MHS has the power to raise revenues through taxes, it has not done so for the past seven years.

2. The Area

MHS is located in the town of Metropolis, which has a population of 50,000. The town has a small college and a modest number of environmentally clean industries.

3. MHS Services

MHS has taken significant steps to reduce hospital stays. It has developed a comprehensive array of services that are accessible, cost-effective, and responsive to the community's needs. These services are wellness oriented in that they strive for prevention rather than treatment. As a result of these steps, inpatient visits have increased overall by only 1,000 per year since 2010 whereas outpatient/same-day surgery visits have had an increase of over 50,000 per year.

A number of programmatic, service, and facility enhancements support this major transition in the community's institutional health care. They are geared to provide the quality, convenience, affordability, and personal care that best suit the health needs of the people whom MHS serves.

- Rehabilitation and Wellness Center—for outpatient physical therapy and return-to-work services, plus cardiac and pulmonary rehabilitation, to get people back to a normal way of living.
- Home Health Services—bringing skilled care, therapy, and medical social services into the home; a comfortable and affordable alternative in longer-term care.
- Same-Day Surgery (SDS)—eliminating the need for an overnight stay. Since 2010 same-day surgery procedures have doubled at MHS.
- Skilled Nursing Facility—inpatient service to assist patients in returning more fully to an independent lifestyle.

- Community Health and Wellness—community health outreach programs that provide educational seminars on a variety of health issues, a diabetes education center, support services for patients with cancer, health awareness events, and a women's health resource center.
- Occupational Health Services—helping to reduce workplace injury costs at over 100 area businesses through consultation on injury avoidance and work-specific rehabilitation services.
- Recovery Services—offering mental health services, including substance abuse programs and support groups, along with individual and family counseling.

4. MHS's Plant

The central building for the hospital is in the center of a two-square-block area. A physicians' office building is to the west. Two administrative offices, converted from former residences, are on one corner. The new ambulatory center, completed two years ago, has an L shape and sits on one corner of the western block. A laundry and maintenance building sits on the extreme back of the property. A four-story parking garage is located on the eastern back corner. An employee parking lot sits beside the laundry and maintenance building. Visitor parking lots fill the front eastern portion of the property. A helipad is on the extreme western edge of the property behind the physicians' office building.

5. MHS Board of Trustees

Eight local community leaders who bring diverse skills to the board govern MHS. The trustees generously volunteer their time to plan the strategic direction of MHS, thus ensuring the system's ability to provide quality comprehensive health care to the community.

6. MHS Management

A chief executive officer manages MHS. Seven senior vice presidents report to the CEO. MHS is organized into 23 major responsibility centers.

7. MHS Employees

All 500 team members employed by MHS are integral to achieving the high standards for which the system strives. The quality improvement program, reviewed and reestablished in 2010, is aimed at meeting client needs sooner, better, and more cost-effectively. Participants in the program are from all areas of the system.

8. MHS Physicians

The MHS medical staff is a key part of MHS's ability to provide excellence in health care. Over 75 physicians cover more than 30 medical specialties. The high quality of their training and their commitment to the practice of medicine are great assets to the health of the community.

The physicians are very much a part of MHS's drive for continual improvement on the quality of healthcare services offered in the community. MHS brings in medical experts from around the country to provide training in new techniques, made possible by MHS's technologic advancements. MHS also ensures that physicians are offered seminars, symposiums, and continuing education programs that permit them to remain current with changes in the medical field.

The medical staff's quality improvement program has begun a care path initiative to track effective means for diagnosis, treatment, and follow-up. This initiative will help avoid unnecessary or duplicate use of expensive medications or technologies.

9. MHS Foundation

Metropolis Health Foundation is presently being created to serve as the philanthropic arm of MHS. It will operate in a separate corporation governed by a board of 12 community leaders and supported by a 15-member special events board. The mission of the foundation will be to secure financial and nonfinancial support for realizing the MHS vision of providing comprehensive health care for the community.

Funds donated by individuals, businesses, foundations, and organizations will be designated for a variety of purposes at MHS, including the operation of specific departments, community outreach programs, continuing education for employees, endowment, equipment, and capital improvements.

10. MHS Volunteer Auxiliary

There are 500 volunteers who provide over 60,000 hours of service to MHS each year. These men and women assist in virtually every part of the system's operations. They also conduct community programs on behalf of MHS.

The auxiliary funds its programs and makes financial contributions to MHS through money it raises on renting televisions and vending gifts and other items at the hospital. In the past, its donations to MHS have generally been designated for medical equipment purchases. The auxiliary has given $250,000 over the last five years.

11. Planning the Future for MHS

The MHS has identified five areas of desired service and programmatic enhancement in its five-year strategic plan:
  I.   Ambulatory Services
  II. Physical Medicine and Rehabilitative Services
  III. Cardiovascular Services
  IV. Oncology Services
  V.   Community Health Services

MHS has set out to answer the most critical health needs that are specific to its community. Over the next five years, the MHS strategic plan will continue a tradition of quality, community-oriented health care to meet future demands.

12. Financing the Future

MHS has established a corporate depreciation fund. The fund's purpose is to ease the financial burden of replacing fixed assets. Presently, it has almost $2 million for needed equipment and renovations.

MHS CASE STUDY

Financial Statements

- Balance Sheet (**Exhibit 33–1**)
- Statement of Revenue and Expense (**Exhibit 33–2**)

- Statement of Cash Flows (**Exhibit 33–3**)
- Statement of Changes in Fund Balance (**Exhibit 33–4**)
- Schedule of Property, Plant, and Equipment (**Exhibit 33–5**)
- Schedule of Patient Revenue (**Exhibit 33–6**)
- Schedule of Operating Expenses (**Exhibit 33–7**)

Exhibit 33–1 Balance Sheet

Metropolis Health System
Balance Sheet
March 31, 2___

Assets		Liabilities and Fund Balance	
Current Assets		Current Liabilities	
Cash and Cash Equivalents	$1,150,000		
Assets Whose Use Is Limited	825,000	Current Maturities of Long-Term Debt	$525,000
Patient Accounts Receivable	7,400,000		
(Net of $1,300,000 Allowance for Bad Debts)		Accounts Payable and Accrued Expenses	4,900,000
		Bond Interest Payable	300,000
Other Receivables	150,000	Reimbursement Settlement Payable	100,000
Inventories	900,000		
Prepaid Expenses	200,000	Total Current Liabilities	5,825,000
Total Current Assets	10,625,000	Long-Term Debt	6,000,000
Assets Whose Use Is Limited		Less Current Portion of Long-Term Debt	(525,000)
Corporate Funded Depreciation	1,950,000	Net Long-Term Debt	5,475,000
Held by Trustee Under Bond Indenture Agreement	1,425,000	Total Liabilities	11,300,000
		Fund Balances	
Total Assets Whose Use Is Limited	3,375,000	General Fund	21,500,000
Less Current Portion	(825,000)	Total Fund Balances	21,500,000
Net Assets Whose Use Is Limited	2,550,000	Total Liabilities and Fund Balances	$32,800,000
Property, Plant, and Equipment, Net	19,300,000		
Other Assets	325,000		
Total Assets	$32,800,000		

Exhibit 33–2 Statement of Revenue and Expense

Metropolis Health System
Statement of Revenue and Expense
for the Year Ended March 31, 2___

Revenue		
Net patient service revenue	$34,000,000	
Other revenue	1,100,000	
Total Operating Revenue		$35,100,000
Expenses		
Nursing services	$5,025,000	
Other professional services	13,100,000	
General services	3,200,000	
Support services	8,300,000	
Depreciation	1,900,000	
Amortization	50,000	
Interest	325,000	
Provision for doubtful accounts	1,500,000	
Total Expenses		33,400,000
Income from Operations		$1,700,000
Nonoperating Gains (Losses)		
Unrestricted gifts and memorials	$20,000	
Interest income	80,000	
Nonoperating Gains, Net		100,000
Revenue and Gains in Excess of Expenses and Losses		$1,800,000

Statistics and Organizational Structure

- Hospital Statistical Data (**Exhibit 33–8**)
- MHS Nursing Practice and Administration Organization Chart (**Figure 33–1**)
- MHS Executive-Level Organization Chart (**Figure 33–2**)

Exhibit 33–3 Statement of Cash Flows

Metropolis Health System
Statement of Cash Flows
for the Year Ended March 31, 2___

Statement of Cash Flows

Operating Activities	
Income from operations	$1,700,000
Adjustments to reconcile income from operations to net cash flows from operating activities	
Depreciation and amortization	1,950,000
Changes in asset and liability accounts	
Patient accounts receivable	250,000
Other receivables	(50,000)
Inventories	(50,000)
Prepaid expenses and other assets	(50,000)
Accounts payable and accrued expenses	(400,000)
Reduction of bond interest payable	(25,000)
Estimated third-party payer settlements	(75,000)
Interest income received	80,000
Unrestricted gifts and memorials received	20,000
Net cash flow from operating activities	$3,350,000
Cash Flows from Capital and Related Financing Activities	
Repayment of long-term obligations	(500,000)
Cash Flows from Investing Activities	
Purchase of assets whose use is limited	(100,000)
Equipment purchases and building improvements	(2,000,000)
Net Increase (Decrease) in Cash and Cash Equivalents	$750,000
Cash and Cash Equivalents, Beginning of Year	400,000
Cash and Cash Equivalents, End of Year	$1,150,000

Exhibit 33–4 Statement of Changes in Fund Balance

Metropolis Health System Statement of Changes in Fund Balance for the Year Ended March 31, 2___	
General Fund Balance April 1, 2____	$19,700,000
Revenue and Gains in Excess of Expenses and Losses	1,800,000
General Fund Balance March 31, 2____	$21,500,000

Exhibit 33–5 Schedule of Property, Plant, and Equipment

Metropolis Health System Schedule of Property, Plant, and Equipment for the Year Ended March 31, 2___	
Buildings and Improvements	$14,700,000
Land Improvements	1,100,000
Equipment	28,900,000
Total	$44,700,000
Less Accumulated Depreciation	(26,100,000)
Net Depreciable Assets	$18,600,000
Land	480,000
Construction in Progress	220,000
Net Property, Plant, and Equipment	$19,300,000

Exhibit 33–6 Schedule of Patient Revenue

Metropolis Health System
Schedule of Patient Revenue
for the Year Ended March 31, 2___

Patient Services Revenue	
Routine revenue	$9,850,000
Laboratory	7,375,000
Radiology and CT scanner	5,825,000
OB–nursery	450,000
Pharmacy	3,175,000
Emergency service	2,200,000
Medical and surgical supply and IV	5,050,000
Operating rooms	5,250,000
Anesthesiology	1,600,000
Respiratory therapy	900,000
Physical therapy	1,475,000
EKG and EEG	1,050,000
Ambulance service	900,000
Oxygen	575,000
Home health and hospice	1,675,000
Substance abuse	375,000
Other	775,000
Subtotal	$48,500,000
Less allowances and charity care	(14,500,000)
Net Patient Service Revenue	$34,000,000

Exhibit 33–7 Schedule of Operating Expenses

Metropolis Health System
Schedule of Operating Expenses
for the Year Ended March 31, 2____

Nursing Services		General Services	
Routine Medical/Surgical	$3,880,000	Dietary	$1,055,000
Operating Room	300,000	Maintenance	1,000,000
Intensive Care Units	395,000	Laundry	295,000
OB–Nursery	150,000	Housekeeping	470,000
Other	300,000	Security	50,000
Total	$5,025,000	Medical Records	330,000
		Total	$3,200,000
Other Professional Services			
Laboratory	$2,375,000	Support Services	
Radiology and CT Scanner	1,700,000	General	$4,600,000
Pharmacy	1,375,000	Insurance	240,000
Emergency Service	950,000	Payroll Taxes	1,130,000
Medical and Surgical Supply	1,800,000	Employee Welfare	1,900,000
Operating Rooms and		Other	430,000
Anesthesia	1,525,000	Total	$8,300,000
Respiratory Therapy	525,000		
Physical Therapy	700,000	Depreciation	1,900,000
EKG and EEG	185,000	Amortization	50,000
Ambulance Service	80,000		
Substance Abuse	460,000	Interest Expense	325,000
Home Health and Hospice	1,295,000		
Other	130,000	Provision for Doubtful	
Total	$13,100,000	Accounts	1,500,000
		Total Operating Expenses	$33,400,000

Exhibit 33–8 Hospital Statistical Data

Metropolis Health System
Schedule of Hospital Statistics
for the Year Ended March 31, 2___

Inpatient Indicators:		Departmental Volume Indicators:	
Patient Days			
Medical and surgical	13,650	Respiratory therapy treatments	51,480
Obstetrics	1,080	Physical therapy treatments	34,050
Skilled nursing unit	4,500	Laboratory workload units	
		(in thousands)	2,750
Admissions		EKGs	8,900
Adult acute care	3,610	CT scans	2,780
Newborn	315	MRI scans	910
Skilled nursing unit	440	Emergency room visits	11,820
		Ambulance trips	2,320
Discharges		Home health visits	14,950
Adult acute care	3,580		
Newborn	315	Approximate number of employees	
Skilled nursing unit	445	(FTE)	510
Average Length of Stay (in days)	4.1		

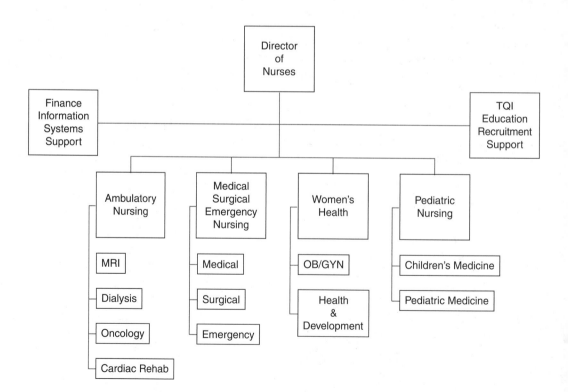

Figure 33–1 MHS Nursing Practice and Administration Organization Chart.
Courtesy of Resource Group, Ltd., Dallas, Texas.

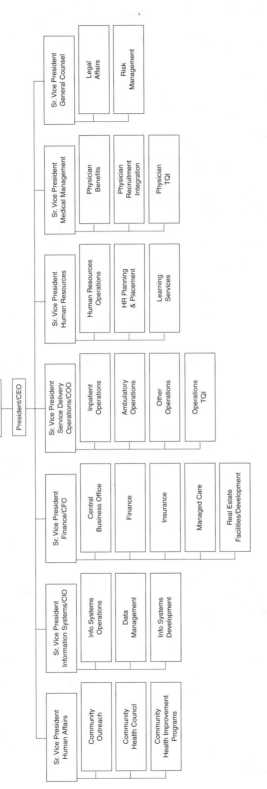

Figure 33–2 MHS Executive-Level Organization Chart.
Courtesy of Resource Group, Ltd., Dallas, Texas.

Metropolis Health System's Financial Statements and Excerpts from Notes

Metropolis Health System
Balance Sheet
March 31, 20X3 and 20X2

Assets

Current Assets		
Cash and cash equivalents	$1,150,000	$400,000
Assets whose use is limited	825,000	825,000
Patient accounts receivable	8,700,000	8,950,000
Less allowance for bad debts	(1,300,000)	(1,300,000)
Other receivables	150,000	100,000
Inventories of supplies	900,000	850,000
Prepaid expenses	200,000	150,000
Total Current Assets	10,625,000	9,975,000
Assets Whose Use Is Limited		
Corporate funded depreciation	1,950,000	1,800,000
Under bond indenture agreements— held by trustee	1,425,000	1,475,000
Total Assets Whose Use Is Limited	3,375,000	3,275,000
Less Current Portion	(825,000)	(825,000)
Net Assets Whose Use Is Limited	2,550,000	2,450,000
Property, Plant, and Equipment, Net	19,300,000	19,200,000
Other Assets	325,000	375,000
Total Assets	$32,800,000	$32,000,000

Metropolis Health System
Balance Sheet
March 31, 20X3 and 20X2

Liabilities and Fund Balance

Current Liabilities		
Current maturities of long-term debt	$525,000	$500,000
Accounts payable and accrued expenses	4,900,000	5,300,000
Bond interest payable	300,000	325,000
Reimbursement settlement payable	100,000	175,000
Total Current Liabilities	5,825,000	6,300,000
Long-Term Debt	6,000,000	6,500,000
Less Current Portion of Long-Term Debt	(525,000)	(500,000)
Net Long-Term Debt	5,475,000	6,000,000
Total Liabilities	11,300,000	12,300,000
Fund Balances		
General Fund	21,500,000	19,700,000
Total Fund Balances	21,500,000	19,700,000
Total Liabilities and Fund Balances	$32,800,000	$32,000,000

Metropolis Health System
Statement of Revenue and Expenses
for the Years Ended March 31, 20X3 and 20X2

Revenue			
Net patient service revenue	$34,000,000		$33,600,000
Other revenue	1,100,000		1,000,000
Total Operating Revenue		35,100,000		34,600,000
Expenses			
Nursing services	5,025,000		5,450,000
Other professional services	13,100,000		12,950,000
General services	3,200,000		3,220,000
Support services	8,300,000		8,340,000
Depreciation	1,900,000		1,800,000
Amortization	50,000		50,000
Interest	325,000		350,000
Provision for doubtful accounts	1,500,000		1,600,000
Total Expenses		33,400,000	33,760,000
Income from Operations		1,700,000	840,000
Nonoperating Gains (Losses)			
Unrestricted gifts and memorials	20,000		70,000
Interest income	80,000		40,000
Nonoperating Gains, Net		100,000	110,000
Revenue and Gains in Excess of Expenses and Losses		$1,800,000	$950,000

Metropolis Health System
Statement of Changes in Fund Balance
for the Years Ended March 31, 20X3 and 20X2

General Fund Balance April 1st	$19,700,000	$18,750,000
Revenue and Gains in Excess of Expenses and Losses	1,800,000	950,000
General Fund Balance March 31st	$21,500,000	$19,700,000

Metropolis Health System
Schedule of Property, Plant, and Equipment
for the Years Ended March 31, 20X3 and 20X2

Buildings and Improvements	$14,700,000	$14,000,000
Land Improvements	1,100,000	1,100,000
Equipment	28,900,000	27,600,000
Total	44,700,000	42,700,000
Less Accumulated Depreciation	(26,100,000)	(24,200,000)
Net Depreciable Assets	18,600,000	18,500,000
Land	480,000	480,000
Construction in Progress	220,000	220,000
Net Property, Plant, and Equipment	$19,300,000	$19,200,000

Metropolis Health System
Schedule of Patient Revenue
for the Years Ended March 31, 20X3 and 20X2

Patient Services Revenue		
Routine revenue	$9,850,000	$9,750,000
Laboratory	7,375,000	7,300,000
Radiology and CT scanner	5,825,000	5,760,000
OB–nursery	450,000	445,000
Pharmacy	3,175,000	3,140,000
Emergency service	2,200,000	2,180,000
Medical and surgical supply and IV	5,050,000	5,000,000
Operating rooms	5,250,000	5,200,000
Anesthesiology	1,600,000	1,580,000
Respiratory therapy	900,000	890,000
Physical therapy	1,475,000	1,460,000
EKG and EEG	1,050,000	1,040,000
Ambulance services	900,000	890,000
Oxygen	575,000	570,000
Home health and hospice	1,675,000	1,660,000
Substance abuse	375,000	370,000
Other	775,000	765,000
Subtotal	48,500,000	48,000,000
Less Allowances and Charity Care	14,500,000	14,400,000
Net Patient Service Revenue	$34,000,000	$33,600,000

Metropolis Health System
Schedule of Operating Expenses
for the Years Ended March 31, 20X3 and 20X2

Nursing Services		
Routine Medical/Surgical	$3,880,000	$4,200,000
Operating Room	300,000	325,000
Intensive Care Units	395,000	430,000
OB–Nursery	150,000	165,000
Other	300,000	330,000
Total	$5,025,000	$5,450,000
Other Professional Services		
Laboratory	$2,375,000	$2,350,000
Radiology and CT Scanner	1,700,000	1,680,000
Pharmacy	1,375,000	1,360,000
Emergency Service	950,000	930,000
Medical and Surgical Supply	1,800,000	1,780,000
Operating Rooms and Anesthesia	1,525,000	1,515,000
Respiratory Therapy	525,000	530,000
Physical Therapy	700,000	695,000
EKG and EEG	185,000	180,000
Ambulance Services	80,000	80,000
Substance Abuse	460,000	450,000
Home Health and Hospice	1,295,000	1,280,000
Other	130,000	120,000
Total	$13,100,000	$12,950,000
General Services		
Dietary	$1,055,000	$1,060,000
Maintenance	1,000,000	1,010,000
Laundry	295,000	300,000
Housekeeping	470,000	475,000
Security	50,000	50,000
Medical Records	330,000	325,000
Total	$3,200,000	$3,220,000
Support Services		
General	$4,600,000	$4,540,000
Insurance	240,000	235,000
Payroll Taxes	1,130,000	1,180,000
Employee Welfare	1,900,000	1,950,000
Other	430,000	435,000
Total	$8,300,000	$8,340,000
Depreciation	$1,900,000	$1,800,000
Amortization	50,000	50,000

Interest Expense	325,000	350,000
Provision for Doubtful Accounts	1,500,000	1,600,000
Total Operating Expenses	$33,400,000	$33,760,000

EXCERPTS FROM METROPOLIS HEALTH SYSTEM NOTES TO FINANCIAL STATEMENTS

Note 1—Nature of Operations and Summary of Significant Accounting Policies

General

Metropolis Hospital System (Hospital) currently operates as a general acute care hospital. The hospital is a municipal corporation and body politic created under the hospital district laws of the state.

Cash and Cash Equivalents

For purposes of reporting cash flows, the hospital considers all liquid investments with an original maturity of three months or less to be cash equivalents.

Inventory

Inventory consists of supplies used for patients and is stated as the lower of cost or market. Cost is determined on the basis of most recent purchase price.

Investments

Investments, consisting primarily of debt securities, are carried at market value. Realized and unrealized gains and losses are reflected in the statement of revenue and expenses. Investment income from general fund investments is reported as nonoperating gains.

Income Taxes

As a municipal corporation of the state, the hospital is exempt from federal and state income taxes under Section 115 of the Internal Revenue Code.

Property, Plant, and Equipment

Expenditures for property, plant, and equipment, and items that substantially increase the useful lives of existing assets are capitalized at cost. The hospital provides for depreciation on the straight-line method at rates designed to depreciate the costs of assets over estimated useful lives as follows:

	Years
Equipment	5 to 20
Land Improvements	20 to 25
Buildings and Improvements	40

Funded Depreciation

The hospital's Board of Directors has adopted the policy of designating certain funds that are to be used to fund depreciation for the purpose of improvement, replacement, or expansion of plant assets.

Unamortized Debt Issue Costs

Revenue bond issue costs have been deferred and are being amortized.

Revenue and Gains in Excess of Expenses and Losses

The statement of revenue and expenses includes revenue and gains in excess of expenses and losses. Changes in unrestricted net assets that are excluded from excess of revenue over expenses, consistent with industry practice, would include such items as contributions of long-lived assets (including assets acquired using contributions that by donor restriction were to be used for the purposes of acquiring such assets) and extraordinary gains and losses. Such items are not present on the current financial statements.

Net Patient Service Revenue

Net patient service revenue is reported as the estimated net realizable amounts from patients, third-party payers, and others for services rendered, including estimated retroactive adjustments under reimbursement agreements with third-party payers. Retroactive adjustments are accrued on an estimated basis in the period the related services are rendered and adjusted in future periods as final settlements are determined.

Contractual Agreements with Third-Party Payers

The hospital has contractual agreements with third-party payers, primarily the Medicare and Medicaid programs. The Medicare program reimburses the hospital for inpatient services under the Prospective Payment System, which provides for payment at predetermined amounts based on the discharge diagnosis. The contractual agreement with the Medicaid program provides for reimbursement based upon rates established by the state, subject to state appropriations. The difference between established customary charge rates and reimbursement is accounted for as a contractual allowance.

Gifts and Bequests

Unrestricted gifts and bequests are recorded on the accrual basis as nonoperating gains.

Donated Services

No amounts have been reflected in the financial statements for donated services. The hospital pays for most services requiring specific expertise. However, many individuals volunteer their time and perform a variety of tasks that help the hospital with specific assistance programs and various committee assignments.

Note 2—Cash and Investments

Statutes require that all deposits of the hospital be secured by federal depository insurance or be fully collateralized by the banking institution in authorized investments. Authorized investments include those guaranteed by the full faith and credit of the United States of America as to principal and interest; or in bonds, notes, debentures, or other similar obligations of the United States of America or its agencies; in interest-bearing savings accounts or interest-bearing certificates of deposit; or in certain money market mutual funds.

At March 31, 20X3, the carrying amount and bank balance of the hospital's deposits with financial institutions were $190,000 and $227,000, respectively. The difference between the carrying amount and the bank balance primarily represents checks outstanding at March 31, 20X3. All deposits are fully insured by the Federal Deposit Insurance Corporation or collateralized with securities held in the hospital's name by the hospital agent.

	Carrying Amount	
	20X3	20X2
U.S. Government Securities or		
U.S. Government Agency Securities	$4,325,000	$3,575,000
Total Investments	4,325,000	3,575,000
Petty Cash	3,000	3,000
Deposits	190,000	93,000
Accrued Interest	7,000	4,000
Total	4,525,000	3,675,000
Consisting of		
Cash and Cash Equivalents—General Fund	1,150,000	400,000
Assets Whose Use Is Limited		
Corporate Funded Depreciation	1,950,000	1,800,000
Held by Trustee Under Bond Indenture Agreements	1,425,000	1,475,000
Total	$4,525,000	$3,675,000

Note 3—Charity Care

The hospital voluntarily provides free care to patients who lack financial resources and are deemed to be medically indigent. Such care is in compliance with the hospital's mission. Because the hospital does not pursue collection of amounts determined to qualify as charity care, they are not reported as revenue.

The hospital maintains records to identify and monitor the level of charity care it provides. These records include the amount of charges forgone for services and supplies furnished under its charity care policy. During the years ended March 31, 20X3 and 20X2, such charges forgone totaled $395,000 and $375,000, respectively.

Note 4—Net Patient Service Revenue

The hospital provides healthcare services through its inpatient and outpatient care facilities. The mix of receivables from patients and third-party payers at March 31, 20X3 and 20X2, is as follows:

	20X3	20X2
Medicare	30.0%	28.5%
Medicaid	15.0	16.0
Patients	13.0	12.5
Other third-party payers	42.0	43.0
Total	100.0%	100.0%

The hospital has agreements with third-party payers that provide for payments to the hospital at amounts different from its established rates. Contractual adjustments under third-party reimbursement programs represent the difference between the hospital's established rates for services and amounts paid by third-party payers. A summary of the payment arrangements with major third-party payers follows.

Medicare

Inpatient acute care rendered to Medicare program beneficiaries is paid at prospectively determined rates-per-discharge. These rates vary according to a patient classification system that is based on clinical, diagnostic, and other factors. Inpatient nonacute care services and certain outpatient services are paid based upon either a cost reimbursement method, established fee screens, or a combination thereof. The hospital is reimbursed for cost reimbursable items at a tentative rate with final settlement determination after submission of annual cost reports by the hospital and audits by the Medicare fiscal intermediary. At the current year end, all Medicare settlements for the previous two years are subject to audit and retroactive adjustments.

Medicaid

Inpatient services rendered to Medicaid program beneficiaries are reimbursed at prospectively determined rates-per-day. Outpatient services rendered to Medicaid program beneficiaries are reimbursed at prospectively determined rates-per-visit.

Blue Cross

Inpatient services rendered to Blue Cross subscribers are reimbursed under a cost reimbursement methodology. The hospital is reimbursed at a tentative rate with final settlement determined after submission of annual cost reports by the hospital and audits by Blue Cross. The Blue Cross cost report for the prior year end is subject to audit and retroactive adjustment.

The hospital has also entered into payment agreements with certain commercial insurance carriers, health maintenance organizations, and preferred provider organizations. The bases for payment under these agreements include discounts from established charges and prospectively determined daily rates.

Gross patient service revenue for services rendered by the hospital under the Medicare, Medicaid, and Blue Cross payment agreements for the years ended March 31, 20X3 and 20X2, is approximately as follows:

	20X3		20X2	
	Amount	%	Amount	%
Medicare	$20,850,000	43.0	$19,900,000	42.0
Medicaid	10,190,000	21.0	10,200,000	21.5
All other payers	17,460,000	36.0	17,300,000	36.5
	$48,500,000	100.0	$47,400,000	100.0

Note 5—Property, Plant, and Equipment

The hospital's property, plant, and equipment at March 31, 20X3 and 20X2, are as follows:

	20X3	20X2
Buildings and improvements	$14,700,000	$14,000,000
Land improvements	1,100,000	1,100,000
Equipment	28,900,000	27,600,000
Total	$44,700,000	$42,700,000
Accumulated depreciation	(26,100,000)	(24,200,000)
Net Depreciable Assets	$18,600,000	$18,500,000
Land	480,000	480,000
Construction in progress	220,000	220,000
Net Property, Plant, Equipment	$19,300,000	$19,200,000

Construction in progress, which involves a renovation project, has not progressed in the last 12-month period because of a zoning dispute. The project will not require significant outlay to reach completion, as anticipated additional expenditures are currently estimated at $100,000.

Note 6—Long-Term Debt

Long-term debt consists of the following:

Hospital Facility Revenue Bonds (Series 1995) at varying interest rates from 4.5% to 5.5%, depending on date of maturity through 2020.	20X3	20X2
	$6,000,000	$6,500,000

The future maturities of long-term debt are as follows:

Years Ending March 31

20X2	$ 475,000
20X3	500,000
20X4	525,000
20X5	550,000
20X6	575,000
20X7	600,000
Thereafter	3,750,000

Under the terms of the trust indenture the following funds (held by the trustee) were established: an interest fund, a bond sinking fund, and a debt service reserve fund.

Interest Fund

The hospital deposits (monthly) into the interest fund an amount equal to one-sixth of the next semi-annual interest payment due on the bonds.

Bond Sinking Fund

The hospital deposits (monthly) into the bond sinking fund an amount equal to one-twelfth of the principal due on the next July 1.

Debt Service Reserve Fund

The debt service reserve fund must be maintained at an amount equal to 10% of the aggregate principal amount of all bonds then outstanding. It is to be used to make up any deficiencies in the interest fund and bond sinking fund.

Assets held by the trustee under the trust indenture at March 31, 20X3 and 20X2, are as follows:

	20X3	20X2
Interest Fund	$ 300,000	$ 325,000
Bond Sinking Fund	525,000	500,000
Debt Service Reserve	600,000	650,000
Total	$1,425,000	$1,475,000

Note 7—Commitments

At March 31, 20X3, the hospital had commitments outstanding for a renovation project at the hospital of approximately $100,000. Construction in progress on the renovation has not progressed in the last 12-month period because of a zoning dispute. Upon resolution of the dispute, remaining construction costs will be funded from corporate funded depreciation cash reserves.

Comparative Analysis Using Financial Ratios and Benchmarking Helps Turn Around a Hospital in the Metropolis Health System

33-B

© L-for/Shutterstock

Sample General Hospital is another facility within the Metropolis Health System. Sample General Hospital has recently been acquired by Metropolis. It is a 100-bed hospital that has been losing money steadily over the last several years. The new chief financial officer (CFO) has decided to use benchmarking as an aid to turn around Sample's financial situation. Benchmarking will illustrate where the hospital stands in relationship to its peer group.

The CFO orders two benchmarking reports: one for the hospitals that are 100 beds or less and one for all hospitals, no matter the size. The 100-beds-or-less report will allow direct comparability for Sample, while the all-hospital report will give a universal or overall view of Sample's standing. Both reports appear at the end of this case study. **Exhibit 33-B–1** is the benchmark data report for Sample General Hospital compared with hospitals less than 100 beds, whereas **Exhibit 33-B–2** is the benchmark data report for Sample General Hospital compared with all hospitals.

When the reports arrive, the CFO writes a description of how the data are arranged so that his managers will better understand the information presented. His description includes the following points:

1. The percentile rankings are intended to present the hospital's performance ranked against all other performers in the comparison group. Whether the hospital's actual performance is good or bad depends on the statistic being evaluated.
2. The first column, labeled "Annual Average Year 1," provides a historical trend of actual performance of the hospital in the previous year. It is provided for reference only so that the reader can see the trend over time.
3. The column labeled "Q1 Year 2" represents the first quarter of the current year. These are the most recent data that this service has been provided for Sample General Hospital and are the data used in the comparison columns that follow.
4. The column labeled "50th %ile" represents the 50th percentile of all of the hospitals in the comparison group that supplied data for the individual line item.
5. The "Variance" column compares the data from Q1 Year 2 of Sample General Hospital with the 50th percentile information from the entire comparison group.
6. The column labeled "%ile Range" indicates where Sample General Hospital's individual score fell within a percentile range.

Exhibit 33-B–1 Hospital Statistical Data

Benchmark Data Report
Sample General Hospital
Compared to Hospitals of Less Than 100 Beds

	Annual Average Year 1	Q1 Year 2	Current Quarter Benchmark		
			50%ile	Variance	%ile Range
Severity/Length of Stay					
Average Length of Stay	3.80	3.91	4.06	–0.15	35–40
Case Mix Index (All Patients)	1.02	1.04	1.04	0.005	50–55
Case Mix Index (Medicare)	1.24	1.26	1.19	0.07	80–85
Productivity/Labor Utilization					
FTE per Adjusted Occupied Bed	5.11	4.68	4.44	0.24	60–65
Paid Hours per Adjusted Patient Day	29.12	26.67	25.3	1.37	60–65
Paid Hours per Adjusted Discharge	110.53	104.19	109.5	–5.32	35–40
Salary Cost per Adjusted Discharge	$2,638	$2,510	$2,510	$0	50–55
Costs & Charges					
Cost per Adjusted Patient Day	$1,704	$1,608	$1,448	$161	70–75
Cost per Adjusted Discharge	$6,467	$6,282	$5,909	$373	55–60
Cost per CMI (All Pat.) Adj. Discharge	$6,328	$6,041	$5,837	$204	50–55
Cost per CMI (All Pat.) Adjusted Patient Day	$1,667	$1,546	$1,408	$139	60–65
Supply Cost per Adjusted Discharge	$1,046	$968	$867	$101	60–65
Supply Cost per CMI (All Pat.) Adj. Discharge	$1,024	$931	$829	$102	60–65
Gross Charges per Adjusted Discharge	$12,987	$14,155	$12,536	$1,620	60–65
Deductions Percentage	0.40%	58.46%	51.04%	7.42%	60–65
Net Charges per Adjusted Discharge	$6,112	$5,880	$5,929	($49)	45–50
Net Charges per Adjusted Patient Day	$1,610	$1,505	$1,424	$82	60–65
Utilization					
Average Daily Census	43.15	46.36	37.69	8.67	65–70
Occupancy Percentage	41.09%	46.36%	57.66%	–11.30%	10–15
Outpatient Charges Percentage	53.15%	54.02%	50.14%	3.88%	55–60
Beds in Use	100	100	66	34	90–95
Adjusted Occupied Beds	92.2	100.82	72.05	28.76	75–80
Total Patient Days Excluding Newborns	3,936	4,172	3,392	780	65–70
Total Discharges Excluding Newborns	1,036	1,068	751	317	80–85
Newborn Days as a % of Total Patient Days	6.95%	5.40%	4.61%	0.79%	60–65

Exhibit 33-B–1 Hospital Statistical Data *(continued)*

	Annual Average Year 1	Q1 Year 2	Current Quarter Benchmark		
			50%ile	Variance	%ile Range
Financial Performance—Profitability Ratios					
Operating Margin	−2.26	−3.18	1.95	−5.13	15–20
Profit Margin	−2.26	−3.18	2.06	−5.24	20–25
Return on Total Assets (Annualized) (%)	−2.37%	−3.58%	1.22%	−4.80%	20–25
Return on Equity (Annualized) (%)	−6.56%	−11.19%	4.61%	−15.80%	15–20
Financial Performance—Liquidity Ratios					
Current Ratio	1.28	1.19	1.9	−0.71	15–20
Quick Ratio	0.54	0.56	1.56	−0.99	15–20
Net Days in Patient AR (Days)	50.73	49	51.86	−2.86	40–45
Financial Performance—Leverage and Solvency Ratios					
Total Asset Turnover—Annualized	1.07	1.13	0.99	0.14	65–70
Current Asset Turnover—Annualized	3.21	3.65	3.57	0.08	50–55
Equity Financing	0.38	0.32	0.47	−0.15	25–30
Long-Term Debt to Equity	0.77	0.85	0.56	0.28	70–75

For example, review the average length of stay information for hospitals less than 100 beds in Exhibit 33-B–1. For the Q1 Year 2, Sample General Hospital has a length of stay of 3.91 versus a benchmark comparison number of 4.06, a favorable performance against the 50th percentile by 0.15 (the −0.15 indicates an amount under the 50th percentile that, in the case of average length of stay, would be favorable). This performance places the hospital's score in the 35th to 40th percentile of all respondents.

As the CFO already knows, Sample General Hospital is in trouble. In most cases, the facility is either at or below (worse than) the 50th percentile information. Most of the labor productivity measures are in the 60th to 65th percentile range, with the cost information in the same relative range. This indicates that Sample is spending more than the peer group for labor and supplies. The utilization statistics also present a dismal picture.

Each statistic has to be evaluated against what it means to the institution before a conclusion can be drawn. For example, the occupancy percentage for Sample is 46.36% versus the 50th percentile of 57.66%. This places Sample in the 10th to 15th percentile range for the comparison group of hospitals less than 100 beds. In terms of utilization, the CFO knows that a facility should be in the 80th to 85th percentile range to use all of its assets effectively.

What other statistics should the CFO review to assure that a higher occupancy percentage is beneficial to the hospital? The answer is average length of stay. Sample General Hospital has a length of stay of 3.91 (as discussed earlier), which is favorable compared with the peer group, but an occupancy rate that is 11.30% below the 50th percentile for the peer group of hospitals less than 100 beds. If these two statistics are observed in combination, one could say that Sample efficiently manages its patients, but just does not have enough of them.

Exhibit 33-B–2 Hospital Statistical Data

Benchmark Data Report
Sample General Hospital
Compared to All Hospitals

	Annual Average Year 1	Q1 Year 2	Current Quarter Benchmark		
			50%ile	Variance	%ile Range
Severity/Length of Stay					
Average Length of Stay	3.80	3.91	4.81	−0.91	10–15
Case Mix Index (All Patients)	1.02	1.04	1.14	−0.103	25–30
Case Mix Index (Medicare)	1.24	1.26	1.38	−0.118	30–35
Productivity/Labor Utilization					
FTE per Adjusted Occupied Bed	5.11	4.68	4.87	−0.19	40–45
Paid Hours per Adjusted Patient Day	29.12	26.67	27.77	−1.1	40–45
Paid Hours per Adjusted Discharge	110.53	104.19	134.6	−30.41	10–15
Salary Cost per Adjusted Discharge	$2,638	$2,510	$2,927	($417)	25–30
Costs & Charges					
Cost per Adjusted Patient Day	$1,704	$1,608	$1,530	$78	60–65
Cost per Adjusted Discharge	$6,467	$6,282	$7,284	($1,001)	30–35
Cost per CMI (All Pat.) Adj. Discharge	$6,328	$6,041	$6,115	($74)	45–50
Cost per CMI (All Pat.) Adjusted Patient Day	$1,667	$1,546	$1,268	$278	80–85
Supply Cost per Adjusted Discharge	$1,046	$968	$1,250	($282)	25–30
Supply Cost per CMI (All Pat.) Adj. Discharge	$1,024	$931	$1,069	($138)	30–35
Gross Charges per Adjusted Discharge	$12,987	$14,155	$17,196	($3,041)	35–40
Deductions Percentage	0.40%	58.46%	56.31%	2.15%	55–60
Net Charges per Adjusted Discharge	$6,112	$5,880	$7,419	($1,539)	20–25
Net Charges per Adjusted Patient Day	$1,610	$1,505	$1,529	($24)	45–50
Utilization					
Average Daily Census	43.15	46.36	142.98	−96.62	15–20
Occupancy Percentage	41.09%	46.36%	69.38%	−23.02%	< 5
Outpatient Charges Percentage	53.15%	54.02%	39.64%	14.38%	85–90
Beds in Use	100	100	206	−106	20–25
Adjusted Occupied Beds	92.2	100.82	225.9	−125.09	15–20
Total Patient Days Excluding Newborns	3,936	4,172	12,868	−8,696	15–20
Total Discharges Excluding Newborns	1,036	1,068	2,506	−1,438	20–25
Newborn Days as a % of Total Patient Days	6.95%	5.40%	4.52%	0.87%	60–65

Exhibit 33-B–2 Hospital Statistical Data *(continued)*

	Annual Average Year 1	Q1 Year 2	Current Quarter Benchmark		
			50%ile	Variance	%ile Range
Financial Performance—Profitability Ratios					
Operating Margin	−2.26	−3.18	4.45	−7.63	10–15
Profit Margin	−2.26	−3.18	4.66	−7.84	10–15
Return on Total Assets (Annualized) (%)	−2.37%	−3.58%	4.04%	−7.62%	10–15
Return on Equity (Annualized) (%)	−6.56%	−11.19%	8.46%	−19.65%	5–10
Financial Performance—Liquidity Ratios					
Current Ratio	1.28	1.19	2.2	−1	10–15
Quick Ratio	0.54	0.56	1.74	−1.18	5–10
Net Days in Patient AR (Days)	50.73	49	55.76	−6.77	25–30
Financial Performance—Leverage and Solvency Ratios					
Total Asset Turnover—Annualized	1.07	1.13	0.93	0.2	70–75
Current Asset Turnover—Annualized	3.21	3.65	3.48	0.18	50–55
Equity Financing	0.38	0.32	0.5	−0.18	20–25
Long-Term Debt to Equity	0.77	0.85	0.59	0.26	65–70

Other statistics bear the same message. The hospital is not profitable, and much of the problem is because the cost of running the institution exceeds the availability of patients to pay the bills. In other words, all institutions have core staffing requirements, and within a certain range of volume, most costs are fixed. Sample has 100 beds in use while the 50th percentile for its peer group shows 66 beds in use. Sample's plant is too big for its patient volume. These circumstances can mean the hospital is heading for disaster.

So what happened to Sample General Hospital? As you can surmise from the data, the previous year (labeled "Year 1" on Exhibits 33-B–1 and 33-B–2) was not favorable. Three years previous, the institution was losing money at a rate of over $1 million per month. The next two years showed improvement (even though the data still show concern), and the improvement trend continued through the year labeled "Year 2" on Exhibits 33-B–1 and 33-B–2. By using benchmarking data (and a lot of other analysis), management was able to determine and address many issues that forced this facility to perform below market averages. By improving quality, managing costs, and controlling productivity, the hospital was able to stabilize its financial position. In addition, with creative management and attention to both clinical quality and customer service, the occupancy percentage rose to above the 50th percentile. Finally, the operating margin improved dramatically. In the first quarter of year 2, the margin was minus 3.18. By the end of year 3, results showed a positive margin of greater than 2.5%, a dramatic turnaround. Benchmarking assisted in this turnaround by showing management where the need for improvement was greatest.

Proposal to Add a Retail Pharmacy to a Hospital in the Metropolis Health System

33-C

Sample General Hospital belongs to the Metropolis Health System. The new chief financial officer (CFO) at Sample Hospital has been attempting to find new sources of badly needed revenue for the facility. Consequently, the CFO is preparing a proposal to add a retail pharmacy within the hospital itself. If the proposal is accepted, this would generate a new revenue stream. The CFO has prepared four exhibits, all of which appear at the end of this case study. **Exhibit 33-C–1**, a three-year retail pharmacy profitability analysis, is the primary document. It is supported by **Exhibit 33-C–2**, the retail pharmacy proposal assumptions. The profitability analysis is further supported by **Exhibit 33-C–3**, a year 1 monthly income statement detail. Finally, **Exhibit 33-C–4** presents the supporting year 1 monthly cash flow detail and assumptions.

When the controller reviewed the exhibits, she asked how the working capital of $49,789 was derived. The CFO explained that it represents 3 months of departmental expense. He also explained that the cost of drugs purchased for the first 60 days was offset by these purchases' accounts payable cycle, so the net effect was 0. In essence, the vendors were financing the drug purchases. Thus, the working capital reconciled as follows:

Working Capital	
Cost of drugs (2 months)	$303,400
Vendor financing (accounts payable)	($303,400)
Departmental expense (3 months)	$49,789
Total Working Capital Required	$49,789

The controller also noticed on Exhibit 33-C–4 that the cost of renovations to the building is estimated at $80,000 and equipment purchases are estimated at $50,000 for a total capital expenditure of $130,000. The building renovations are depreciated on a straight-line basis over a useful life of 15 years, whereas the equipment purchases are depreciated on a straight-line basis over a useful life of 5 years. The required capital is proposed to be obtained from hospital sources, and no borrowing would be necessary. In addition, the total capital expenditure is projected to be retrieved through operating cash flows before the end of year 1.

Exhibit 33-C–1 Sample General Hospital 3-Year Retail Pharmacy Profitability Analysis

	Year 1	Year 2	Year 3
Rx Sales	2,587,613	2,692,152	2,828,375
Cost of Goods Sold	2,047,950	2,088,909	2,151,576
Gross Margin	539,663	603,243	676,799
GM %	20.9%	22.4%	23.9%
Expenses			
Salaries and Wages	192,000	197,760	203,693
Benefits	38,400	39,552	40,739
Materials and Supplies	12,000	14,400	17,280
Contract Services and Fees	14,400	17,280	20,736
Depreciation and Amortization	15,333	15,333	15,333
Interest	—	—	—
Provision for Bad Debts	25,876	26,922	28,284
Misc. Expenses	3,600	4,320	5,184
Total Expense	301,609	315,567	331,248
Net Income	238,053	287,676	345,550
Operating Margin	9.2%	10.7%	12.2%

Cash Flow

	Year 1	Year 2	Year 3
Sources			
Net Income	238,053	287,676	345,550
Depreciation	15,333	15,333	15,333
Borrowing	—	—	—
Total Sources	253,386	303,010	360,884
Uses			
Capital Purchasing	130,000	—	—
Working Capital	49,789	—	—
Total Uses	179,789	—	—
Cash at Beginning of Period	—	73,597	376,607
Net Cash Activities	73,597	303,010	360,884
Cash at Ending of Period	73,597	376,607	737,490

Volume

	Year 1	Year 2	Year 3
Number of Prescriptions Sold	55,350	56,457	58,151

Courtesy of Resource Group, Ltd., Dallas, Texas.

Exhibit 33-C–2 Sample General Hospital Retail Pharmacy Proposal Assumptions

		Prescriptions	
1. Annual Prescription Estimates—Rate of Growth/Capture		Per Day	Annual
Year 1		225	55,350
Year 2	2.0%	230	56,457
Year 3	3.0%	236	58,151
2. Average Net Revenue per Prescription—Yearly Increases			
Year 1			$ 46.75
Year 2	2.0%		$ 47.69
Year 3	2.0%		$ 48.64
3. Bad Debt Percentage	1.0%		
4. Average Cost per Prescription—Yearly Increases			
Year 1			$ 37.00
Year 2	3.0%		$ 38.11
Year 3	3.0%		$ 39.25
5. Inflation Rates—Per Year			
Salary and Wages			3.0%
Other Than Prescriptions			2.0%
Benefits as a % of Salaries			20.0%
6. Initial Capital Requirements			
Building			80,000
Equipment			50,000
Working Capital			49,789
Total			179,789

	Year 1	Year 2	Year 3
Gross Margin	539,663	603,243	676,799
Net Income before Taxes	238,053	287,676	345,550

	Year 1	Year 2	Year 3
Beginning Cash Balance	—	73,597	376,607
Net Cash Activity	73,597	303,010	360,884
Ending Cash Balance	73,597	376,607	737,490

Courtesy of Resource Group, Ltd., Dallas, Texas.

Exhibit 33-C-3 Sample General Hospital Retail Pharmacy Proposal Year 1 Monthly Income Statement Detail

Return on Investment Analysis	Month 1	Month 2	Month 3	Month 4	Month 5	Month 6	Month 7	Month 8	Month 9	Month 10	Month 11	Month 12
Average Rx Sales Price	$47	$47	$47	$47	$47	$47	$47	$47	$47	$47	$47	$47
Average Rx Cost	$37	$37	$37	$37	$37	$37	$37	$37	$37	$37	$37	$37
Gross Margin	21%	21%	21%	21%	21%	21%	21%	21%	21%	21%	21%	21%
Scripts per Day	225	225	225	225	225	225	225	225	225	225	225	225
	7.4%	7.4%	7.4%	7.8%	7.8%	8.3%	8.3%	8.7%	9.1%	9.3%	9.3%	9.3%
Business Days in the Month	20.5	20.5	20.5	20.5	20.5	20.5	20.5	20.5	20.5	20.5	20.5	20.5
Monthly Scripts	4,100	4,100	4,100	4,305	4,305	4,612.5	4,612.5	4,817.5	5,022.5	5,125	5,125	5,125
Rx Sales	$191,675	$191,675	$191,675	$201,259	$201,259	$215,634	$215,634	$225,218	$234,802	$239,594	$239,594	$239,594
COG Sold	$151,700	$151,700	$151,700	$159,285	$159,285	$170,663	$170,663	$178,248	$185,833	$189,625	$189,625	$189,625
Gross Margin	$39,975	$39,975	$39,975	$41,974	$41,974	$44,972	$44,972	$46,971	$48,969	$49,969	$49,969	$49,969
GM %	21%	21%	21%	21%	21%	21%	21%	21%	21%	21%	21%	21%
Expenses												
Salaries and Wages	$16,000	$16,000	$16,000	$16,000	$16,000	$16,000	$16,000	$16,000	$16,000	$16,000	$16,000	$16,000
Benefits	$3,200	$3,200	$3,200	$3,200	$3,200	$3,200	$3,200	$3,200	$3,200	$3,200	$3,200	$3,200
Materials and Supplies	$1,000	$1,000	$1,000	$1,000	$1,000	$1,000	$1,000	$1,000	$1,000	$1,000	$1,000	$1,000
Contract Services and Fees	$1,200	$1,200	$1,200	$1,200	$1,200	$1,200	$1,200	$1,200	$1,200	$1,200	$1,200	$1,200
Depreciation and Amortization	$1,278	$1,278	$1,278	$1,278	$1,278	$1,278	$1,278	$1,278	$1,278	$1,278	$1,278	$1,278
Interest	$0	$0	$0	$0	$0	$0	$0	$0	$0	$0	$0	$0
Provision for Bad Debts	$1,917	$1,917	$1,917	$2,013	$2,013	$2,156	$2,156	$2,252	$2,348	$2,396	$2,396	$2,396
Misc. Expenses	$300	$300	$300	$300	$300	$300	$300	$300	$300	$300	$300	$300
Total Expenses	$24,895	$24,895	$24,895	$24,991	$24,991	$25,134	$25,134	$25,230	$25,326	$25,374	$25,374	$25,374
Net Income	$15,080	$15,080	$15,080	$16,983	$16,983	$19,838	$19,838	$21,740	$23,643	$24,595	$24,595	$24,595
Accumulated Profits	$15,080	$30,161	$45,241	$62,224	$79,207	$99,045	$118,882	$140,623	$164,266	$188,861	$213,456	$238,050

Courtesy of Resource Group, Ltd., Dallas, Texas.

Exhibit 33-C–4 Sample General Hospital Retail Pharmacy Proposal Year 1 Monthly Cash Flow Detail and Assumptions

Depreciation	Years		Month 1	Month 2	Month 3	Month 4	Month 5	Month 6	Month 7	Month 8	Month 9	Month 10	Month 11	Month 12
Renovations	15	80,000	444	444	444	444	444	444	444	444	444	444	444	444
Equipment	5	50,000	833	833	833	833	833	833	833	833	833	833	833	833
Total Depreciation		130,000	1,278	1,278	1,278	1,278	1,278	1,278	1,278	1,278	1,278	1,278	1,278	1,278

Cash Flow

	Month 1	Month 2	Month 3	Month 4	Month 5	Month 6	Month 7	Month 8	Month 9	Month 10	Month 11	Month 12
Beginning Balance	$0	($163,431)	($147,073)	($130,714)	($112,453)	($94,192)	($73,076)	($51,961)	($28,942)	($4,021)	$21,852	$47,725
Sources												
Net Income	$15,080	$15,080	$15,080	$16,983	$16,983	$19,838	$19,838	$21,741	$23,644	$24,595	$24,595	$24,595
Depreciation	1,278	1,278	1,278	1,278	1,278	1,278	1,278	1,278	1,278	1,278	1,278	1,278
Borrowing	0	0	0	0	0	0	0	0	0	0	0	0
Total Sources	$16,358	$16,358	$16,358	$18,261	$18,261	$21,116	$21,116	$23,018	$24,921	$25,873	$25,873	$25,873
Uses												
Capital Purchasing	130,000	0	0	0	0	0	0	0	0	0	0	0
Working Capital	49,789	0	0	0	0	0	0	0	0	0	0	0
Total Uses	179,789	0	0	0	0	0	0	0	0	0	0	0
Net Cash Activities	($163,431)	$16,358	$16,358	$18,261	$18,261	$21,116	$21,116	$23,018	$24,921	$25,873	$25,873	$25,873
Ending Balance	($163,431)	($147,073)	($130,714)	($112,453)	($94,192)	($73,076)	($51,961)	($28,942)	($4,021)	$21,852	$47,725	$73,597

Courtesy of Resource Group, Ltd., Dallas, Texas.

So how was the proposal received by the hospital's board of trustees? They first asked for a small market study to test the amount of prescription sales projected within the proposal. When the market study results came back positive, the board approved the project, and renovations are about to commence.

# PART XII

Mini-Case Studies

Mini-Case Study 1

The Economic Significance of Resource Misallocation: Client Flow Through the Women, Infants, and Children Public Health Program*

Billie Ann Brotman, Mary Bumgarner, and Penelope Prime

CONFRONTING THE OPERATIONAL PROBLEM

The Women, Infants, and Children (WIC) Program, a federal program managed by the county boards of health, provides a mandated health service under strict federal guidelines to women and young children. In this chapter, we analyze how a WIC clinic, located in the Atlanta metropolitan area, can serve its clientele more efficiently in an environment of constraints. We focus on achieving shorter waiting times for WIC clients through better management of the flow of clients through the clinic. We apply the peak-load framework from economics to this basic operations research problem.

THE ENVIRONMENT

The WIC program provides nutrition counseling, limited physical examinations, and food vouchers for low-income pregnant women and for children with nutritional deficiencies who are five years old or less. WIC represents just one part of the integrated services provided to women and children by the county clinic. Other services include inoculations, medical visits with the nurse, and a variety of social services. Providing more than one health service at the county clinic is advantageous because it reinforces good health practices, provides intervention where necessary, and is convenient for the clients. However, it also complicates the management of service provision and makes it more difficult to improve the delivery of WIC's services.

To participate in the WIC program, a certification of income and health status is required. The first step for a client is to schedule an appointment for certification with a clinic nurse. Once certified, the client is immediately eligible to receive food vouchers and can return to the clinic to pick up her vouchers for up to a year without revisiting a nurse. Vouchers may also be picked up when a client comes to the clinic for nutritional classes, which are required periodically.

From the providers' point of view, several activities directly related to the WIC program are managed simultaneously. They include the scheduling of appointments for certification, meeting previously scheduled certification appointments by the nurses, accommodating unscheduled clients who walk in seeking certification, and distributing food

---

*B. A. Brotman, M. Bumgarner, and P. Prime, "Client Flow through the Women, Infants, and Children Public Health Program," *Journal of Health Care Finance* 25, no. 1 (1998): 72–77.

vouchers to eligible clients. (Eligible clients include those certified by the county clinic as well as those who have been certified by Kennestone Hospital and Home Visits, and Child Health.)

In principle, the appointment system is designed to regulate these activities. In practice, several factors, none of which are within the control of the clinic staff, undermine it. First, because clients come to the clinic for other services as well, they often are delayed for their WIC appointments. Second, of those that make appointments, 40 to 50% of them do not keep them because they either arrive late or simply do not come. Understanding the obstacles many of the clients face when arranging work schedules, getting transportation to the clinic, and arranging for child care, the clinic's management has instituted a policy of waiting 20 minutes for a client to arrive before rescheduling the appointment. Third, walk-ins are common and, according to federal guidelines, must be accommodated. In addition, the clinic has difficulty retaining qualified staff, and its physical space is limited. The end result is that women and children are often in the clinic for hours, are uncomfortable, and are unable to adequately care for their children during this time.

THE PEAK-LOAD PROBLEM

The economic problem faced by the clinic is one of demand exceeding capacity, leading to excessive wait times for the clinic's patrons as well as inefficient use of clinic nurses and clerks. The problem arises because the clinic's services are beneficial to the health of expectant mothers and children, and are provided without fee to the patient. Without a price mechanism to ration demand, quantity demanded exceeds quantity supplied. This problem is not uncommon. It is encountered often in the public or quasi-public sector, when the price of the good or service does not adequately reflect the benefits of the good or service as perceived by the public.

In this case, the problem of disequilibrium between demand and supply is exacerbated by the fact that demand for the clinic's services is unpredictable. Clients often do not keep their appointments or arrive at unscheduled times. As a result, appointments may go unfilled, or two or more clients may seek the same appointment time.

On the supply side, capacity constraints, coupled with a persistent lack of sufficient numbers of experienced clerks and nurses, hamper the clinic's ability to respond to unexpected demand shifts. Moreover, due to employee turnover experienced by the clinic, few employees become sufficiently skilled to work as part-time clerks during periods of peak demand.

The economic significance of the problem is one of resource misallocation. In this case, too many resources are employed in the production of WIC services. The market solution is to increase the price of the service, thereby matching demand with capacity. But because that option is not available, efficiently managing demand and supply is necessary if the amount of resources used in providing WIC services is to be reduced.

Federal guidelines for the WIC program leave little maneuvering room to improve the delivery of services. For example, the clinic cannot refuse to see unscheduled walk-ins, all clients must see a nurse for certification, all clients must attend nutrition classes, and vouchers must be closely monitored. Based on the data and information provided by the clinic, we determined that the fundamental cause of the queuing problem was the time spent by clients waiting to see clerks and nurses. Our hypothesis is that the flow of traffic through the clinic can be managed more efficiently by changing the current policy of waiting 20 minutes before filling a broken appointment with a "walk-in," to a new policy of filling the appointment immediately.

METHOD

We began by collecting information on the average daily client volume, the pattern of client flow through various services, the waiting points and times, and services rendered to the clients.

The data were collected by clinic personnel, recorded in a chart throughout the day in periodic intervals, and included nine items:

1. Number of clerks available
2. Number of nurses available
3. Waiting time to see clerks for walk-ins and appointments
4. Waiting time to see nurses for walk-ins and appointments
5. Total time in the clinic for walk-ins and appointments
6. Waiting time to get vouchers
7. Number of nutrition classes
8. Number of appointments met
9. Number of appointments missed

The actual flow of traffic through the clinic is depicted in **Figure 34–1**.

Clients visit the clinic to keep an appointment with the nurse, attend a nutrition class, or as an unscheduled walk-in. All clients first see a clerk to arrange for their records to be pulled. They then check in and wait to be called to their class or appointment. At the completion of the appointment, they see a clerk to pick up vouchers. Vouchers are also distributed at the end of the nutrition classes.

The General Purpose Simulation System for personal computer model simulates the average flow of traffic through the clinic. Estimation of traffic flow through the clinic is initiated when the client signs in and continues as the client meets with the clerks and the nurses. The model estimates the average amount of time a client spends in the clinic as well as average waiting times at each station. Clerk and nurse utilization rates are also generated assuming a variety of staffing levels. For comparison purposes, each version of the model is run with a 20-minute time lag before a late appointment is filled and then run with a 1-minute lag.

Six versions of the model are estimated using different combinations of numbers of clerks and nurses. Model A assumes that the clinic is staffed with three nurses and three clerks, Model B with two clerks and three nurses, and Model C with two clerks and two nurses.

RESULTS

Models A, B, and C present the results of all the computer simulations.

Model A: Three Nurses and Three Clerks

A comparison of the results generated changing a 20-minute wait to a 1-minute wait show that reducing the time before an appointment is filled results in the following:

1. A decrease in the total time in the clinic for the client from 3 hours and 16 minutes to 1 hour and 11 minutes

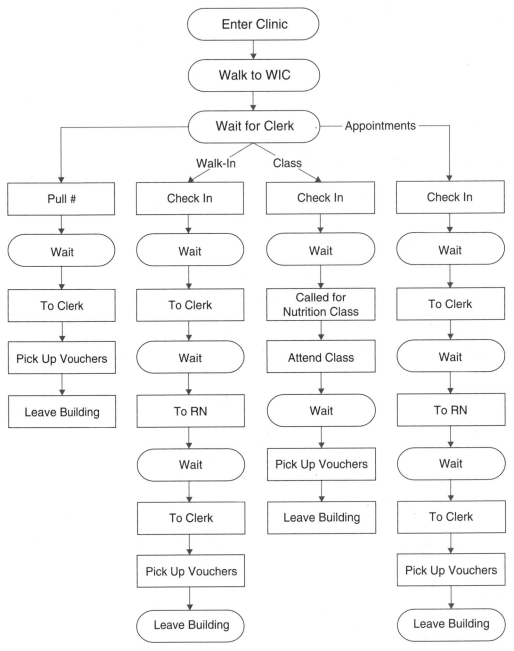

Figure 34–1 Traffic Flow.
Republished with permission of Wolters Kluwer Law & Business, from Brotman et al. Client Flow through the Women, Infants, and Children Public Health Program, *Journal of Health Care Finance 25*, no. 1 (1998): 72–77.

2. A decrease in the time spent waiting for the clerk from 1 hour and 9 minutes to approximately 3 minutes

3. An increase in time spent waiting for a nurse from 3 minutes to 10 minutes

4. A decrease in the utilization of clerks from 91.6% to 53.2%
5. An increase in the utilization of nurses from 46.7% to 61.2%

Model B: Three Nurses and Two Clerks

1. A decrease in the total time in the clinic for the client from 3 hours and 13 minutes to 1 hour and 27 minutes
2. A decrease in the time spent waiting for the clerk from 1 hour and 19 minutes to approximately 1 minute
3. An increase in time spent waiting for a nurse from 8 minutes to 43 minutes
4. A decrease in the utilization of clerks from 91.6% to 46.8%
5. An increase in the utilization of nurses from 51.2% to 73.3%

Model C: Two Nurses and Two Clerks

1. A decrease in the total time in the clinic for the client from 1 hour and 50 minutes to 1 hour and 9 minutes
2. A decrease in the time spent waiting for the clerk from 19 minutes to less than 1 minute
3. A decrease in time spent waiting for a nurse from 18 minutes to 13 minutes
4. A decrease in the utilization of clerks from 76.6% to 30.3%
5. A decrease in the utilization of nurses from 64.6% to 53.7%

In all three versions of the model that were estimated, the results of the simulations reveal that reducing the time before a late appointment is filled significantly decreases the time spent in the clinic by the client, on average, for all clients. Furthermore, the time spent waiting for both clerks and nurses decreases, the utilization of the clerks decreases, and the utilization of the nurses increases in two of the three estimations.

Greater decreases in waiting time occur when the clinic is staffed with three nurses and either three or two clerks. Smaller decreases occur when only two nurses and two clerks are available. This suggests that the clinic has little to no scheduling flexibility on days when it is understaffed, and a policy of filling late appointments immediately should be particularly beneficial.

The utilization of clerks and the time spent waiting for a clerk decreases in all three models when appointments are filled within one minute, and in every case but one, the utilization rate of nurses increases when appointments are filled immediately. This suggests that the flow of clients through the clinic is improved by filling appointments quickly. Utilization rates of nurses decreases only when the clinic is staffed with three nurses and three clerks. One explanation for this result is that the clinic is overstaffed with this combination of nurses and clerks. A supporting piece of evidence for this conclusion is that the change in rates of utilization for both nurses and clerks is the smallest when three of each are employed.

Another implication of these results is that if the clinic does not implement the expedited scheduling policy, it makes little difference to time spent in the clinic whether it is staffed with two nurses and two clerks or three nurses and two clerks. Both scenarios result in clients spending approximately 3.25 hours in the clinic. With the 20-minute wait before rescheduling, the clinic must be staffed with three nurses and three clerks if the time spent in the clinic by the client is to fall below 2 hours.

In summary, our results suggest that following a policy of immediately rescheduling missed appointments reduces the misallocation of resources employed in the clinic and thus permits the clinic to respond to its clients' needs more efficiently. Although this approach cannot duplicate the increase in efficiency that could be realized through the use of a price mechanism, it does improve the overall welfare of the clinic's clients. Filling appointments immediately results in shorter wait times for all clients, so no client is made worse off by the new policy. Moreover, as the patients realize that timeliness is important, more will arrive on time, further increasing the clinic's ability to monitor demand and provide services for its clients.

Mini-Case Study 2
Technology in Health Care: Automating Admissions Processes*

CHAPTER

35

Eric Christ

Alexander Bain was a clever fellow. He invented the electric clock and the first electric printing telegraph. He also invented the fax machine, the device that many long-term care providers rely on for patient referral and admissions communications. That was in 1843.

That's right, the technology at the core of the referral and admissions process for many continuing care providers is more than 150 years old.

Needless to say, a lot has changed since then. Providers can benefit from these changes by looking at their patient intake processes and considering ways to use the Internet and other technological advances to automate and accelerate admissions and referral management.

ASSESS ADMISSIONS PROCESS

The first step for providers who are considering improved tools for patient intake is to assess current processes. Here are some good questions to start with:

- How many referrals are received per day or per month?
- How many sources (hospitals, physicians, liaisons, other long-term care providers) send referrals?
- How many pages of documents are associated with each referral?
- How are patient review and approval tasks assigned and tracked?
- How are referral and intake activities collected and reported?

Many providers do not realize what vast mountains of paper they manage. Results from a 2007 survey of about 400 skilled nursing facilities and home health agencies indicate the average provider receives 4 referrals per day, each with 22 pages of related documents. That's 1,460 referrals and 32,120 pages of documents per year—an 8-foot stack of paper for the average provider to process, review, and manage.

In a study conducted by a Canadian health policy organization, nursing facility admissions processes were found to involve 160 steps, including 69 handling steps, 36 forms to complete, 4 family trips to the facility that involved 53 steps and 5 staff members, and 9 forms.

---

*E. Christ, "Technology in Health Care: Automating Admissions Processes," *Provider Magazine* (Oct. 2008): 81–84. Reprinted with permission from *Provider Magazine.*

AREAS TO AUTOMATE

Clearly, providers have many opportunities to streamline the admissions process. For example, there are typically four to five steps between an initial inquiry and a response to the referral source, after which insurance must be verified before a final decision to admit is made.

Once a provider has identified the steps in its admissions process, it can evaluate ways to apply messaging, management, and workflow technologies that can improve admissions in the following areas: fax and document management, communications, referral tracking and approval, and reporting.

FAX AND DOCUMENT MANAGEMENT

"Any solution that doesn't address the fax challenges will typically fall short," says Felicia Wilson, a licensed nursing facility administrator and director of the human services program at Shorter College in Rome, Georgia. "Experience has shown that providers must take steps to minimize receipt and management of faxed paper documents to make referral management more efficient."

Providers also may not realize how frequently fax errors occur that could delay or block inbound referrals. Typically, about 8% of outbound faxes do not reach their intended destination on the first try.

One option for providers is to convert faxed documents into an electronic format. Fax servers can provide this capability at a reasonable cost.

Providers may also benefit from software that helps organize and manage those electronic documents, which helps facilitate a smooth transition away from paper-filing processes.

It is important to note that providers should not let discussions about waiting for universal healthcare data standards for electronic medical records sidetrack attempts to automate. Just storing and managing documents in a common electronic document format, such as the ubiquitous PDF, is a huge incremental improvement over paper filing.

COMMUNICATION IS IMPORTANT

Both internal and external communications are critical to a responsive, efficient admissions team. In the May 2008 *Provider* cover story, Donna Shaw, administrator of Woodbine Rehabilitation Health Care in Alexandria, Virginia, summed up the critical need for responsive communications with referral sources: "Relationships with social workers and discharge planners at the hospitals are key," she said. "In an effort to move patients out quickly, hospitals are now expediting their placing process, which, in many cases, means a patient is referred to the facility that has the first available bed."

That urgency means providers cannot afford to miss calls or play phone tag with referral sources. Messaging and alerting systems can help providers know immediately when a referral comes in and send automated e-mails or faxes back to the referral source to update the status.

There are also emerging technologies to instantly confirm patient information, such as insurance verification—a step that typically requires multiple phone calls and can delay an admissions decision.

Some hospitals have adopted e-referral solutions that facilitate faster exchange of referral communications. These e-referrals still represent a small percentage of inbound referrals, however—about 6% according to the 2007 admissions survey. About 80% of new referral inquiries still arrive by fax or phone.

Providers should adopt tools and processes to effectively manage all inbound referrals, from all sources or methods, and communicate instantly with those referral sources.

REFERRAL TRACKING AND APPROVAL

Referral tracking and approval often remains a decidedly low-tech operation. A hospital or other source faxes in a referral request. The intake coordinator receives the fax, captures it in a handwritten log book or spreadsheet, makes copies of the paper documents, and distributes them to the appropriate clinical and management staff for review, with sticky notes affixed providing further instructions.

While this process may ultimately work, it is slow and inefficient. It also does not provide any mechanism for viewing the status of multiple active referral cases.

Some providers have adopted workflow automation software that can enable the admissions team to do several things:

- Notify staff when a new referral arrives
- Set review tasks for multiple staff members
- Capture and share notes related to the referrals
- Provide a quick update of referral status

"In an area where every second counts, workflow automation can make the difference between winning or losing a qualified patient referral," says Wilson.

ANALYZING REFERRAL ACTIVITY

Admissions staff often must report referral activity to management weekly or even daily. Much like the typical referral review process, this effort usually involves manually capturing information from multiple sources and compiling it into a written report or spreadsheet.

These manual processes make it extremely difficult to analyze referral activity, capacities, and win-loss data and create a particular challenge for multi-location providers that seek to view and analyze referral activity across all locations. They struggle to identify and deliver the services that are most in demand, prioritize and measure marketing programs, and keep admissions at peak levels.

One of the greatest advantages of automating admissions and referral processes is the enhanced ability to see and analyze referral activity. If a provider adopts a system that helps manage referral documents and workflows, by nature, that system will be capturing information that can help the provider make more informed decisions related to the admissions process.

There are several things a provider can expect to get a better view of with an automated system, including wins and losses; referral sources, types, and methods; reasons for decline; referral status and performance across locations; and acceptance rates.

Any provider considering solutions for automating admissions should evaluate up front what data it wants to report.

HOURS SAVED

One six-location skilled nursing provider implemented a web automation solution for centralized admissions and has seen the potential for tremendous gains in responsiveness and efficiency. An analysis that examined the time the provider spent on daily referral management processes revealed that the provider will save an estimated 1,175 hours, or 29.5 work weeks per year, by expediting referral review and communications processes.

This helps the provider meet goals to improve responsiveness to referral sources and maintain a competitive advantage in its marketplace.

The good news for providers seeking similar results is that many of the associated technologies are fairly simple, such as fax servers, e-mail messaging and alerting tools, and electronic document formats.

Providers may also benefit from web-based subscription solutions. Accessing a program through a web portal that is utilized as a monthly or annual subscription can eliminate upfront investments, such as software and hardware, as well as the need to install upgrades.

Providers simply need to assess their current admission processes and identify and apply the right mix to make admissions faster, smarter, and more effective.

Checklists

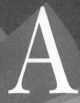

Checklist A-1 Reviewing a Budget

1. Is this budget static (not adjusted for volume) or flexible (adjusted for volume during the year)?

2. Are the figures designated as fixed or variable?

3. Is the budget for a defined unit of authority?

4. Are the line items within the budget all expenses (and revenues, if applicable) that are controllable by the manager?

5. Is the format of the budget comparable with that of previous periods so that several reports over time can be compared if so desired?

6. Are actual and budget for the same period?

7. Are the figures annualized?

8. Test one line-item calculation. Is the math for the dollar difference computed correctly? Is the percentage properly computed based on a percentage of the budget figure?

Checklist A-2   Building a Budget

1. What is the proposed volume for the new budget period?

2. What is the appropriate inflow (revenues) and outflow (cost of services delivered) relationship?

3. What will the appropriate dollar cost be?

   (Note: this question requires a series of assumptions about the nature of the operation for the new budget period.)

   3a. Forecast service-related workload.

   3b. Forecast non-service-related workload.

   3c.. Forecast special project workload if applicable.

   3d. Coordinate assumptions for proportionate share of interdepartmental projects.

4. Will additional resources be available?

5. Will this budget accomplish the appropriate managerial objectives for the organization?

Checklist A-3   Balance Sheet Review

1. What is the date on the balance sheet?

2. Are there large discrepancies in balances between the prior year and the current year?

3. Did total assets increase over the prior year?

4. Did current assets increase, decrease, or stay about the same?

5. Did current liabilities increase, decrease, or stay about the same?

6. Did land, plant, and equipment increase or decrease significantly over the prior year?

7. Did long-term debt increase or decrease significantly over the prior year?

Courtesy of J.J. Baker and R.W. Baker, Dallas, Texas.

Checklist A-4 Review of the Statement of Revenue and Expense

1. What is the period reported on the statement of revenue and expense?

2. Is it one year or a shorter period? If it is a shorter period, why is that?

3. Are there large discrepancies in balances between the prior year operations and the current year operations?

4. Did total operating revenue increase over the prior year?

5. Did total operating expenses increase, decrease, or stay about the same? Is any particular line item unusually large or small?

6. Did income from operations increase, decrease, or stay about the same?

7. Are there unusual nonoperating gains or losses?

8. Did the current year result in an excess of revenue over expense? Is it as much as that of the prior year?

9. Did long-term debt increase or decrease significantly over the prior year?

Checklist A-5 Considerations for Forecasting Equipment Acquisition

- Only one location?
- Equipment—single purpose or multi-purpose?
- Technology—new, middle-aged, old (obsolete vs. untested)?
- Equipment compatibility
- Medical supply cost
- High or low capital investment?
- Buy new or used (refurbished)?
- Buy or lease?
- Lease for a number of years or lease on a pay-per-procedure deal?
- How much staff training is required?
- Certification required?
- Square footage required for equipment?
- Is the required square footage available?
- Cleaning methods and equipment (and staff level required)?
- Repairs and maintenance expense (high, medium, low)?

Checklist A-6   Checklist for Assessing ICD-10 Progress: Key Performance Indicators

- Number of days to final bill
- Number of days to payment
- Claims acceptance/rejection rates
- Claims denial rate
- Payment amounts
- Reimbursement rate
- Coder productivity
- Volume of coder questions
- Payer requests for additional information
- Daily charges/claims
- Incomplete or missing charges
- Incomplete or missing diagnosis codes
- Use of unspecified codes
- Clearinghouse edits
- Payer edits
- RTP/FISS volumes
- Medical necessity pass rate
- Use of ICD-10 codes on prior authorizations and referrals

Modified from CMS, "ICD-10: Next Steps for Providers—Assessment & Maintenance Toolkit."

Glossary

Accountable Care Organization (ACO): An organization consisting of a group of providers who have joined together voluntarily to provide coordinated, quality care to patients.

Alternative Payment Model (APM): Provides new methods of payment by Medicare for physicians and other eligible professionals (a.k.a. eligible clinicians).

Accounting Rate of Return: See Unadjusted Rate of Return.

Accounting System: Records the evidence that some event has occurred in the healthcare financial system.

Accrual Basis Accounting: Revenue is recorded when it is earned, not when payment is received. Expenses are recorded when they are incurred, not when they are paid. The opposite of accrual basis is cash basis accounting.

Action Plan: A detailed plan of operations that shows how one part of a particular objective will be accomplished.

Annualize: To convert data to an annual (12-month) period.

Assets: The net value of what an organization owns.

Balance Sheet: One of the four basic financial statements. Generally speaking, the balance sheet records what an organization owns, what it owes, and what it is worth at a particular point in time.

Base Year: A 12-month unit of time (one year) used as a basis for comparison.

Baseline Period: A unit of time (period) used as a basis for comparison.

Benchmarking: The continuous process of measuring products, services, and activities against the best levels of performance. Best levels may be found inside or outside of the organization.

Big Data: A very large data set that is typically used for analysis to reveal patterns and/or trends.

Book Value: The book value (also known as net book value) of a fixed asset is a balance sheet figure that represents the remaining undepreciated portion of the fixed asset cost.

Break-Even Point: The point when the contribution margin (i.e., net revenues less variable costs) equals the fixed costs.

Budget: The organization-wide instrument through which activities are quantified in financial terms.

Business Plan: A document that is typically prepared in order to obtain funding and/or financing.

Capital: Represents the financial resources of the organization. Generally considered to be a combination of debt and equity.

Capital Expenditure Budget: A budget usually intended to plan, monitor, and control long-term financial issues.

Capital Structure: Means the proportion of debt versus equity within the organization. The phrase "capital structure" actually refers to the debt–equity relationship.

Case Mix Adjusted: A performance measure that has been adjusted for the acuity level of the patient and, presumably, the resource level required to provide care.

Cash Basis Accounting: A transaction does not enter the books until cash is either received or paid out. The opposite of cash basis is accrual basis accounting.

Cash Flow Analysis: This type of analysis illustrates how the project's cash is expected to move over a period of time.

Certificate of Need (CON) Program: A program to control excess capacity in the form of facility overbuilding.

Certified EHR Technology: An electronic health record (EHR) that has been specially certified for use in the EHR Incentive Programs.

Chart of Accounts: Maps out account titles in a uniform manner through a method of numeric coding.

Code Users: Any individual who needs to have some level of understanding of the coding system, but does not actually assign codes.

Common Sizing: A process of converting dollar amounts to percentages to put information on the same relative basis. Also known as vertical analysis.

Common Stock: Stocks represent equity, or net worth, in a company. Common stock typically pays a proportionate share of net income out as a dividend to its investors.

Composite Performance Score: See also Composite Score.

Composite Score: An overall score assembled from multiple scores, or parts.

Contribution Income Statement: Specifically identifies the contribution margin within the income statement format.

Contribution Margin: Called this because it contributes to fixed costs and to profits. Computed as net revenues less variable costs.

Controllable Expenses: Subject to a manager's own decision making and thus "controllable."

Controlling: Making sure that each area of the organization is following the plans that have been established.

Core Objectives: EHR Incentive Program criteria that is necessary to achieve meaningful use. Core objectives are mandatory; thus the provider must meet all applicable core objectives. See also Menu Objective.

Cost: The amount of cash expended (or property transferred, services performed, or liability incurred) in consideration of goods or services received or to be received.

Cost-Profit-Volume: A method of illustrating the break-even point, whereby the three elements of cost, profit, and volume are accounted for within the computation.

Cost Object: Any unit for which a separate cost measurement is desired.

Critical Access Hospitals (CAHs): Certain rural providers qualify as CAHs under the Medicare program. These eligible CAHs are a separate provider type and are reimbursed using a separate payment method.

Cross-cutting (measure): A measure that crosses among different types of facilities (thus "cuts across").

Cross-setting: Allowing information to flow back and forth among different types of facilities (thus "across-settings").

Cumulative Cash Flow: The accumulated effect of cash inflows and cash outflows are added and/or subtracted to show the overall net accumulated result.

Current Ratio: A liquidity ratio considered to be a measure of short-term debt-paying ability. Computed by dividing current assets by current liabilities.

Data: Factual information typically used to measure and/or calculate, although data may also be used for reasoning and/or discussion.

Data Analytics: The process of mining data to discover patterns, correlations, and other related information, primarily in order to make better decisions.

Database (also Data Base): A particular set of computerized data organized in a manner designed for efficient retrieval.

Data Mining: The process used by organizations to turn raw data into useful information.

Data Set: A group of data (a set) gathered together for a like purpose.

Days Cash on Hand Ratio: A liquidity ratio that indicates the number of days of operating expenses represented in the amount of unrestricted cash on hand. Computed by dividing unrestricted cash and cash equivalents by the cash operating expenses divided by number of days in the period.

Days Receivables Ratio: A liquidity ratio that represents the number of days in receivables. Computed by dividing net receivables by net credit revenues divided by number of days in the period.

Debentures: Bonds that are unsecured. Debentures are backed by revenues that the issuing organization can earn.

Debt Service Coverage Ratio: A solvency ratio universally used in credit analysis to measure ability to pay debt service. Computed by dividing change in unrestricted net assets (net income) plus interest, depreciation, and amortization by maximum annual debt service.

Decile: A distribution into 10 classes, each of which contains one-tenth of the whole; any one of the 10 classes is a decile.

Decision Making: Making choices among available alternatives.

Deflation: A contraction in the volume of available money and credit that results in a general decline in prices.

Denominator: The bottom part of a fraction. The denominator indicates the total number of parts available to be divided. See also Numerator.

Depreciation: Depreciation expense spreads, or allocates, the cost of a fixed asset over the useful life of that asset.

Diagnoses: A common method of grouping healthcare expenses for purposes of planning and control. Such a grouping may be by major diagnostic categories or by diagnosis-related groups.

Digital Media: Information that may be stored digitally, such as in a computer or mobile device, or online.

Direct Costs: These costs are incurred for the sole benefit of a particular operating unit. They can therefore be specifically associated with a particular unit or department or patient. Laboratory tests are an example of a direct cost.

Discounted Fee-for-Service: The provider of services is paid according to an agreed-upon contracted discount and after the service is delivered.

Dispenser: Either a person or other legal entity who provides drug products for human use on prescription in the course of professional practice, and who is licensed, registered, or otherwise permitted by the jurisdiction in which the person practices, or the entity is located, to do so.

Electronic Data Interchange: The electronic transfer of information such as electronic media claims. The transfer is made in a standard format between trading partners.

Electronic Health Record (EHR): A health-related electronic record of an individual that includes patient demographic and clinical information and that has the capacity to provide clinical decision support, support physician order entry, capture and query quality information, and exchange and integrate electronic health information. It is possible for this digital record to contain information about a patient's total health status across all providers. See also Electronic Medical Record (EMR).

Electronic Medical Record (EMR): The digital version of the traditional paper chart as recorded by a single provider. See also Electronic Health Record (EHR).

Electronic Prescribing (E-Prescribing): Transmitting a prescription or prescription-related information using electronic media between a prescriber, dispenser, PBM, or health plan.

The transmission may be either direct or through an intermediary, including an e-prescribing network.

Electronic Transaction Standards: Standards that are adopted and used to facilitate the electronic transmission of healthcare information and related business transactions.

Eligible Clinician: Another term for Eligible Professional.

Eligible Professional: In this context, physicians, practitioners, and other professionals who are eligible for payment in certain incentive programs.

Equity: Claims held by the owners of the business because they have invested in the business; what the business is worth on paper, net of liabilities.

Estimates: A judgment that takes the place of actual measurement.

Expenses: Actual or expected cash outflows incurred in the course of doing business. Expenses are the costs that relate to the earning of revenue. An example is salary expense for labor performed.

Expired Costs: Costs that are used up in the current period and are matched against current revenues.

Fee-for-Service: The provider of services is paid according to the service performed and after the service is delivered.

FIFO: The First-In, First-Out inventory costing method recognizes the first costs placed into inventory as the first costs moved out into cost of goods sold when a sale occurs.

Financial Accounting: Is generally for outside, or third-party, use and thus emphasizes external reporting.

Financial Forecast: "Forecasted" prospective financial statements. Forecasts are based on assumptions that are expected to exist, and that reflect actions that are expected to occur.

Financial Lease: A formal agreement that may be called a lease but is actually a contract to purchase. This type of lease must meet certain criteria.

Financial Projection: "Projected" prospective financial statements that are often prepared to answer "what-if" questions. The statements "project" a view of future events, projects, or operations using a set of presumed, or hypothetical, assumptions.

Fixed Costs: Those costs that do not vary in total when activity levels or volume of operations change. Rent expense is an example of fixed cost.

Flexible Budget: A budget based on a range of activity or volume. The flexible budget is adjusted, or flexed (thus "flexible") to the actual level of output achieved or expected to be achieved during the budget period.

Forecasts: Information used for purposes of planning for the future. Forecasts can be short, intermediate, or long range.

For-Profit Organization: A proprietary organization that is generally subject to income tax.

Full-Time Equivalent (FTE): A measure to express the equivalent of an employee (annualized) or a position (staffed) for the full time required.

Fund Balance: The difference between net assets and net liabilities; a term generally used by not-for-profit organizations.

General Ledger: A document in which all transactions for the period reside.

General Services Expenses: This type of expense provides services necessary to maintain the patient, but the service is not directly related to patient care. Examples of general services expenses are laundry and dietary.

Goal: A statement of aim or purpose that is part of a strategic plan.

Gross Domestic Product (GDP): A measure of the output of goods and services produced by labor and property located in the United States. The Bureau of Economic Analysis (BEA) is responsible for releasing quarterly estimates of the GDP.

Healthcare Analytics: Data analytics applied to the healthcare industry.

Health Delivery System: A health system containing varying levels of care and multiple sites of service that deliver care under one integrated system.

Health Information Exchange (HIE): The electronic movement, or transmission, of health-related information between and among organizations using nationally recognized standards.

Health Information Technology (HIT): Technology that is designed for, or supports use by, healthcare entities or patients. Includes hardware, software, integrated technologies or related licenses, intellectual property, upgrades, or packaged solutions.

Horizontal Analysis: The process of comparing and analyzing figures over several time periods. Also known as trend analysis.

ICD-10 Codes: The International Classification of Diseases (ICD) is the international standard for diagnostic disease classifications. ICD-10 indicates the tenth revision.

IMPACT Act: A legislative act that requires standardized patient assessment data be reported by four types of post-acute care facilities. Its full name is the "Improving Medicare Post-Acute Care Transformation Act of 2014."

Indirect Cost: These costs are incurred on behalf of the overall operation and therefore cannot be associated with the provision of specific health services. The finance office is an example of an indirect cost. Also known as joint costs.

Inflation: An increase in the volume of money and credit relative to available goods and services resulting in a continuing rise in the general price level.

Information System: Gathers the evidence that some event has occurred in the healthcare financial system.

Information Technology (IT): Computer and telecommunications technology that organizes, processes, stores, retrieves, secures, and transmits information.

Innovation: An idea, practice, or object that is perceived as new.

Internal Rate of Return: A return on investment method, defined as the rate of interest that discounts future net inflows (from the proposed investment) down to the amount invested.

Interoperability: The ability to operate, or transmit, across data systems used by different types of facilities.

Inventory: All the items ("goods") that an organization has for sale in the normal course of its business.

Inventory Turnover: A ratio that shows how fast inventory is sold, or "turns over."

Joint Costs: These costs are incurred on behalf of the overall operation and therefore cannot be associated with the provision of specific health services. The finance office is a typical example of a joint cost. Also known as indirect cost.

Liabilities: What the organization owes.

Liabilities to Fund Balance Ratio: A solvency ratio used as a quick indicator of debt load. Computed by dividing total liabilities by unrestricted net assets. Also known as Debt to Net Worth Ratio.

LIFO: The Last-In, First-Out inventory costing method recognizes the latest, or last, costs placed into inventory as the first costs moved out into cost of goods sold when a sale occurs.

Liquidity Ratios: Ratios that reflect the ability of the organization to meet its current obligations. Liquidity ratios are measures of short-term sufficiency.

Loan Costs: Those costs necessary to close a loan.

MACRA: A legislative act that reformed Medicare payment to physicians and certain eligible professionals (a.k.a. eligible clinicians). Its full name is the "Medicare Access and CHIP Reauthorization Act of 2015."

Managed Care: A means of providing healthcare services within a network of healthcare providers. The central concept is coordination of all healthcare services for an individual.

Managerial Accounting: Is generally for inside, or internal, use and thus emphasizes information useful for managerial employees.

Mean: An average of numbers or values.

Meaningful Use: Providers must show that they are "meaningfully using" their certified EHR technology by meeting thresholds, or minimums, for certain program objectives.

Meaningful User: To be a meaningful user of electronic health records, the provider must be using EHR in a meaningful manner, be connected in a way that allows electronic exchange of health information, and be reporting on measures using EHR.

Measure Development Plan (MDP): A plan to develop quality measures that support the transition to new payment methods for physicians and certain other professionals.

Median: The median occupies a position in a ranked series of values (numbers) in which the same number of values appears above the median as appear below it (or, in the case of an even number of values, the average of the two middle-ranked values).

Medicaid Program: A federal and state matching entitlement program intended to provide medical assistance to eligible needy individuals and families. The program was established under Title XIX of the Social Security Act.

Medicare Program: A federal health insurance program for the aged (and, in certain instances, for the disabled) intended to complement other federal benefits. The program was established under Title XVIII of the Social Security Act.

Menu Objective: EHR Incentive Program criteria that is necessary to achieve meaningful use. Menu objectives provide a choice; thus the provider must meet a certain number of applicable menu objectives, but not all of them. See also Core Objectives.

Merit-Based Incentive Program (MIPS): A value-based program that combines certain parts of existing quality reporting programs for physicians and certain eligible professionals (a.k.a. eligible clinicians).

Mission Statement: A Mission Statement explains the purpose of the organization. It explains "what we are now."

Mixed Cost: Those costs that contain an element of variable cost and an element of fixed cost.

Mode: The number or value that appears the most frequently within a series of numbers or values.

Monetary Unit: A measure of units of currency, such as the dollar. Monetary units should be comparable when reporting financial results.

Mortgage Bonds: Bonds that are backed, or secured, by certain real property.

Municipal Bonds: Long-term obligations that are typically used to finance capital projects.

Net Worth: See Equity.

Noncontrollable Expenses: Outside the manager's power to make decisions, and thus "noncontrollable."

Nonproductive Time: Paid-for time when the employee is not on duty—that is, not producing. Paid-for vacation days and holidays are examples of nonproductive time.

Nonprofit Organization: Indicates the taxable status of the organization. A nonprofit (or voluntary) organization is exempt from paying income taxes.

Not-for-Profit Organization: See Nonprofit Organization.

Numerator: The top part of a fraction. The numerator indicates the total number of parts of the denominator taken. See also Denominator.

Operating Budget: A budget that generally deals with actual short-term revenues and expenses necessary to operate the facility.

Operating Lease: A lease that is considered an operating expense and thus is treated as an expense of current operations. This type of lease does not meet the criteria to be treated as a financial lease.

Operating Margin: A profitability ratio generally expressed as a percentage, the operating margin is a multipurpose measure. It is used for a number of managerial purposes and also sometimes enters into credit analysis. Computed by dividing operating income (loss) by total operating revenues.

Operations Expenses: This type of expense provides service directly related to patient care. Examples of operations expenses are radiology expense and drug expense.

Organization Chart: Indicates the formal lines of communication and reporting and how responsibility is assigned to managers.

Organizational Values: Organizational values express the philosophy of the organization, most often expressed in a Values Statement.

Organizing: Deciding how to use the resources of the organization to most effectively carry out the plans that have been established.

Original Records: Provide evidence that some event has occurred in the healthcare financial system.

Overhead: Refers to the remaining expenses of operation that are necessary to produce the service but that are not directly attributable to that service.

Pareto Analysis: An analytical tool employing the Pareto principle, also known as the 80/20 rule. The Pareto principle states that 80% of an organization's problems are caused by 20% of the possible causes.

Patient Engagement: A patient who is an active partner in his or her own health care.

Patient Mix: A term indicating the mix of payers; thus, whether the individual is a Medicare patient, a Medicaid patient, a patient covered by private insurance, or a private pay patient varies the patient mix proportions. Patient mix information allows estimated payment levels to be associated with the service utilization assumptions.

Pay-for-Performance (P4P): Providers receive payment incentives when meeting performance measures that show they are delivering and promoting improvements in high-quality, efficient care.

Payback Period: The length of time required for the cash coming in from an investment to equal the amount of cash originally spent when the investment was acquired.

Payer Mix: The proportion of revenues realized from different types of payers. A measure often included in the profile of a healthcare organization.

Payment Adjustment: Term used for the downward adjustment of a provider's payment. A payment adjustment is usually viewed as a penalty.

Performance Measures: Measures that compare and quantify performance. Performance measures may be financial, nonfinancial, or a combination of both types.

Performance Period: A unit of time during which performance is measured.

Period Cost: For purposes of healthcare businesses, period cost is necessary to support the existence of the organization itself, rather than actual delivery of a service. Period costs are matched with revenue on the basis of the period during which the cost is incurred. The term originated with the manufacturing industry.

Planning: Identifying objectives of the organization and identifying the steps required to accomplish the objectives.

Population Health: Health care concerned with the outcomes of an entire population instead of a single patient.

Predictive Analytics: An advanced analytical method used to extract value from data.

Preferred Stock: Stock that has preference over common stock in certain issues such as payment of dividends.

Prescriber: A physician, dentist, or other person who issues prescriptions for drugs for human use, and who is licensed, registered, or otherwise permitted by the United States or the jurisdiction in which he or she practices to do so.

Present Value Analysis: A concept based on the time value of money. The value of a dollar today is more than the value of a dollar in the future.

Private Sector Organizations: Those organizations that are not part of the government.

Procedures: A common method of grouping healthcare expenses for purposes of planning and control. Such a grouping will generally be by Current Procedural Terminology (or CPT) codes, which list descriptive terms and identifying codes for medical services and procedures performed.

Product Cost: For the purposes of healthcare businesses, product cost is necessary to actually deliver the service. The term originated with the manufacturing industry.

Productive Time: Equates to the employee's net hours on duty when performing the functions in his or her job description.

Profit Center: Makes a manager responsible for both the revenue/volume (inflow) side and the expense (outflow) side of a department, division, unit, or program. Also known as a responsibility center.

Profitability Ratios: Ratios that reflect the ability of the organization to operate with an excess of operating revenue over operating expense.

Profit-Oriented Organization: Indicates the taxable status of the organization. A profit-oriented (or proprietary) organization is responsible for paying income taxes.

Profit-Volume (PV) Ratio: The contribution margin (i.e., net revenues less variable costs) expressed as a percentage of net revenue.

Proprietary Organization: Indicates the taxable status of the organization. A proprietary (or profit-oriented) organization is responsible for paying income taxes.

Prospective Analytics: A subset of predictive analytics that is used as a decision-making tool.

Quartile: A distribution into four classes, each of which contains one-quarter of the whole; any one of the four classes is a quartile.

Quick Ratio: A liquidity ratio considered the most severe test of short-term debt-paying ability (even more severe than the current ratio). Computed by dividing cash and cash equivalents plus net receivables by current liabilities. Also known as the acid-test ratio.

Reimbursement: A method of paying (reimbursing) a healthcare provider for services or procedures provided.

Reporting System: Produces reports of an event's effect in the healthcare financial system.

Responsibility Centers: Makes a manager responsible for both the revenue/volume (inflow) side and the expense (outflow) side of a department, division, unit, or program. Also known as a profit center.

Retrospective Analytics: Identifies trends and problems by looking at historical information and drawing empirical conclusions.

Return on Total Assets: A profitability ratio generally expressed as a percentage, this is a broad measure of profitability in common use. Computed by dividing earnings before interest and taxes, or EBIT, by total assets. This ratio is known by its acronym, EBIT, in credit analysis circles.

Revenue: Actual or expected cash inflows due to the organization's major business. Revenues are amounts earned in the course of doing business. In the case of health care, revenues are mostly earned by rendering services to patients.

Revenue Amount: Refers to how much each payer is expected to pay for the service and/or drug or device.

Revenue Sources: Refers to how many payers will pay for the service and/or drug and device, and in what proportion.

Revenue Type: A designation as to whether, for example, revenue is derived entirely from services or whether part of the revenue is derived from drugs and devices.

Salvage Value: Also known as residual value or scrap value, represents any expected cash value of the asset at the end of its useful life.

Semifixed Costs: Those costs that stay fixed for a time when activity levels or volume of operations change; rises will occur, but not in direct proportion.

Semivariable Costs: Those costs that vary when activity levels or volume of operations change, but not in direct proportion. A supervisor's salary is an example of a semivariable cost.

Situational Analysis: Management tool that reviews, assesses, and analyzes the organization's internal operations for strengths and weaknesses and the organization's external environment for opportunities and threats.

Social Media: Online technology and content whose original purpose was that of enhancing social communication and collaboration. Current examples of social media include Facebook and Twitter.

Solvency Ratios: Ratios that reflect the ability of the organization to pay the annual interest and principal obligations on its long-term debt. These ratios determine ability to "be solvent."

Space Occupancy: Within the context of a forecast or projection, refers to the overall cost of occupying the space required for the service or procedure. Considered to be an indirect cost.

Staffing: A term that means the assigning of staff to fill scheduled positions.

Stakeholder: A person or entity that has an interest in a service, program, and/or outcome.

Standardized Data: Data that are both uniform and comparable.

Statement of Cash Flows: One of the four basic financial statements, this statement reports the current period cash flow by taking the accrual basis statements and converting them to an effective cash flow. This is accomplished by a series of reconciling adjustments that account for the noncash amounts.

Statement of Fund Balance/Net Worth: One of the four basic financial statements, this statement reports the excess of revenue over expenses (or vice versa) for the period as the excess flows into equity (or reduces equity, in the case of a loss for the period).

Statement of Revenue and Expense: One of the four basic financial statements, this statement reports the inflow of revenue and the outflow of expense over a stated period of time. The net result is also reported, either as excess of revenue over expense or, in the case of a loss for the period, excess of expense over revenue.

Static Budget: A budget based on a single level of operations, or volume. After it is approved and finalized, the single level of operations (volume) is never adjusted; thus, the budget is "static" or unchanging.

Stock Warrants: Warrants allow the owner of the warrant to purchase additional shares of stock in the company, generally at a particular price and prior to an expiration date.

Strategic Objective: A strategic objective further defines intended outcomes in order to achieve a goal.

Structured Data: Data that adheres to standards that allow patient information to be easily retrieved and transferred.

Subsidiary Journals: Documents that contain specific sets of transactions and that support the general ledger.

Subsidiary Reports: Reports that support, and thus are subsidiary to, the four major financial statements.

Supplies: Within the context of a forecast or projection, refers to the necessary supplies that are required to perform a procedure or service. Considered to be a direct expense.

Support Services Expenses: This type of expense provides support to both general services expenses and to operations expenses. It is necessary for support, but it is neither directly related to patient care nor is it a service necessary to maintain the patient. Examples of support services are insurance and payroll taxes.

Sustainable Growth Rate (SGR): A method to ensure that the yearly increase in expense per Medicare beneficiary does not exceed the growth in the GDP.

SWOT Analysis: Acronym for a method of situational analysis assessing an organization's strengths-weaknesses-opportunities-threats; thus "SWOT."

Target Operating Income: Allows the manager to determine, or target, how many units must be sold in order to yield a particular operating income.

Three-Variance Method: A method of variance analysis that compares volume variance to use (or quantity) variance and to spending (or price) variance.

Threshold: A minimum number, or percentage, to be met.

Time Value of Money: The present value concept, which is that the value of a dollar today is more than the value of a dollar in the future.

Trend Analysis: The process of comparing and analyzing figures over several time periods. Also known as horizontal analysis.

Trial Balance: A document used to balance the general ledger accounts and to produce financial statements.

Two-Variance Method: A method of variance analysis that compares volume variance to budgeted costs (defined as standard hours for actual production)—thus the "two-variance" method.

Unadjusted Rate of Return: An unsophisticated return on investment method, the answer for which is an estimate containing no precision.

Unexpired Costs: Costs that are not yet used up and will be matched against future revenues.

Useful Life: The useful life of a fixed asset determines the period over which the fixed asset's cost will be spread.

Value-Based Concept: In finance, a combination of cost and quality. Value-based concepts may be applied to purchasing, payment, pricing, strategy, and/or patient care.

Values Statement: See Organizational Values.

Variable Costs: Those costs that vary in direct proportion to changes in activity levels of volume of operations. Food for meal preparation is an example of variable cost.

Variance Analysis: A variance is the difference between standard and actual prices and quantities. Variance analysis analyzes these differences.

Version 5010 of Transmission Standards: The current version of electronic transmission standards at the time of this writing. See Electronic Transmission Standards.

Vertical Analysis: A process of converting dollar amounts to percentages to put information on the same relative basis. Also known as common sizing.

Vision Statement: The Vision Statement explains "what we want to be." It is a look further into the future.

Voluntary Organization: Indicates the taxable status of the organization. A voluntary (or nonprofit) organization is exempt from paying income taxes.

Examples and Exercises, Supplemental Materials, and Solutions

The following examples and exercises include examples, practice exercises, and assignment exercises. Solutions to the practice exercises are found at the end of this section. Exercises are designated by chapter number.

EXAMPLES AND EXERCISES

CHAPTER 1

Assignment Exercise 1–1

Review the chapter text about types of organizations and examine the list in Exhibit 1–1.

Required

1. Obtain listings of healthcare organizations from the yellow pages of a telephone book.
2. Set up a worksheet listing the classifications of organizations found in Exhibit 1–1.
3. Enter the organizations you found in the yellow pages onto the worksheet.
4. For each organization indicate the type of organization.
5. If some cannot be identified by type, comment on what you would expect them to be; that is, proprietary, voluntary, or government owned.

Assignment Exercise 1–2

Review the chapter text about organization charts. Also examine the organization charts appearing in Figures 1–2 and 1–3.

Required

1. Refer to the Metropolis Health System (MHS) case study appearing in Chapter 33 and read about the various types of services offered by MHS.
2. The MHS organization chart has seven major areas of responsibility, each headed by a senior vice president. Select one of the seven areas and design additional levels of detail that indicate the managers. If you have considerable detail you may choose one

department (such as ambulatory operations) instead of the entire area of responsibility for that senior vice president.

3. Do you believe your design of the detailed organization chart indicates centralized or decentralized lines of authority for decision making? Can you explain your approach in one to two sentences?

CHAPTER 2

Assignment Exercise 2–1: Health System Flowsheets

Review the chapter text about information flow and Figures 2–2 and 2–3.

Required

1. Find an information flowsheet from a healthcare organization. It can be from a published source or from an actual organization.
2. Based on this flowsheet, comment on what the structure of the organization's information system appears to be.
3. If you were a manager (at this organization), would you want to change the structure? If so, why? If not, why not?

Assignment Exercise 2–2: Chart of Accounts

Review the chapter text about the chart of accounts and how it is a map of the company elements. Also review Exhibits 2–1, 2–2, and 2–3.

Required

1. Find an excerpt from a healthcare organization's chart of accounts. It can be from a published source or from an actual organization.
2. Based on this chart of accounts excerpt, comment on what the structure of the organization's reporting system appears to be.
3. If you were a manager (at this organization), would you want to change the system? If so, why? If not, why not?

CHAPTER 3

Assignment Exercise 3–1

Review the chapter text concerning the engaged patient.

Required

1. Find a source that discusses one of the patient engagement digital impact areas mentioned in the chapter text (patient portals, telemedicine, remote monitoring, etc.).
2. Based on the source that you find, comment on how effective you believe this type of patient engagement would be.

3. Would you want to use this type of patient engagement digital connection in your organization? If so, why? If not, why not?

Assignment 3–2

Review the chapter text concerning population health.

Required

1. Find a source of information from a healthcare organization that claims to be addressing population health.
2. Review the organization's information and answer the following: Does it define the population? Does it describe the care the population is receiving? Does it describe the delivery system that is providing this care?
3. Can you tell from this information whether there is a gap between the care required for this population and the care that is provided? If so, what do you think could be done to bridge this gap?

CHAPTER 4

Example 4A: Assets and Liabilities

Study the chapter text concerning examples of assets and liabilities. Is the difference between short-term and long-term assets and liabilities clear to you?

Practice Exercise 4–I

Place an "X" in the appropriate classification for each balance sheet item listed below.

	Short-Term Asset	*Long-Term Asset*	*Short-Term Liability*	*Long-Term Liability*
Payroll taxes due				
Accounts receivable				
Land				
Mortgage payable (noncurrent)				
Buildings				
Note payable (due in 24 months)				
Inventory				
Accounts payable				
Cash on hand				

Assignment Exercise 4–1: Balance Sheet

Locate a healthcare-related balance sheet. The source of the balance sheet can be internal (within a healthcare facility of some type) or external (from a published article or from a company's annual report, for example). Write your impressions and/or comments about the assets, liabilities, and net worth found on your balance sheet. Would you have preferred more detail in this statement? If so, why?

Assignment Exercise 4–2: Balance Sheet

Locate a second healthcare-related balance sheet. Again, the source of the balance sheet can be either internal or external. Compare the balance sheet you acquired for Assignment Exercise 4-1 with the second balance sheet you have now obtained. What is the same? What is different? Which one do you find more informative? Why?

CHAPTER 5

Example 5A: Contractual Allowances

Contractual allowances represent the difference between the full established rate and the agreed-upon contractual rate that will be paid. An example was given in the text of Chapter 5 by which the hospital's full established rate for a certain procedure is $100, but Giant Health Plan has negotiated a managed care contract whereby the plan pays only $90 for that procedure. The contractual allowance is $10 ($100 less $90 = $10). Assume instead that Near-By Health Plan has negotiated its own managed care contract whereby this plan pays $95 for that procedure. In this case the contractual allowance is $5 ($100 less $95 = $5).

Assignment Exercise 5–1: Contractual Allowances

Physician office revenue for visit code 99214 has a full established rate of $72.00. Of 10 different payers, there are 9 different contracted rates, as follows:

Payer	Contracted Rate (in dollars)
FHP	35.70
HPHP	58.85
MC	54.90
UND	60.40
CCN	70.20
MO	70.75
CGN	10.00
PRU	54.90
PHCS	50.00
ANA	45.00

Rates for illustration only.

Required

1. Set up a worksheet with four columns: Payer, Full Rate, Contracted Rate, and Contractual Allowance.
2. For each payer, enter the full rate and the contracted rate.
3. For each payer, compute the contractual allowance.

The first payer has been computed below:

Payer	Full Rate	(less)	Contracted Rate	(equals)	Contractual Allowance
FHP	$72.00		$35.70		$36.30

Example 5B: Revenue Sources and Grouping Revenue

Sources of healthcare revenue are often grouped by payer. Thus, services might be grouped as follows:

Revenue from the Medicare Program (payer = Medicare)
Revenue from the Medicaid Program (payer = Medicaid)
Revenue from Blue Cross Blue Shield (payer = Commercial Insurance)
or
Revenue from Blue Cross Blue Shield (payer = Managed Care Contract)

Assignment Exercise 5–2: Revenue Sources and Grouping Revenue

The Metropolis Health System (MHS) has revenue sources from operations, donations, and interest income. The revenue from operations is primarily received for services. MHS groups its revenue first by cost center. Within each cost center the services revenue is then grouped by payer.

Required

1. Set up a worksheet with individual columns across the top for six revenue sources (payers): Medicare, Medicaid, Other Public Programs, Patients, Commercial Insurance, and Managed Care Contracts.
2. Certain situations concerning the Intensive Care Unit and the Laboratory are described below.

    Set up six vertical line items on your worksheet, numbered 1 through 6. Six situations are described below. For each of the six situations, indicate its number (1 through 6) and enter the appropriate cost center (either Intensive Care Unit or Laboratory). Then place an X in the column(s) that represents the correct revenue source(s) for the item. The six situations are as follows:

    (1) ICU stay billed to employee's insurance program.
    (2) Lab test paid for by an individual.
    (3) Pathology work performed for the state.
    (4) ICU stay billed to member's health plan.

(5) ICU stay billed for Medicare beneficiary.

(6) Series of allergy tests run for eligible Medicaid beneficiary.

Headings for your worksheet:

	Medicare	Medicaid	Other Public Programs	Patients	Commercial Insurance	Managed Care Contracts
(1)						
(2)						
(3)						
(4)						
(5)						
(6)						

CHAPTER 6

Example 6A: Grouping Expenses by Cost Center

Cost centers are one method of grouping expenses. For example, a nursing home may consider the Admitting department as a cost center. In that case the expenses grouped under the Admitting department cost center may include:

- Administrative and Clerical Salaries
- Admitting Supplies
- Dues
- Periodicals and Books
- Employee Education
- Purchased Maintenance

Practice Exercise 6–I: Grouping Expenses by Cost Center

The Metropolis Health System groups expenses for the Intensive Care Unit into its own cost center. Laboratory expenses and Laundry expenses are likewise grouped into their own cost centers.

Required

1. Set up a worksheet with individual columns across the top for the three cost centers: Intensive Care Unit, Laboratory, and Laundry.
2. Indicate the appropriate cost center for each of the following expenses:
   - Drugs Requisitioned
   - Pathology Supplies
   - Detergents and Bleach
   - Nursing Salaries
   - Clerical Salaries
   - Uniforms (for Laundry Aides)
   - Repairs (parts for microscopes)
     (Hint: One of the expenses will apply to more than one cost center.)

Headings for your worksheet:

      Intensive Care Unit   Laboratory   Laundry

Assignment Exercise 6–1: Grouping Expenses by Cost Center

The Metropolis Health System's Rehabilitation and Wellness Center offers outpatient therapy and return-to-work services plus cardiac and pulmonary rehabilitation to get people back to a normal way of living. The Rehabilitation and Wellness Center expenses include the following:

- Nursing Salaries
- Physical Therapist Salaries
- Occupational Therapist Salaries
- Cardiac Rehab Salaries
- Pulmonary Rehab Salaries
- Patient Education Coordinator Salary
- Nursing Supplies
- Physical Therapist Supplies
- Occupational Therapist Supplies
- Cardiac Rehab Supplies
- Pulmonary Rehab Supplies
- Training Supplies
- Clerical Office Supplies
- Employee Education

Required

1. Decide how many cost centers should be used for the above expenses at the Rehabilitation and Wellness Center.
2. Set up a worksheet with individual columns across the top for the cost centers you have chosen.
3. For each of the expenses listed above, indicate to which of your cost centers it should be assigned.

Example 6B

Study the chapter text concerning grouping expenses by diagnoses and procedures. Refer to Exhibits 6–3 and 6–4 (about major diagnostic categories), Exhibit 6–5 (about DRGs and MDCs), and Table 6–1 (about procedure codes) for examples of different ways to group expenses by diagnoses and procedures.

Assignment Exercise 6–2

Required

Find a listing of expenses by diagnosis or by procedure. The source of the list can be internal (within a healthcare facility of some type) or external (such as a published article, report, or survey). Comment upon whether you believe the expense grouping used is appropriate. Would you have grouped the expenses in another way?

CHAPTER 7

Example 7A: Direct and Indirect Costs

Review the chapter text regarding direct and indirect costs. In particular, review the example of ambulance direct costs (Exhibit 7–1) and indirect costs (Exhibit 7–2). Remember that indirect costs are shared and are sometimes called joint costs or common costs. Because such costs are shared they must be allocated. Also, remember that one test of a direct cost is to ask: "If the operating unit (such as a department) did not exist, would this cost not be in existence?"

Practice Exercise 7–I: Identifying Direct and Indirect Costs

Make a worksheet with two columns: Direct Cost and Indirect Cost. Place each of the following items in the appropriate column:

- Managed care marketing expense
- Real estate taxes
- Liability insurance
- Clinic telephone expense
- Utilities (for the entire facility)
- Emergency room medical supplies

Assignment Exercise 7–1: Allocating Indirect Costs

Study Table 7–1, Table 7–2, and review the chapter text describing how the indirect cost is allocated. This assignment will change the allocation bases input for (A) Number of Visits (Volume), (B) Proportion of Direct Costs, and (C) Number of Computers in Service.

Required

1. Compute the costs allocated to cost centers "Clerical Salaries," "Administrative Salaries," and "Computer Services" using the new allocation bases shown below. Use worksheet #1 that replicates the set up in Table 7–2. Total the new results.
   The new allocation bases are:

   A = # Visits (Volume): PT = 9,600; OT = 4,000; ST = 2,400; Total = 16,000
   (16,000 × $3.50 = $56,000)
   B = Proportion of Direct Costs: PT = 60%; OT = 25%; ST = 15%; Total = 100%
   (% × $55,000 total)
   C = # Computers in Service: PT = 10; OT = 3; ST = 3; Total = 16
   (16 × $5,000 each = $80,000)

2. Using worksheet #2 that replicates the set up in Table 7–1, enter the new direct cost and the new totals for indirect costs resulting from your work. Total the new results.

Practice Exercise 7–II: Responsibility Centers

The Metropolis Health System has one director who supervises the areas of Security, Communications, and Ambulance Services. This director also supervises the medical records relevant to Ambulance Services, the educational training for Security and Ambulance Services personnel, and the human resources for Security, Communications, and Ambulance Services personnel.

Required

Of the duties and services described, all of which are supervised by one director, which areas should be responsibility centers and which areas should be support centers? Draw them in a visual and indicate the reporting requirements.

Assignment Exercise 7–2: Responsibility Centers

Choose among the strategic financial planning Case Study in Chapter 32, the public health clinic Mini-Case Study in Chapter 34, or the Metropolis Health System information as contained in its Chapter 33 Case Study and the Chapter 33-A Appendix that contains its comparative financial statements. Designate the responsibility centers and the support centers for the organization selected. Prepare a rationale for the structure you have designed.

CHAPTER 8

Example 8A: Fixed, Variable, and Semivariable Distinction

Review the chapter text for the distinction between fixed, variable, and semivariable costs. Pay particular attention to the accompanying Figures 8–1 through 8–5.

Practice Exercise 8–I: Analyzing Mixed Costs

The Metropolis Health System (MHS) has a system-wide training course for nurse aides. The course requires a packet of materials that MHS calls the training pack. Due to turnover and because the course is system-wide, there is a monthly demand for new packs. In addition, the local community college also obtains the training packs used in their credit courses from MHS.

The education coordinator needs to know how much of the cost is fixed and how much of the cost is variable for these training packs. She decides to use the high–low method of computation.

Required

Using the monthly utilization information presented below, find the fixed and variable portion of costs through the high–low method.

Month	Number of Training Packs	Cost
January	1,000	$ 6,200
February	200	1,820
March	250	2,350
April	400	3,440

May	700	4,900
June	300	2,730
July	150	1,470
August	100	1,010
September	1,100	7,150
October	300	2,850
November	250	2,300
December	100	1,010

Assignment Exercise 8–1: Analyzing Mixed Costs

The education coordinator decides that the community college packs may be unduly influencing the high–low computation. She decides to rerun the results, omitting the community college volume.

Required

1. Using the monthly utilization information presented here, and omitting the community college training packs, find the fixed and variable portion of costs through the high–low method. Note that the college only acquires packs in three months of the year: January, May, and September. These dates coincide with the start dates of their semesters and summer school.
2. The reason the education coordinator needs to know how much of the cost is fixed is because she is supposed to collect the appropriate variable cost from the community college for their packs. For her purposes, which computation do you believe is better? Why?

Month	Total Number of Training Packs	Total Cost	Community College Number Packs	Community College Cost (in dollars)
January	1,000	$ 6,200	200	1,240
February	200	1,820		
March	250	2,350		
April	400	3,440		
May	700	4,900	300	2,100
June	300	2,730		
July	150	1,470		
August	100	1,010		
September	1,100	7,150	300	1,950
October	300	2,850		
November	250	2,300		
December	100	1,010		

Example 8B: Contribution Margin

Computation of a contribution margin is simplified if the fixed and variable expense has already been determined. Examine Table 8–1, which contains Operating Room fixed and variable costs.

We can see that the total costs are $1,217,756. Of this amount, $600,822 is designated as variable cost and $616,934 is designated as fixed ($529,556 plus $87,378 equals $616,934). For purposes of our example, assume the Operating Room revenue amounts to $1,260,000. The contribution margin is computed as follows:

	Amount
Revenue	$1,260,000
Less Variable Cost	(600,822)
Contribution Margin	$659,178

Thus, $659,178 is available to contribute to fixed costs and to profit. (In this example fixed costs amount to $616,934, so there is an amount left to contribute toward profit.)

Practice Exercise 8–II: Calculating the Contribution Margin

Greenside Clinic has revenue totaling $3,500,000. The clinic has costs totaling $3,450,000. Of this amount, 40% is variable cost and 60% is fixed cost.

Required

Compute the contribution margin for Greenside Clinic.

Assignment Exercise 8–2: Calculating the Contribution Margin

The Mental Health program for the Community Center has just completed its fiscal year end. The program director determines that his program has revenue for the year of $1,210,000. He believes his variable expense amounts to $205,000 and he knows his fixed expense amounts to $1,100,000.

Required

1. Compute the contribution margin for the Community Center Mental Health Program.
2. What does the result tell you about the program?

Example 8C: Cost-Volume-Profit (CVP) Ratio and Profit-Volume (PV) Ratio

Closely review the examples of ratio calculations in the chapter text. Also note that examples are presented in visuals as well as text.

Practice Exercise 8–3: Calculating the PV Ratio

The profit-volume (PV) ratio is also known as the contribution margin (CM) ratio. Use the same assumptions for the Community Center Mental Health Program. In addition to the contribution margin figures already computed, now compute the PV ratio (also known as the CM ratio).

Assignment Exercise 8–3: Calculating the PV Ratio and the CVP Ratio

Use the same assumptions for the Greenside Clinic. One more assumption will be added: The clinic had 35,000 visits.

Required

1. In addition to the contribution margin figures already computed, now compute the PV ratio (also known as the CM ratio).
2. Add another column to your worksheet and compute the clinic's per-visit revenue and costs.
3. Create a Cost-Volume-Profit chart. Refer to the chapter text along with Figure 8–6.

CHAPTER 9

Assignment Exercise 9–1: FIFO and LIFO Inventory

Study the FIFO and LIFO explanations in the chapter.

Required

1. Use the format in Exhibit 9–1 to compute the ending FIFO inventory and the cost of goods sold, assuming $90,000 in sales; beginning inventory 500 units @ $50; purchases of 400 units @ $50; 100 units @ $65; 400 units @ $80.
   a. Also compute the cost of goods sold percentage of sales.
2. Use the format in Exhibit 9–2 to compute the ending LIFO inventory and the cost of goods sold, using same assumptions.
   a. Also compute the cost of goods sold percentage of sales.
   b. Comment on the difference in outcomes.

Assignment Exercise 9–2: Inventory Turnover

Study the "Calculating Inventory Turnover" portion of the chapter closely, whereby the cost of goods sold divided by the average inventory equals the inventory turnover.

Required

Compute two inventory turnover calculations as follows:

1. Use the LIFO information in the previous assignment to first compute the average inventory and then to compute the inventory turnover.
2. Use the FIFO information in the previous assignment to first compute the average inventory and then to compute the inventory turnover.

Example 9A: Depreciation Concept

Assume that Metropolis Health System (MHS) purchased equipment for $200,000 cash on April 1 (the first day of its fiscal year). This equipment has an expected life of 10 years. The salvage value is 10% of cost. No equipment was traded in on this purchase.

Straight-line depreciation is a method that charges an equal amount of depreciation for each year the asset is in service. In the case of this purchase, straight-line depreciation would amount to $18,000 per year for 10 years. This amount is computed as follows:

Step 1. Compute the cost net of salvage or trade-in value: 200,000 less 10% salvage value or 20,000 equals 180,000.

Step 2. Divide the resulting figure by the expected life (also known as estimated useful life): 180,000 divided by 10 equals 18,000 depreciation per year for 10 years.

Accelerated depreciation represents methods that are speeded up, or accelerated. In other words a greater amount of depreciation is taken earlier in the life of the asset. One example of accelerated depreciation is the double-declining balance method. Unlike straight-line depreciation, trade-in or salvage value is not taken into account until the end of the depreciation schedule. This method uses *book value*, which is the net amount remaining when cumulative previous depreciation is deducted from the asset's cost. The computation is as follows:

Step 1. Compute the straight-line rate: 1 divided by 10 equals 10%.
Step 2. Now double the rate (as in *double-declining method*): 10% times 2 equals 20%.
Step 3. Compute the first year's depreciation expense: 200,000 times 20% equals 40,000.
Step 4. Compute the carry-forward book value at the beginning of the second year: 200,000 book value beginning Year 1 less Year 1 depreciation of 40,000 equals book value at the beginning of the second year of 160,000.
Step 5. Compute the second year's depreciation expense: 160,000 times 20% equals 32,000.
Step 6. Compute the carry-forward book value at the beginning of the third year: 160,000 book value beginning Year 2 less Year 2 depreciation of 32,000 equals book value at the beginning of the third year of 128,000.
—Continue until the asset's salvage or trade-in value has been reached.
—Do not depreciate beyond the salvage or trade-in value.

Practice Exercise 9–I: Depreciation Concept

Assume that MHS purchased equipment for $600,000 cash on April 1 (the first day of its fiscal year). This equipment has an expected life of 10 years. The salvage value is 10% of cost. No equipment was traded in on this purchase.

Required

1. Compute the straight-line depreciation for this purchase.
2. Compute the double-declining balance depreciation for this purchase.

Assignment Exercise 9–3: Depreciation Concept

Assume that MHS purchased two additional pieces of equipment on April 1 (the first day of its fiscal year), as follows:

1. The laboratory equipment cost $300,000 and has an expected life of 5 years. The salvage value is 5% of cost. No equipment was traded in on this purchase.
2. The radiology equipment cost $800,000 and has an expected life of 7 years. The salvage value is 10% of cost. No equipment was traded in on this purchase.

Required

For both pieces of equipment:

1. Compute the straight-line depreciation.
2. Compute the double-declining balance depreciation.

Example 9B: Depreciation

This example shows straight-line depreciation computed at a five-year useful life with no salvage value. Straight-line depreciation is the method commonly used for financing projections and funding proposals.

Depreciation Expense Computation: Straight Line

Five-year useful life; no salvage value

Year #	Annual Depreciation	Remaining Balance
Beginning Balance =		60,000
1	12,000	48,000
2	12,000	36,000
3	12,000	24,000
4	12,000	12,000
5	12,000	–0

Example 9C: Depreciation

This example shows straight-line depreciation computed at a five-year useful life with a remaining salvage value of $10,000. Note the difference in annual depreciation between Example 9B and Example 9C.

Depreciation Expense Computation: Straight Line

Five-year useful life; $10,000 salvage value

Year #	Annual Depreciation	Remaining Balance
Beginning Balance =		60,000
1	10,000	50,000
2	10,000	40,000
3	10,000	30,000
4	10,000	20,000
5	10,000	10,000

Example 9D: Depreciation

This example shows double-declining depreciation computed at a five-year useful life with no salvage value. As is often the case with a five-year life, the double-declining method is used for the first three years and the straight-line method is used for the remaining two years. The double-declining method first computes what the straight-line percentage would be. In this case 100% divided by five years equals 20%. The 20% is then doubled. In this case 20% times 2 equals 40%. Then the 40% is multiplied by the remaining balance to be depreciated. Thus 60,000 times 40% for year one equals 24,000 depreciation, with a remaining balance of 36,000.

Then 36,000 times 40% for year two equals 14,400 depreciation, and 36,000 minus 14,400 equals 21,600 remaining balance, and so on.

Now note the difference in annual depreciation between Example 9B, using straight-line for all five years, and Example 9D, using the combined double-declining and straight-line methods.

Depreciation Expense Computation: Double-Declining-Balance

Five-year useful life; $10,000 salvage value

Year #	Annual Depreciation	Remaining Balance
Beginning Balance =		60,000
1	24,000*	36,000
2	14,400*	21,600
3	8,640*	12,960
4	6,480**	6,480
5	6,480**	6,480

*double-declining balance depreciation
** straight-line depreciation for remaining two years (12,960 divided by 2 = 6,480/yr)

Practice Exercise 9–II: Depreciation

Compute the straight-line depreciation for each year for equipment with a cost of $50,000, a five-year useful life, and a $5,000 salvage value.

Assignment Exercise 9–4: Depreciation

Set up a purchase scenario of your own and compute the depreciation with and without salvage value.

Assignment Exercise 9–5: Depreciation Computation: Units-of-Service

Study the "Units of Service" portion of the chapter closely.

Required

1. Using the format in Table 9–A-5, compute units of service depreciation using the following assumptions:

> Cost to be depreciated = $50,000
> Salvage value = zero
> Total units of service = 10,000
> Units of service per year: Year 1 = 2,200; Year 2 = 2,100;
> Year 3 = 2,300; Year 4 = 2,200; Year 5 = 200

2. Using the same format, compute units of service depreciation using adjusted assumptions as follows:

> Cost to be depreciated = $50,000
> Salvage value = $5,000
> Total units of service = 10,000
>   Units of service per year: Year 1 = 2,200; Year 2 = 2,100;
>   Year 3 = 2,300; Year 4 = 2,200; Year 5 = 200

CHAPTER 10

Example 10A

Review the chapter text about annualizing positions. In particular review Exhibit 10–2, which contains the annualizing calculations.

Practice Exercise 10–I: FTEs to Annualize Staffing

The office manager for a physicians' group affiliated with Metropolis Health System (MHS) is working on her budget for next year. She wants to annualize her staffing plan. To do so she needs to convert her staff's net paid days worked to a factor. Their office is open and staffed seven days a week, per their agreement with two managed care plans.

The office manager has the MHS worksheet, which shows 9 holidays, 7 sick days, 15 vacation days, and 3 education days, equaling 34 paid days per year not worked. The physicians' group allows 8 holidays, 5 sick days, and 1 education day. An employee must work one full year to earn 5 vacation days. An employee must have worked full time for three full years before earning 10 annual vacation days. Because the turnover is so high, nobody on staff has earned more than 5 vacation days.

Required

1. Compute net paid days worked for a full-time employee in the physicians' group.
2. Convert net paid days worked to a factor so the office manager can annualize her staffing plan.

Assignment Exercise 10–1: FTEs to Annualize Staffing

The Metropolis Health System managers are also working on their budgets for next year. Each manager must annualize his or her staffing plan, and thus must convert staff net paid days worked to a factor. Each manager has the MHS worksheet, which shows 9 holidays, 7 sick days, 15 vacation days, and 3 education days, equaling 34 paid days per year not worked.

The Laboratory is fully staffed 7 days per week and the 34 paid days per year not worked is applicable for the lab. The Medical Records department is also fully staffed 7 days per week. However, Medical Records is an outsourced department so the employee benefits are somewhat different. The Medical Records employees receive 9 holidays plus 21 personal leave days, which can be used for any purpose.

Required

1. Compute net paid days worked for a full-time employee in the Laboratory and in Medical Records.
2. Convert net paid days worked to a factor for the Laboratory and for Medical Records so these MHS managers can annualize their staffing plans.

Example 10B

Review the chapter text about staffing requirements to fill a position. In particular review Exhibit 10–4, which contains (at the bottom of the exhibit) the staffing calculations. Remember this method uses a basic work week as the standard.

Practice Exercise 10–II: FTEs to Fill a Position

Metropolis Health System (MHS) uses a basic work week of 40 hours throughout the system. Thus, one full-time employee works 40 hours per week. MHS also uses a standard 24-hour scheduling system of three 8-hour shifts. The Admissions manager needs to compute the staffing requirements to fill his departmental positions. He has more than one Admissions office staffed within the system. The West Admissions office typically has two Admissions officers on duty during the day shift, one Admissions officer on duty during the evening shift, and one Admissions officer on duty during the night shift. The day shift also has one clerical person on duty. Staffing is identical for all seven days of the week.

Required

1. Set up a staffing requirements worksheet, using the format in Exhibit 10–4.
2. Compute the number of FTEs required to fill the Admissions officer position and the clerical position at the West Admissions office.

Assignment Exercise 10–2: FTEs to Fill a Position

Metropolis Health System (MHS) uses a basic work week of 40 hours throughout the system. Thus, one full-time employee works 40 hours per week. MHS also uses a standard 24-hour scheduling system of three 8-hour shifts. The Director of Nursing needs to compute the staffing requirements to fill the Operating Room (OR) positions. Since MHS is a trauma center, the OR is staffed 24 hours a day, 7 days a week. At present, staffing is identical for all 7 days of the week, although the Director of Nursing is questioning the efficiency of this method.

The Operating Room department is staffed with two nursing supervisors on the day shift and one nursing supervisor apiece on the evening and night shifts. There are two technicians on the day shift, two technicians on the evening shift, and one technician on the night shift. There are three RNs on the day shift, two RNs on the evening shift, and one RN plus one LPN on the night shift. In addition, there is one aide plus one clerical worker on the day shift only.

Required

1. Set up a staffing requirements worksheet, using the format in Exhibit 10–4.
2. Compute the number of FTEs required to fill the Operating Room staffing positions.

CHAPTER 11

Practice Exercise 11–I: Components of Balance Sheet and Statement of Net Income

Financial statements for Doctors Smith and Brown are provided here. Use the doctors' balance sheet, statement of revenue and expenses, and statement of capital for this assignment.

Required

Identify the following doctors' balance sheet and statement of net income components. List the name of each component and its amount(s) from the appropriate financial statement.

    Current Liabilities
    Total Assets
    Income from Operations
    Accumulated Depreciation
    Total Operating Revenue
    Current Portion of Long-Term Debt
    Interest Income
    Inventories

Assignment Exercise 11–1: Components of Balance Sheet and Statement of Net Income

Refer to the Metropolis Health System (MHS) financial statements contained in Appendix 33-A. Use the MHS comparative balance sheet, statement of revenue and expenses, and statement of fund balance for this assignment.

Required

Identify the following MHS balance sheet components. List the name of each component and its amount(s) from the appropriate MHS financial statement.

    Current Liabilities
    Total Assets
    Income from Operations
    Accumulated Depreciation
    Total Operating Revenue
    Current Portion of Long-Term Debt
    Interest Income
    Inventories

Doctors Smith and Brown:
Statement of Net Income
for the Three Months Ended March 31, 2___

Revenue

Net patient service revenue	180,000	
Other revenue	-0-	
Total Operating Revenue		180,000

Expenses

Nursing/PA salaries	16,650	
Clerical salaries	10,150	
Payroll taxes/employee benefits	4,800	
Medical supplies and drugs	15,000	
Professional fees	3,000	
Dues and publications	2,400	
Janitorial service	1,200	
Office supplies	1,500	
Repairs and maintenance	1,200	
Utilities and telephone	6,000	
Depreciation	30,000	
Interest	3,100	
Other	5,000	
Total Expenses		100,000
Income from Operations		80,000

Nonoperating Gains (Losses)

Interest Income		-0-
Nonoperating Gains, Net		-0-
Net Income		80,000

Doctors Smith and Brown
Balance Sheet
March 31, 2____

Assets

Current Assets

Cash and cash equivalents	25,000	
Patient accounts receivable	40,000	
Inventories—supplies and drugs	5,000	
Total Current Assets		70,000

Property, Plant, and Equipment

Buildings and Improvements	500,000	
Equipment	800,000	
Total	1,300,000	
Less Accumulated Depreciation	(480,000)	
Net Depreciable Assets	820,000	
Land	100,000	
Property, Plant, and Equipment, Net		920,000
Other Assets		10,000
Total Assets		1,000,000

Liabilities and Capital

Current Liabilities

Current maturities of long-term debt	10,000	
Accounts payable and accrued expenses	20,000	
Total Current Liabilities		30,000
Long-Term Debt	180,000	
Less Current Portion of Long-Term Debt	(10,000)	
Net Long-Term Debt		170,000
Total Liabilities		200,000
Capital		800,000
Total Liabilities and Capital		1,000,000

Doctors Smith and Brown
Statement of Changes in Capital
for the Three Months Ended March 31, 2____

Beginning Balance	$720,000
Net Income	80,000
Ending Balance	$800,000

Example 11A: Components of Balance Sheet and Income Statement

The "Accounts Receivable (net)" in Exhibit 11–1 means the accounts receivable figure of $250,000 on the balance sheet is net of the allowance for bad debts. If the allowance for bad debts is raised on the balance sheet, then bad debt expense (a.k.a. provision for doubtful accounts) on the income statement (a.k.a. statement of revenue and expense) also rises. Think of these two accounts as a pair.

Practice Exercise 11–II: Components of Balance Sheet and Income Statement

Refer to Doctors Smith and Brown's balance sheet, where patient accounts receivable is stated at $40,000. Do you think this figure is net of an allowance for bad debts?

Assignment Exercise 11–2: Components of Balance Sheet and Income Statement

Refer to the Metropolis Health System (MHS) balance sheet and statement of revenue and expense in the MHS Case Study appearing in Chapter 33. Patient accounts receivable of $7,400,000 is shown as net of $1,300,000 allowance for bad debts (8,700,000 − 1,300,000 = 7,400,000). (1) What percentage of gross accounts receivable is the allowance for bad debts? (2) If the allowance for bad debts is raised to $1,500,000, where does the extra $200,000 go?

Example 11B: Components of Balance Sheet and Income Statement

Refer to Exhibit 11–1 and Exhibit 11–2's Westside Clinic statements. The "Property, Plant, and Equipment (net)" total in Exhibit 11–1 means the property, plant, and equipment figure of $360,000 on the balance sheet is net of the reserve for depreciation. If the reserve for depreciation is raised on the balance sheet, then the depreciation expense on the income statement (a.k.a. statement of revenue and expense) also rises. Think of these two accounts as another pair.

Practice Exercise 11–III: Components of Balance Sheet and Income Statement

Refer to Doctors Smith and Brown's balance sheet, where buildings and equipment are both stated as net (the $820,000 figure), but land is not. Do you recall why this is so?

Assignment Exercise 11–3: Components of Balance Sheet and Income Statement

Refer to the Metropolis Health System (MHS) balance sheet and statement of revenue and expense in the MHS Case Study appearing in Chapter 33. Property, plant, and equipment of $19,300,000 is shown as "net," meaning net of the reserve for depreciation. If the $19,300,000 is reduced by $200,000 (meaning the reserve for depreciation has risen), what happens on the income statement?

CHAPTER 12

Example 12A

To better understand how the information for the numerator and the denominator of each calculation is obtained, Figure 12–1 illustrates the process. This figure takes the balance sheet and the statement of revenue and expense that were discussed in the preceding chapter and illustrates the source of each figure in the four liquidity ratios. The multiple computations in days cash on hand and in days receivables are further broken out into a three-step process to better illustrate sources of information.

Practice Exercise 12–I: Liquidity Ratios

Two of the liquidity ratios are illustrated in this practice exercise. Refer to Doctors Smith and Brown's financial statements appearing in the preceding exercises for Chapter 11.

Required

1. Set up a worksheet for the current ratio and the quick ratio.
2. Compute the ratios for Doctors Smith and Brown.

Assignment Exercise 12–1: Liquidity Ratios

Refer to the Metropolis Health System (MHS) case study appearing in Chapter 33.

Required

1. Set up a worksheet for the liquidity ratios.
2. Compute the four liquidity ratios using the MHS financial statements appearing in Chapter 33.

Example 12B

To better understand how the information for the numerator and the denominator of each calculation is obtained, Figure 12–2 illustrates the process. This figure takes the balance sheet and the statement of revenue and expense that were discussed in the preceding chapter and illustrates the source of each figure in the two solvency ratios. Any multiple computations are further broken out to better explain sources of information.

Practice Exercise 12–II: Solvency Ratios

Refer to Doctors Smith and Brown's financial statements appearing in the preceding exercises for Chapter 11.

Required

1. Set up a worksheet for the solvency ratios.
2. Compute these ratios for Doctors Smith and Brown. To do so, you will need one additional piece of information that is not present on the doctors' statements: their maximum annual debt service is $22,200.

Assignment Exercise 12–2: Solvency Ratios

Refer to the Metropolis Health System (MHS) case study appearing in Chapter 33.

Required

1. Set up a worksheet for the liquidity ratios.
2. Compute the solvency ratios using the Chapter 33 MHS financial statements.

Example 12C

To better understand how the information for the numerator and the denominator of each calculation is obtained, study Figure 12–2. This figure takes the balance sheet and the statement of revenue and expense that were discussed in the preceding chapter and illustrates the source of each figure in the two profitability ratios. Any multiple computations are further broken out to better explain sources of information.

Practice Exercise 12–III: Profitability Ratios

Refer to Doctors Smith and Brown's financial statements appearing in the preceding exercises for Chapter 11.

Required

1. Set up a worksheet for the profitability ratios.
2. Compute these ratios for Doctors Smith and Brown. All the necessary information is present on the doctors' statements.
   [Hint: "Operating Income (Loss)" is also known as "Income from Operations."]

Assignment Exercise 12–3: Profitability Ratios

Refer to the Metropolis Health System (MHS) case study appearing in Chapter 33.

Required

1. Set up a worksheet for the liquidity ratios.
2. Compute the profitability ratios using the Chapter 33 MHS financial statements.

CHAPTER 13

Example 13A: Unadjusted Rate of Return

Assumptions

- Average annual net income = $100,000
- Original investment amount = $1,000,000
- Unrecovered asset cost at the end of useful life (salvage value) = $100,000

Calculation using original investment amount:

$$\frac{\$100,000}{\$1,000,000} = 10\% \text{ Unadjusted Rate of Return}$$

Calculation using average investment amount:

Step 1: Compute average investment amount for total unrecovered asset cost.

At beginning of estimated useful life	=	$1,000,000
At end of estimated useful life	=	$ 100,000
	Sum	$1,100,000

Divided by 2 = $550,000 average investment amount

Step 2: Calculate unadjusted rate of return.

$$\frac{\$100,000}{\$550,000} = 18.2\% \text{ Unadjusted Rate of Return}$$

Practice Exercise 13–I: Unadjusted Rate of Return

Assumptions

- Average annual net income = $100,000
- Original investment amount = $500,000
- Unrecovered asset cost at the end of useful life (salvage value) = $50,000

Required

1. Compute the unadjusted rate of return using the original investment amount.
2. Compute the unadjusted rate of return using the average investment method.

Assignment Exercise 13–1: Unadjusted Rate of Return

Metropolis Health Systems' Laboratory Director expects to purchase a new piece of equipment. The assumptions for the transaction are as follows:

- Average annual net income = $70,000
- Original investment amount = $410,000
- Unrecovered asset cost at the end of useful life (salvage value) = $41,000

Required

1. Compute the unadjusted rate of return using the original investment amount.
2. Compute the unadjusted rate of return using the average investment method.

Example 13B: Finding the Future Value (with a Compound Interest Table)

Betty Dylan is Director of Nurses at Metropolis Health System. Her oldest son will be entering college in five years. Today Betty is trying to figure what his college fund will amount to in five more years. (Hint: Compound interest means interest is not only earned on the principal, but also is earned on the previous interest earnings that have been left in the account. Interest is thus compounded.)

The college fund savings account presently has a balance of $9,000 and any interest earned over the next five years will be left in the account. Betty assumes the annual interest rate will be 6%. How much money will be in the account at the end of five more years?

Solution to Example

Step 1.   Refer to the Compound Interest Table appearing in Appendix 13-B at the back of this chapter. Reading across, or horizontally, find the 6% column. Reading down, or vertically, find Year 5. Trace across the Year 5 line item to the 6% column. The factor is 1.338.

Step 2.   Multiply the current savings account balance of $9,000 times the factor of 1.338 to find the future value of $12,042. In five years at compound interest of 6%, the college fund will have a balance of $12,042.

Practice Exercise 13–II: Finding the Future Value (with a Compound Interest Table)

Assume the college savings fund in the preceding example presently has a balance of $11,000 and any interest earned will be left in the account. Assume the annual interest rate will be 7%.

Required

Compute how much money will be in the account at the end of six more years. (Use the compound interest table appearing in Appendix 13-B.)

Assignment Exercise 13–2: Finding the Future Value (with a Compound Interest Table)

John Whitten is one of the physicians on staff at Metropolis Health System. His practice is six years old. He has set up an office savings account to accumulate the funds to replace equipment in his practice. Today John is trying to figure what his equipment fund will amount to in four more years.

The equipment fund savings account presently has a balance of $63,500 and any interest earned over the next four years will be left in the account. John assumes the annual interest rate will be 5%. How much money will be in the account at the end of four more years?

Required

Compute how much money will be in the account at the end of four more years. (Use the compound interest table appearing in Appendix 13-B.)

Example 13C: Finding the Present Value (with a Present-Value Table)

Betty Dylan is taking an adult education night course in personal finance at the community college. The class is presently studying retirement planning. Each student is to estimate the amount of funds (in addition to pension plans and social security) they believe will be needed at retirement. Then they are to make a retirement plan.

Betty has estimated she would need $100,000 fifteen years from now. In order to complete her assignment, she needs to know the present value of the $100,000. Betty further assumes an interest rate of 6%.

Solution to Example

Step 1. Refer to the Present-Value Table appearing in Appendix 13-A at the back of this chapter. Reading across, or horizontally, find the 6% column. Reading down, or vertically, find Year 15. Trace across the Year 15 line item to the 6% column. The factor is 0.4173.

Step 2. Multiply $100,000 times the factor of 0.4173 to find the present value of $41,730.

Practice Exercise 13–III: Finding the Present Value (with a Present-Value Table)

Betty isn't finished with her assignment. Now she wants to find the present value of $150,000 accumulated fifteen years from now. She further assumes a better interest rate of 7%.

Required

Compute the present value of $150,000 accumulated fifteen years from now. Assume an interest rate of 7%. (Use the Present-Value Table appearing in Appendix 13-A at the back of this chapter.)

Assignment Exercise 13–3: Finding the Present Value (with a Present-Value Table)

Part 1—Dr. John Whitten is still figuring out his equipment fund. According to his calculations he needs $250,000 to be accumulated six years from now. John is now trying to find the present value of the $250,000. He continues to assume an interest rate of 5%.

Required

Compute the present value of $250,000 accumulated fifteen years from now. Assume an interest rate of 5%. (Use the Present-Value Table appearing in Appendix 13-A at the back of this chapter.)

Part 2—John doesn't like the answer he gets. What if he can raise the interest rate to 7%? How much difference would that make?

Required

Compute the present value of $250,000 accumulated fifteen years from now assuming an interest rate of 7%. Compare the difference between this amount and the present value at 5%.

Example 13D: Internal Rate of Return

Review the chapter text to follow the steps set out to compute the internal rate of return.

Practice Exercise 13–IV: Internal Rate of Return

Metropolis Health System (MHS) is considering purchasing a tractor to mow the grounds. It would cost $16,950 and have a 10-year useful life. It will have zero salvage value at the end of

10 years. The head of the MHS grounds crew estimates it would save $3,000 per year. He figures this savings because just one of the present maintenance crew would be driving the tractor, replacing the labor of several men now using small household-type lawn mowers. Compute the internal rate of return for this proposed acquisition.

Assignment Exercise 13–4: Computing an Internal Rate of Return

Dr. Whitten has decided to purchase equipment that has a cost of $60,000 and will produce a pretax net cash inflow of $30,000 per year over its estimated useful life of six years. The equipment will have no salvage value and will be depreciated by the straight-line method. The tax rate is 50%. Determine Dr. Whitten's approximate after-tax internal rate of return.

Example 13E: Payback Period

Review the chapter text and follow the Doctor Green detailed example of payback period computation.

Practice Exercise 13–V: Payback

The MHS Chief Financial Officer is considering a request by the Emergency Room department for purchase of new equipment. It will cost $500,000. There is no trade-in. Its useful life would be 10 years. This type of machine is new to the department but it is estimated that it will result in $84,000 annual revenue and operating costs would be one-quarter of that amount. The CFO wants to find the payback period for this piece of equipment.

Assignment Exercise 13–5: Payback Period

The MHS Chief Financial Officer is considering alternate proposals for the hospital Radiology department. The Director of Radiology has suggested purchasing one of two pieces of equipment. Machine A costs $15,000 and Machine B costs $12,000. Both machines are estimated to reduce radiology operating costs by $5,000 per year.

Required

Which machine should be purchased? Make your payback calculations to provide the answer.

CHAPTER 14

Example 14A: Common Sizing

Common sizing converts numbers to percentages so that comparative analysis can be performed. Reread the chapter text about common sizing and examine the percentages shown in Table 14–1.

Practice Exercise 14–I: Common Sizing

The worksheet below shows the assets of two hospitals.

Required

Perform common sizing for the assets of the two hospitals.

	Same Year for Both Hospitals	
	Hospital A	Hospital B
Current Assets	$ 2,000,000	$ 8,000,000
Property, Plant, & Equipment	7,500,000	30,000,000
Other Assets	500,000	2,000,000
Total Assets	$10,000,000	$40,000,000

Assignment Exercise 14–1: Common Sizing

Refer to the Metropolis Health System (MHS) comparative financial statements appearing in Appendix 33-A.

Required

Common size the MHS statement of revenue and expenses.

Example 14B: Trend Analysis

Trend analysis allows comparison of figures over time. Reread the chapter text about trend analysis and examine the difference columns shown in Table 14–3.

Practice Exercise 14–II: Trend Analysis

The worksheet below shows the assets of Hospital A over two years.

Required

Perform trend analysis for the assets of Hospital A.

	Hospital A	
	Year 1	Year 2
Current Assets	$1,600,000	$ 2,000,000
Property, Plant, & Equipment	6,000,000	7,500,000
Other Assets	400,000	500,000
Total Assets	$8,000,000	$10,000,000

Assignment Exercise 14–2: Trend Analysis

Refer to the Metropolis Health System (MHS) comparative financial statements appearing in Appendix 33-A.

Required

Perform trend analysis on the MHS statement of revenue and expenses.

Practice Exercise 14–III: Contractual Allowance

Assumptions:

1. Your unit's gross charges for the period to date amount to $200,000.
2. The uniform gross charge for each procedure in your unit is $100.
3. The unit receives revenue from four major payers. For purposes of this exercise, assume the revenue volume from each represents 25% of the total. (The equal proportion is unrealistic, but serves the purpose for this exercise.)
4. The following contractual payment arrangements are in effect for the current period. The percentage of the gross charge that is currently paid by each payer is as follows:
   Payer 1 = 90%
   Payer 2 = 80%
   Payer 3 = 70%
   Payer 4 = 50%

Q: How many procedures has your unit recorded for the period to date?

Q: Of these, how many procedures are attributed to each payer?

Q: How much is the net revenue per procedure for each payer, and how much is the contractual allowance per procedure for each payer?

Assignment Exercise 14–3

As a follow-up to the previous Practice Exercise, new assumptions are as follows:

1. Your unit's gross charges for the period to date amount to $200,000.
2. The uniform gross charge for each procedure in your unit is $100.
3. The unit receives revenue from four major payers. The number of procedures performed for the period totals 2,000. Of that total, the number of procedures per payer (stated as a percentage) is as follows:
   Payer 1 = 30%
   Payer 2 = 40%
   Payer 3 = 20%
   Payer 4 = 10%
4. The following contractual payment arrangements are in effect for the current period. The percentage of the gross charge that is currently paid by each payer is as follows:
   Payer 1 = 80% [Medicare]
   Payer 2 = 70% [Commercial managed care plans]
   Payer 3 = 50% [Medicaid]
   Payer 4 = 90% [Self-pay]

Q: How many procedures are attributed to each payer?

Q: How much is the net revenue per procedure for each payer, and how much is the contractual allowance per procedure for each payer?

Q: How much is the total net revenue for each payer, and how much is the total contractual allowance for each payer?

Assignment Exercise 14–4.1: Forecast Capacity Levels

Review the information in Exhibit 14–1. The exhibit assumes three chairs and one 40-hour RN, for a realistic capacity level of seven patients infused per day.

Required

Prepare another Infusion Center Capacity Level Forecast as follows:

Assume the same three infusion chairs, but add another nurse for either four or six hours per day. How would this change the daily capacity level for number of patients infused per day?

Assignment Exercise 14–4.2

Required

Prepare another Infusion Center Capacity Level Forecast as follows:

Increase the number of infusion chairs to four, and add another nurse for either four or six hours per day. How would this change the daily capacity level for number of patients infused per day?

CHAPTER 15

Assignment Exercise 15–1: Comparable Data in a Graph

Review Figures 15–1 through 15–5. Each of the five figures presents a graph depicting some type of comparative data.

Required

Locate healthcare information that can reasonably be compared. (1) Prepare your comparative data. (2) Using your data, create one or more graphs similar to those found in Figures 15–1 through 15–5.

Assignment Exercise 15–2: Cumulative Inflation Factor for Comparable Data

Review Table 15–3 and the accompanying text.

Assumptions

Two hospitals report their annual projected revenue for five years to the local newspaper for a story on the area's future economic outlook. However, Hospital 1 has applied a cumulative inflation factor of 5% per year while Hospital 2 has not applied any inflation factor. Thus the information is not properly comparable.

	Projected Revenue				
	Year 1	Year 2	Year 3	Year 4	Year 5
Hospital 1	$20,000,000	$22,500,000	$27,500,000	$27,500,000	$30,000,000
Hospital 2	$20,000,000	$21,000,000	$25,000,000	$24,000,000	$26,000,000

Required

Revise Hospital 2's projections by applying a cumulative inflation factor of 5% per year.

Assignment Exercise 15–3

The head of your department is a prominent researcher. A health research foundation has asked him travel to London to give an important speech at a conference. He will then travel to Paris to tour a research facility before returning home. Although his travel expenses are being funded by the foundation, he will still need to take along some personal money. Consequently, he asks you to figure the exchange rates for $500 and for $1,000 in both pounds and euros. He explains that he is trying to judge the spending power of U.S. dollars when converted to the other currencies so he can decide how much personal money to take on the trip.

Required

Locate the current exchange rates for pounds and euros and compute the currency conversion for $500 and for $1,000.

Assignment Exercise 15–4: The Discovery

The Chief Financial Officer at Sample General Hospital has just discovered that the hospital's Chief of the Medical Staff's son Jason, a student at the local community college, is paid $100 per week year-round for grounds maintenance at the hospital's Outpatient Center.

The CFO, no fan of the Chief of Medical Staff, now wants you to prepare a report that compares the relative costs of lawn care at each of three locations: the hospital itself, the outpatient center, and the hospital-affiliated nursing home down the block.

Required

Review the available information for grounds maintenance at the three facilities. Decide how to convert this information into comparable data. Then prepare a report, based on your assumptions, that presents comparable costs of grounds care. Also provide your assessment of what the best future course of action should be.

Relevant Information

So far you have assembled the following information. Now you need to decide how it can be converted into comparable data.

Introduction to the Three Facilities

Sample General Hospital is an older 100-bed hospital. The new Outpatient Center, built last year, is across the street and the Golden Age Nursing Facility is down one block, on the corner. All three facilities are part of the Metropolis Health System. (The Case Study about Comparative Analysis Using Financial Ratios and Benchmarking appearing in Appendix 33-B contains some financial details about Sample Hospital.) The hospital is located in the Midwestern sun-belt; there is occasional frost in the winter but no snow.

Grounds Maintenance Tasks That Should Be Performed at All Three Sites

- Mowing and edging
- Walk sweeping
- Raking leaves
- Blowing off parking lot
- Flower bed maintenance (where necessary)
- Hedge trimming and minor tree pruning (major tree trimming is performed by a contractor on an as-needed basis and thus should be disregarded)

Figure Ex–1 provides a map that illustrates the layout of the grounds for each facility and their proximity to each other.

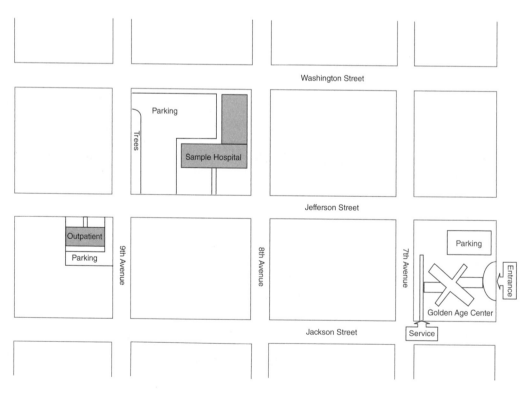

Figure Ex–1 Sample Hospital Map.

Grounds Maintenance Arrangements for the Three Facilities

The current grounds maintenance arrangements vary among the three facilities as follows:

1. Sample General Hospital uses its Maintenance department employees for grounds care. The hospital pays these employees $15 per hour plus 15% employee benefits; it is estimated they spend 1,000 hours per year on grounds maintenance work. Another estimated 120 hours per year are spent on maintaining the lawn care equipment. The employees use a riding lawn mower, edger, and blower, all owned by the hospital. The hospital just bought a new mower for $2,995 less a 10% discount. It is expected that the mower should last for five years.

2. The hospital's Chief of the Medical Staff's son Jason, a student at the local community college, is paid $100 per week year-round for grounds maintenance at the hospital's Outpatient Center. A friend sometimes helps, but when that happens Jason pays him out of his weekly $100. It takes about 1.5 hours to mow, edge, and blow. Jason uses his dad's riding mower and blower, but Jason recently bought his own edger. Jason also buys fertilizer for the grass twice a year.

3. The Nursing Facility contracts with a landscape service on a seasonally adjusted sliding scale. The landscape service is paid $600 per month from April to October (mowing season); $400 per month for February, March, and November; and $200 per month for November, December, and January. The landscape service provides all their own equipment. They also provide fertilizer and provide annuals to plant in the flower beds every quarter.

Sample General Hospital Property Description

The grounds to be maintained are as follows:

- The front lawn is grass in two sections on either side of the front entrance. Each section is about 50 feet by 60 feet.
- There is a hedge along the front of the building that is about 50 feet on either side of the front entrance.
- There are two small matching flower beds on either side of the front entrance.
- Another strip of grass alongside of the building is 30 feet by 100 feet.
- A third small strip of grass about 5 feet by 25 feet is by the Emergency entrance.
- The walkway dimensions are as follows: about 50 feet of front walk; about 30 feet of staff entrance walk, both of which are 5 feet wide.
- The Emergency Department's paved patient drop-off area is about 25 feet by 30 feet.
- The parking lot surface is about 200 feet by 250 feet. Along one side are overhanging trees that drop leaves and debris and are a constant sweeping problem. These are the only trees on the hospital site.

Outpatient Center Property Description

The grounds to be maintained are as follows:

- There is a strip of grass at the front of the building that is 12 feet wide and 65 feet long, split in the middle by a walkway 5 feet wide.
- There is a strip of grass at the back of the building between the building and the parking lot that is 5 feet wide and 50 feet long
- All the rest of the property is paved.

Nursing Center Property Description

Golden Age Nursing Center occupies one whole block. The grounds have many large trees. Flower beds have been planted around the trees as well as along the front walk and entrance. There are also two secured patio areas at the side of the building, screened by hedges, and each has a small bed of annuals. Because of the unique design of the building, grounds maintenance requires considerable handwork such as edging with a weed eater.

CHAPTER 16

Example 16A: Budgeting

A static budget is based on a single level of operations that is never adjusted. Therefore, the static budgeted expense amounts will not change, even though actual volume does change during the year.

The computation of a static budget variance only requires one calculation, as follows:

$$\begin{array}{ccccc} \text{Actual} & & \text{Static Budget} & & \text{Static Budget} \\ \text{Results} & \text{minus} & \text{Amount} & \text{equals} & \text{Variance} \end{array}$$

We can set up the example in the chapter text in this format as follows:

Use patient days as an example of level of volume, or output. Assume that the budget anticipated 40,000 patient days this year at an average of $600 revenue per day, or $2,400,000. Further assume that expenses were budgeted at $560 per patient day, or $22,400,000. The budget would look like this:

	As Budgeted
Revenue	$24,000,000
Expenses	22,400,000
Excess of Revenue over Expenses	$1,600,000

Now assume that only 36,000, or 90%, of the patient days are going to actually be achieved for the year. The average revenue of $600 per day will be achieved for these 36,000 days (thus 36,000 times $600 equals $21,600,000). Further assume that, despite the best efforts of the Chief Financial Officer, the expenses will amount to $22,000,000. The actual results would look like this:

	Actual
Revenue	$21,600,000
Expenses	22,000,000
Excess of Expenses over Revenue	$ (400,000)

The budgeted revenue and expenses still reflect the original expectation of 40,000 patient days; the budget report would look like this:

	Actual	Budget	Static Budget Variance
Revenue	$21,600,000	$24,000,000	$(2,400,000)
Expenses	22,000,000	22,400,000	(400,000)
Excess of Expenses over Revenue	$ (400,000)	$ 1,600,000	$(2,000,000)

(Note: The negative actual result of (400,000) combined with the positive budget expectation of 1,600,000 amounts to the negative net variance of [(2,000,000].)

This example has shown a static budget, geared toward only one level of activity and remaining constant or static.

Practice Exercise 16–I: Budgeting

Budget assumptions for this exercise include both inpatient and outpatient revenue and expense. Assumptions are as follows:
As to the initial budget:

- The budget anticipated 30,000 inpatient days this year at an average of $650 revenue per day.
- Inpatient expenses were budgeted at $600 per patient day.
- The budget anticipated 10,000 outpatient visits this year at an average of $400 revenue per visit.
- Outpatient expenses were budgeted at $380 per visit.

As to the actual results:

- Assume that only 27,000, or 90%, of the inpatient days are going to actually be achieved for the year.
- The average revenue of $650 per day will be achieved for these 270,000 inpatient days.
- The outpatient visits will actually amount to 110%, or 11,000 for the year.
- The average revenue of $400 per visit will be achieved for these 11,000 visits.
- Further assume that, due to the heroic efforts of the Chief Financial Officer, the actual inpatient expenses will amount to $11,600,000 and the actual outpatient expenses will amount to $4,000,000.

Required

1. Set up three worksheets that follow the format of those in Example 16A. However, in each of your worksheets make two lines for revenue; label one as Revenue—Inpatient and the other Revenue—Outpatient. Add a Revenue Subtotal line. Likewise, make two lines for expense; label one as Expense—Inpatient and the other Expense— Outpatient. Add an Expense Subtotal line.
2. Using the new assumptions, complete the first worksheet for "As Budgeted."
3. Using the new assumptions, complete the second worksheet for "Actual."
4. Using the new assumptions, complete the third worksheet for "Static Budget Variance."

Assignment Exercise 16–1: Budgeting

Select an organization: either from the Case Studies appearing in Chapters 31, 32, 33, 33-A, 33-B or 33-C or from one of the Mini-Case Studies appearing in Chapters 34 and 35.

Required

1. Using the organization selected, create a budget for the next fiscal year. Set out the details of all assumptions you needed in order to build this budget.
2. Use the "Checklist for Building a Budget" (Exhibit 16–2) and critique your own budget.

Assignment Exercise 16–2: Budgeting

Find an existing budget from a published source. Detail should be extensive enough to present a challenge.

Required

1. Using the existing budget, create a new budget for the next fiscal year. Set out the details of all the assumptions you needed in order to build this budget.
2. Use the "Checklist for Building a Budget" (Exhibit 16–2) and critique your own effort.
3. Use the "Checklist for Reviewing a Budget" (Exhibit 16–3) and critique the existing budget.

Assignment Exercise 16–3: Transactions Outside the Operating Budget

Review Figure 16–2 and the accompanying text.

Metropolis Health System (MHS) has received a wellness grant from the charitable arm of an area electronics company. The grant will run for 24 months, beginning at the first of the next fiscal year. Two therapists and two registered nurses will each be spending half of their time working on the wellness grant. All four individuals are full-time employees of MHS. The electronics company has only recently begun to operate the charitable organization that awarded the grant. While they have gained all the legal approvals necessary, they have not yet provided the manuals and instructions for grant transactions that MHS usually receives when grants are awarded. Consequently, guidance about separate accounting is not yet forthcoming from the grantor.

Required

How would you handle this issue on the MHS operating budget for next year?

Assignment Exercise 16–4: Identified Versus Allocated Costs in Budgeting

Review Figure 16–3 and the accompanying text.

Metropolis Health System is preparing for a significant upgrade in both hardware and software for its information systems. As part of the project, the Chief of Information Operations (CIO) has indicated that the Information Systems (IS) department can change the format of the MHS operating budgets and related reports before the operating budget is constructed for the coming fiscal year. The Chief Financial Officer (CFO) has long wanted to modify what costs are identified and what costs are allocated (along with the method of allocation). This is a golden opportunity to do so. To gain ammunition for the change, the CFO is preparing to conduct a survey. The survey will obtain a variety of suggestions for potential changes in allocation methods for the new operating budget report formats. You have been selected as one of the employees who will be surveyed.

Required

You may choose your role for this assignment, as follows:

Refer to the "MHS Executive-Level Organization Chart" (appearing as Figure 33–2 in the MHS Case Study). (1) Either (a) choose any type of patient service that would be under the direction of the Senior Vice President of Service Delivery Operations or (b) choose any other function shown on the organization chart. (Your function could be a whole department or a division or unit of that department. For example, you might choose Community Outreach or Human Resources Operations or the Emergency department, etc.) (2) Make up your own organization chart for other employee levels within the function you have chosen. (3) Now make up another chart that indicates the operating budget costs you think would be mostly identifiable for the department or unit or division you have chosen and what other operating budget costs you think would be mostly allocated to it. (You may use Figure 16–3 as a rough guide, but do not let it limit your imagination. Model the detail on your "identifiable versus allocated costs" chart after a real department if you so choose.) Use MHS hospital statistics appearing in Exhibit 33–8 of the MHS Case Study as a basis for allocation if these statistics are helpful. If they are not, make a note of what other statistics you would like to have.

(Note: As an alternative approach, you may choose a function from the MHS "Nursing Practice and Administration Organization Chart" appearing in Figure 33–1 of the MHS Case Study instead of choosing from the Executive-Level Organization Chart.)

CHAPTER 17

Example 17A: Description of Capital Expenditure Proposals Scoring System

Worthwhile Hospital has a total capital expenditure budget for next year of five million dollars. Of this amount, three million is already committed as spending for capital assets that have already been acquired and are in place. The remaining two million dollars is available for new assets and for new projects or programs.

Worthwhile Hospital typically divides the available capital expenditure funds into monies available for inpatient purposes and monies available for outpatient purposes. This year the split is proposed to be 50-50.

The hospital's CFO is also proposing that a scoring system be used to evaluate this year's proposals. She has set up a scoring system that allows a maximum of five points. Thus the low is a score of one point and the high is a score of five points.

In addition to the points earned by a funding proposal, the CFO will allow one "bonus point" for upgrading existing equipment and one "bonus point" for funding expansion of existing programs.

Practice Exercise 17–I: Capital Expenditure Proposals

Jody Smith, the director who supervises the Intensive Care Units, wants to secure as much of the one million dollars available for inpatient purposes as is possible for the ICU. At the same time

Ted Jones, the director who supervises the Surgery Unit, also wants to secure as much of the one million dollars available for inpatient purposes as is possible for his Surgery Unit.

Given the CFO's new scoring system, how should Jody go about choosing exactly what to request?

Assignment Exercise 17–1: Capital Expenditure Proposals

Ted Jones, the Surgery Unit Director, is about to choose his strategy for creating a capital expenditure funding proposal for the coming year. Ted's unit needs more room. The Surgery Unit is running at over 90% capacity. In addition, a prominent cardiology surgeon on staff at the hospital wants to create a new cardiac surgery program that would require extensive funding for more space and for new state-of-the-art equipment. The surgeon has been campaigning with the hospital board members.

Required

What should Ted decide to ask for? How should he go about crafting a strategy to justify his request, given the hospital's new scoring system?

CHAPTER 18

Example 18A: Variance Analysis

Our variance analysis example and practice exercise use the flexible budget approach. A flexible budget is one that is created using budgeted revenue and/or budgeted cost amounts. A flexible budget is adjusted, or flexed, to the actual level of output achieved (or perhaps expected to be achieved) during the budget period. A flexible budget thus looks toward a range of activity or volume (versus only one level in the static budget).

Examples of how the variance analysis works are contained in Figure 18–1 (the elements), in Figure 18–2 (the composition), and in Figures 18–3 and 18–4 (the calculations). Study these examples before undertaking the Practice Exercise.

We have restated Exhibit 18–2 in a worksheet format for purposes of this example. The new format appears as follows. (The numbers have not changed.)

Actual Cost	$920,000
Less: Flexible Budget	990,000
Price Variance (favorable)	$ 70,000
Budgeted Cost	$937,500
Less: Flexible Budget	990,000
Quantity Variance (unfavorable)	$(52,500)
Net Variance (favorable)	$ 17,500

Assumptions (*refer to Exhibit 18–2*)

	Overhead Cost	divided by	# Therapy Minutes (Activity Level)	equals	Cost per Therapy Minute
Actual	(1) $920,000		(3) 330,000		(5) $2.79
Budgeted	(2) $937,500		(4) 312,500		(6) $3.00

Practice Exercise 18–1

Exhibit 18–2 presents the Variance Analysis for hospital rehab services for the third quarter. For our practice exercise we will duplicate this report for the fourth quarter. We are able to reformat the information in Exhibit 18–2 into a worksheet as follows. The fourth quarter assumptions appear below the worksheet.

Actual Cost	
Less: Flexible Budget	
Price Variance (favorable)	
Budgeted Cost	
Less: Flexible Budget	
Quantity Variance (unfavorable)	
Net Variance (unfavorable)	

Assumptions

	Overhead Cost	divided by	# Therapy Minutes (Activity Level)	equals	Cost per Therapy Minute
Actual	(1) $950,000		(3) 350,000		(5) $2.71
Budgeted	(2) $930,000		(4) 310,000		(6) $3.00

Required

1. Set up a worksheet for the fourth quarter like that shown in Exhibit 18–2 for the third quarter.
2. Insert the Fourth Quarter Input Data (per assumptions given above) on the worksheet.
3. Complete the "Actual Cost," "Flexible Budget," and "Budgeted Cost" sections at the top of the worksheet.
4. Compute the Price Variance and the Quantity Variance in the middle of the worksheet.
5. Indicate whether the Price and the Quantity Variances are favorable or unfavorable for the fourth quarter.

Optional

Can you compute how the $950,000 actual overhead costs and the $930,000 budgeted overhead costs were calculated?

Assignment Exercise 18–1: Variance Analysis

Greenview Hospital operated at 120% of normal capacity in two of its departments during the year. It operated 120% times 20,000 normal capacity direct labor nursing hours in routine services and it operated 120% times 20,000 normal capacity equipment hours in the laboratory. The lab allocates overhead by measuring minutes and hours the equipment is used; thus equipment hours.

Assumptions

For Routine Services Nursing:

- 20,000 hours × 120% = 24,000 direct labor nursing hours.
- Budgeted Overhead at 24,000 hours = $42,000 fixed plus $6,000 variable = $48,000 total.
- Actual Overhead at 24,000 hours = $42,000 fixed plus $7,000 variable = $49,000 total.
- Applied Overhead for 24,000 hours at $2.35 = $56,400.

For Laboratory:

- 20,000 hours × 120% = 24,000 equipment hours.
- Budgeted Overhead at 24,000 hours = $59,600 fixed plus $11,400 variable = $71,000 total.
- Actual Overhead at 24,000 hours = $59,600 fixed plus $11,600 variable = $71,200 total.
- Applied Overhead for 24,000 hours at $3.455 = $82,920.

Required

1. Set up a worksheet for applied overhead costs and volume variance with a column for Routine Services Nursing and a second column for Laboratory.
2. Set up a worksheet for actual overhead costs and budget variance with a column for Routine Services Nursing and a second column for Laboratory.
3. Set up a worksheet for volume variance and budget variance totaling net variance with a column for Routine Services Nursing and a second column for Laboratory.
4. Insert input data from the Assumptions.
5. Complete computations for all three worksheets.

Example 18B

Review the "Sensitivity Analysis Overview" section and Figure 18–5 in Chapter 18.

Assignment Exercise 18–2: Three-Level Revenue Forecast

Three eye-ear-nose-and-throat physicians decide to hire an experienced audiologist in order to add a new service line to their practice.* They ask the practice manager to prepare a three-level volume forecast as a first step in their decision making.

Assumptions: For the base level (most likely) revenue forecast, assume $200 per procedure times 4 procedures per day times 5 days equals 20 procedures per week times 50 weeks per year equals 1,000 potential procedures per year.

For the best-case revenue forecast, assume an increase in volume of one procedure per day average, for an annual increase of 250 procedures (5 days per week times 50 weeks equals 250). (The best case is if the practice gains a particular managed care contract.)

For the worst case revenue forecast, assume a decrease in volume of 2 procedures per day average, for an annual decrease of 500 procedures. (The worst case is if the practice loses a major payer.)

*Assume audiologists were designated as "eligible for physician and other prescriber incentives." Thus the new service line was a logical move.

Required

Using the above assumptions, prepare a three-level forecast similar to the example in Figure 18–5 and document your calculations.

Practice Exercise 18–II

Closely study the chapter text concerning target operating income.
  The necessary inputs for target operating income include the following:

- Desired (target) operating income amount = $20,000
- Unit price for sales = $500
- Variable cost per unit = $300
- Total fixed cost = $10,000

Compute the required revenue to achieve the target operating income and compute a contribution income statement to prove the totals.

Assignment Exercise 18–3: Target Operating Income

Acme Medical Supply Company desires a target operating income amount of $100,000, with assumption inputs as follows:

- Desired (target) operating income amount = $100,000
- Unit price for sales = $80
- Variable cost per unit = $60
- Total fixed cost = $60,000

Compute the required revenue to achieve the target operating income and compute a contribution income statement to prove the totals.

CHAPTER 19

Assignment Exercise 19–1: Estimate of Loss

You are the practice manager for a four-physician office. You arrive on Monday morning to find the entire office suite flooded from overhead sprinklers that malfunctioned over the weekend. Water stands ankle-deep everywhere. The computers are fried and the contents of all the filing cabinets are soaked. Your own office, where most of the records were stored, has the worst damage.
  The practice carries valuable papers insurance coverage for an amount up to $250,000. It is your responsibility to prepare an estimate of the financial loss so that a claim can be filed with

the insurance company. How would you go about it? What would your summary of the losses look like?

Assignment Exercise 19–2: Estimate of Replacement Cost

The landlord carries contents insurance that should cover the damage to the furnishings, equipment, and to the computers, and the insurance company adjuster will come tomorrow to assess the furnishings and equipment damage. However, your boss is sure that the insurance settlement will not cover replacement costs. Consequently, you have been instructed to prepare an estimate of what has been lost and/or damaged plus an estimate of what the replacement cost might be. How would you go about it? What would your summary of these losses look like?

Assignment Exercise 19–3: Benchmarking

Review the chapter text about benchmarking.

Required

1. Select an organization: either from the Case Studies appearing in Chapters 31, 32, 33, 33-A, 33-B or 33-C or from one of the Mini-Case Studies appearing in Chapters 34 and35.
2. Prepare a list of measures that could be benchmarked for this organization. Comment on why these items are important for benchmarking purposes.
3. Find another example of benchmarking for a healthcare organization. The example can be an organization report or it can be taken from a published source such as a journal article.

Assignment Exercise 19–4: Pareto Rule

Review the chapter text about the Pareto rule and examine Figure 19–4. Note that the text says Pareto diagrams are often drawn to reflect before and after results.

Assume that Figure 19–4 is the before diagram for the Billing department. Further assume that the after results are as follows:

Activity	Activity Code	Number
Process Denied Bills	PDB	12
Review with Supervisor	RWS	10
Locate Documentation	LD	6
Copy Documentation	CD	5
		33

Required

1. Redo the Pareto diagram with the after results. (Use Figure 19–4 as a guide.)
2. Comment on the before and after results for the Billing department.

Assignment Exercise 19–5: Quartiles

Review the chapter text about quartiles and study Table 19–1, which indicates results in quartiles.

Required

1. Locate healthcare information (such as bed days, number of visits, payment amounts, etc.) that contains a list of no less than twelve numerical amounts.
2. Divide the list you have found into quartiles.
3. Enter your results on a worksheet with the highest quartile first and the lowest quartile last. Include an explanation of your computations.

CHAPTER 20

Assignment 20–1

Study the chapter text that discusses retrospective versus predictive data analytics.

Required

1. Locate an article that presents a healthcare study of some sort that has used data analytics.
2. Write a review of the article. Your review should identify whether retrospective or predictive analytics have been used to obtain the study results.
3. If you had designed this study, would you have used the same type of analysis? If so, explain why. If not, explain why not.

Assignment 20–2

Review the chapter text about big data, especially the section about big data in the healthcare industry.

Required

1. Find a healthcare organization's description of how it, in its organization, utilizes big data.
2. Review their description of this usage: For what purpose? Who performs the actual analysis; can you tell if the analysis is done internally or externally? Are the results current? Are the results useful in some way, and is that usefulness described?
3. If you were employed by this organization and you had been assigned to write this description, what would you do differently? Do you think you would use the data differently? If so, describe how. If not, explain why not.

CHAPTER 21

Assignment Exercise 21–1

Review the information about public companies and stock exchanges in the Chapter 21 text.

Required

Obtain a copy of the *Wall Street Journal.* Locate the "Stock Tables" section of the *Journal.* Review the column headings in the tables and locate the names of various stock exchanges that are included in the findings. See if you can find the abbreviated names and the stock exchange symbols for healthcare companies that are publicly held.

Alternatively, explore the websites of three or four publicly held healthcare organizations. Somewhere on the website they should identify their stock exchange symbol. Then go onto a web-based stock exchange listing of the market for the day, locate the symbols, and determine their current stock prices according to the listing.

Assignment 21–2

Review the chapter text about mean, median, and mode and refer to the illustration in Table 21–1.

Required

Locate an article that reports results expressed as the mean, the median, or the mode. Can you tell why the particular method was used to report results? (For example, why was the mean used instead of the median?) If so, describe your conclusions. Alternatively, locate a series of numbers such as scores and find the mean, the median, and the mode. Illustrate them as is shown in Table 21–1.

CHAPTER 22

Example 22A: Loan Amortization

This example illustrates the initial monthly payments of a loan with a principal balance of $50,000, an interest rate of 10%, and a payment period of 3 years or 36 months.

Loan Amortization Schedule
Principal borrowed: $50,000
Total payments: 36
Annual interest rate 10.00% (monthly rate = 0.8333%)

Payment #	Total Payment	Principal Portion of Payment	Interest Expense Portion of Payment	Remaining Principal Balance
			Beginning balance =	$50,000.00
1	$1,613.36	$1,196.69	$416.67	$48,403.31
2	1,613.36	1,206.67	406.69	47,596.64
3	1,613.36	1,216.72	396.64	46,379.92
4	1,613.36	1,226.86	386.50	45,153.06
5	1,613.36	1,237.08	376.28	43,915.98
6	1,613.36	1,247.39	365.97	42,668.58

Practice Exercise 22–I: Loan Amortization

This exercise illustrates a different principal amount than Example 22A, but computed at the same monthly interest rate and the same number of payments.

Required

Compute the first 6 months of a loan amortization schedule with a principal balance of $60,000, an interest rate of 10%, and a payment period of 3 years or 36 months.

Loan Amortization Schedule
Principal borrowed: $60,000
Total payments: 36
Annual interest rate 10.00% (monthly rate = 0.8333%)

Payment #	Total Payment	Principal Portion of Payment	Interest Expense Portion of Payment	Remaining Principal Balance
			Beginning balance =	$60,000.00
1				
2				
3				
4				
5				
6				

Assignment Exercise 22–1: Financial Statement Capital Structures

Required

Find three different financial statements that have varying capital structures. Write a paragraph about each that explains the debt–equity relationship and that computes the percentage of debt and the percentage of equity represented.

Also note whether the percentage of annual interest on debt is revealed in the notes to the financial statements. If so, do you believe the interest rate is fair and equitable? Why?

CHAPTER 23

Practice Exercise 23–I: Cost of Leasing

A cost of leasing table is reproduced below.

Required

Using the appropriate table from the Time Value of Money Appendices appearing as 13-A, 13-B, and 13-C, record the present-value factor at 6% for each year and compute the present-value cost of leasing.

Cost of Leasing: Suburban Clinic—Comparative Present Value

Not-for-Profit Cost of Leasing:	Year 0	Year 1	Year 2	Year 3	Year 4	Year 5
Net Cash Flow	(11,000)	(11,000)	(11,000)	(11,000)	(11,000)	—
Present-value factor (at 6%)						
Present-value answer =						
Present-value cost of leasing =						

Assignment Exercise 23–1: Cost of Owning and Cost of Leasing

Cost of owning and cost of leasing tables are reproduced below.

Required

Using the appropriate table from the Chapter 13 Time Value of Money Appendices appearing as 13-A, 13-B, and 13-C, record the present-value factor at 10% for each year and compute the present-value cost of owning and the present value of leasing. Which alternative is more desirable at this interest rate? Do you think your answer would change if the interest rate was 6% instead of 10%?

Cost of Owning: Anywhere Clinic—Comparative Present Value

For-Profit Cost of Owning:	Year 0	Year 1	Year 2	Year 3	Year 4	Year 5
Net Cash Flow	(48,750)	2,500	2,500	2,500	2,500	5,000
Present-value factor						
Present-value answers =						
Present-value cost of owning =						

Cost of Leasing: Anywhere Clinic—Comparative Present Value

Line	For-Profit Cost of Leasing:	Year 0	Year 1	Year 2	Year 3	Year 4	Year 5
19	Net Cash Flow	(8,250)	(8,250)	(8,250)	(8,250)	(8,250)	—
20	Present-value factor						
21	Present-value answers =						
22	Present-value cost of leasing =						

Assignment Exercise 23–2

Great Docs, a three-physician practice with two office sites, is considering whether to buy or lease a new computer system. Currently they own a low-tech (and low-cost) information system. The new system will have to meet all government specifications for an electronic health record system and will also have to connect the two office sites. It will be considerably more sophisticated than the current hardware and software and thus will require training for office staff, clinical staff, and the physicians. Everyone agrees there will be a learning curve in order to reach the system's full potential.

Doctor Smith, the majority owner of the practice, wants to buy a medical records system from Sam's Club. He argues that the package is supposed to electronically prescribe, track billings, set appointments, and keep records, so it should meet their needs. The cost of the first installed system is supposed to be $25,000, plus $10,000 for each additional system. The doctors are not sure if this means $25,000 for one office site plus $10,000 for the (connected) second office site for a total of $35,000, or if this means $25,000 for the first installed system plus $10,000 each for three more doctors, for a total of $55,000. There is also supposed to be $4,000 to $5,000 in maintenance costs each year as part of the purchased package. Doctor Smith proposes to pay 20% down and obtain a five-year installment loan from the local bank for the remaining 80% at an interest rate of 8%.

Doctor Jones, the youngest of the three physicians, has been recently added to the practice. A computer nerd, he wants to lease a complete system from the small company his college room-mate began last year. While he has received a quote of $20,000 for the entire system including first year maintenance, it does not meet the government requirements for an electronic health record system. Consequently, the other two doctors have outvoted Doctor Jones and this system will not be seriously considered.

Doctor Brown, the usual peace-maker between Doctor Smith and Doctor Jones, wants to lease a system. He argues that leasing will place the responsibility for upgrades and main-tenance upon the lessor company, and that removing the responsibilities of ownership is advantageous. He has received a quote of $20,000 per year for a five-year lease that includes hardware and software for both offices, that meets the government requirements for an elec-tronic health record system, and that includes training, maintenance, and upgrades.

Required

Summarize the costs to the practice of owning a system (per Doctor Smith) versus leasing (per Doctor Brown). Include a computation of comparative present value. (Refer to Assignment 23–1 for setting up a comparative present-value table.)

Assignment Exercise 23–3

Metropolis Health System has to do something about their ambulance situation. They have to (1) buy a new ambulance, (2) lease a new one, or (3) renovate an existing ambulance that MHS already owns. Rob Lackey, the Assistant Controller, has been asked to gather pertinent informa-tion in order to make a decision. So far Rob has found these facts:

1. It will cost at least $250,000 to purchase a new ambulance, although the cost varies widely depending upon the quantity and sophistication of the emergency equipment contained on the vehicle.
2. In order to renovate the existing vehicle, it will cost at least $100,000 to purchase and install a new "box." (In other words, a new emergency-equipped body is installed on the existing chassis.) Rob has found this existing ambulance has an odometer reading of 80,000 miles. The vehicle will also need a new fuel pump and new tires, but he believes these items would be recorded as repair and maintenance operating expenses and thus would not be included in his calculations.
3. Lease terms for ambulances also vary widely, but so far Rob believes a cost of $60,000 per year is a ballpark figure.

Required

How much more information should Rob have before he begins to make any calculations? Make a list. Which alternative do you believe would be best? Give your reasons.

CHAPTER 24

Assignment Exercise 24–1

This group project assignment concerns situational analysis.

Create a hypothetical organization, complete with an IT department and financial, clinical, and administrative staff levels. This IT department is tasked with adopting and implementing EHR.

Required

Step 1. Using your hypothetical organization's personnel, assign a variety of scores to a Scoring Summary Sheet such as that shown in Exhibit 24–A-1 appearing in the chapter Appendix 24-A.

Step 2. Summarize the scores and place the net scores in a SWOT matrix such as the one shown in Figure 24–6.

Step 3. Create a report to the organization's CEO that summarizes the (good or bad) results.

Optional Additional Assignment

Required

Locate several healthcare organizations' mission, value, and vision statements. Use public sources with no privacy concerns.

Then fit the statements you have discovered into the chapter's categories of recognizing a special status or focus within the statements; financial emphasis within the statements; and/or relaying the message.

CHAPTER 25

Example 25A: Assumptions

Types of assumptions required for the financial portion of a business plan typically include answers to the following questions:

- What types of revenue?
- How many services will be offered to produce the revenue (by month)?
- How much labor will be required (FTEs)?
- What will the labor cost?
- How many and what type of supplies, drugs, and/or devices will be required to offer the service?
- What will the supplies, drugs, and/or devices cost?
- How much space will be required?
- What will the required space occupancy cost?
- Is special equipment required?
- If so, how much will it cost?
- Is staff training required to use the special equipment?
- If so, how much time is required, and what will it cost?

Practice Exercise 25–I: Assumptions

Refer to the Case Study proposal to add a retail pharmacy appearing in Chapter 33–C.

Required

Identify how many of the assumption items listed in the example above can be found in the retail pharmacy proposal worksheets.

Assignment Exercise 25–1: Business Plan

Refer to the Case Study proposal to add a retail pharmacy appearing in Chapter 33–C.

Required

Build a business plan for this proposal. Prepare the service description using your consumer knowledge of a retail pharmacy (if necessary). Of course this retail pharmacy will be located within the hospital, but its purpose is to dispense prescriptions to carry off-site and use at home. Thus, it operates pretty much like the neighborhood retail pharmacy that you use yourself.

Use the information provided in the MHS Case Study appearing in Chapter 33 to prepare the financial section of the business plan. Use your imagination to create the marketing segment and the organization segment.

CHAPTER 26

Assignment Exercise 26–1

Review the chapter text that defines a health delivery system.

Required

1. First, define a geographic area for healthcare delivery purposes. If you live in a city, it could be your metropolitan area. If you live in a more rural area, it could be an area of so many square miles.
2. Next, using the definition of a health delivery system within the chapter, list all the health delivery systems that presently exist within the geographic area defined above. Make a chart that shows the services and care settings that each system provides.
3. Research how many mergers or other types of consolidation have occurred within the past five years that have affected the systems on your list. Have any facilities closed in your geographic area within past five years? Are there rumors about possible future mergers?
4. Do you see a pattern of strategic plans and/or strategic thinking within your geographic area's health delivery system relationships? If so, please describe. If not, what are your reasons for so believing?

Assignment Exercise 26–2

Study the chapter text concerning stakeholders in health delivery systems.

Required

1. Review the section about internal and external stakeholders and choose one example to study. (Internal stakeholders deliver care, support the care deliverers, or receive the care, while Figure 26–1 lists 12 different types of external stakeholders.)

2. Research your chosen example. Write a report about what part your chosen entity plays within the system. What strategic relationships can you identify for your research subject? Can you make a map of those relationships?

3. How much strategic power do you think your chosen example has within the overall internal and external players within a system? Do you think that power is increasing or decreasing? Explain why within your report.

CHAPTER 27

Assignment Exercise 27–1

Review the chapter text about value-based financial outcomes, including examples.

Required

This assignment may be a group project. If so, divide the groups into two or more teams; each team should choose a different example to report.

1. Choose one value-based financial outcomes example from the text, such as the documented positive financial outcomes of Intermountain Health or the investment dollars required by Duke and Kaiser Permanente.
2. Find a similar type of value-based financial outcome as reported by some other healthcare entity. Research both information about the outcome and information about the entity that is reporting this financial outcome.
3. Write a report about the findings of your research. Present your report to the class and hold a Q&A session afterward.

Alternative Assignment Exercise 27–1

Review the chapter text about value-based digital outcomes, including examples.

Required

This assignment may also be a group project. If so, divide the groups into two or more teams; each team to choose a different example to report.

1. Choose one value-based digital outcomes example from the text, such as how digital outcomes would benefit a particular organization (the example in the text was a physician practice), or what value-based digital outcomes might be reported by a large healthcare system (the examples in the text were Duke and Kaiser Permanente).
2. Find a similar type of value-based digital outcome as reported by some other healthcare entity. Research both information about the outcome and information about the entity that is reporting this digital outcome.
3. Write a report about the findings of your research. Present your report to the class and hold a Q&A session afterward.

Assignment Exercise 27–2

Review the chapter text about value-based strategic planning.

Required

1. Find information about value-based strategic planning by either a private-sector or public-sector healthcare organization.
2. See if you can determine the focus of this organization's value-based strategic planning. (The chapter text recognized long-term goals, patient-centered views, and a population-health focus; there are others as well.) Describe this focus in as much depth as is possible.
3. Do you believe this organization's focus is appropriate for value-based planning? If so, why? Or is it too broad, too narrow, or deficient in some other manner? If so, why?

CHAPTER 28

Assignment Exercise 28–1

Review the chapter text about physician incentives under MACRA within the chapter text. See also the maximum incentive payments an eligible professional can receive under MIPS (Figure 28–5). Also review those professionals who are included and excluded, per Exhibits 28–1 and 28–2.

Required

1. Locate additional information about electronic systems (or add-ons) that are being sold to physicians based on implementation of MACRA/MIPS requirements. Attempt to determine what the net cost of hardware, software, and installation would be for an average physician practice. Compare this cost with the payment adjustments that an eligible physician would receive over a five-year period. Determine the approximate net technology cost to the physician after such incentive payments.
2. Also determine the cost to the physician practice if the practice does not comply and is penalized through a negative payment adjustment over a five-year period. Compare this negative payment adjustment against the approximate net technology cost to the physician if implementation were to occur.
3. As an extension of this assignment, you might also determine what start-up costs, other than the technology costs, may be incurred by the physician.

Assignment Exercise 28–2

Review the entire chapter text.

Required

Assume you are an employee of a health delivery system. You are assigned to write a training plan about MACRA, MIPS, and APMs. Training content is to be at three different levels (basic, intermediate, advanced), depending upon who is receiving the training.

1. Decide which employees should receive which level of training, and create a list.
2. Decide what essential subjects should be included and create a basic training list.
3. Determine what additional detail should be included at the intermediate level and create an intermediate training list.
4. Determine what extra detail should be included at the advanced level and create an advanced training list.

5. Determine who should serve as trainers for the different levels and create a list.
6. Assemble your lists into a draft training plan.

CHAPTER 29

Assignment Exercise 29–1

This assignment may be a group project.
    Review the chapter text about standardized data and interoperability.

Assumptions

First choose one type of care setting: either a skilled nursing facility (SNF) or a home health agency (HHA). Assume that, in the near future, this hypothetical SNF or HHA must (1) make the necessary changes to forms, processes, and scheduling in order to implement standardized data, and (2) invest in additional electronics that are necessary to implement cross-setting interoperability. Not all details about required changes are available at this point in time. Nevertheless, a task force has been assembled to begin planning for the transition and to produce a draft implementation plan. You are part of the task force.

Required

1. List the organization's departments that will be directly affected by the transition and those that will be indirectly affected.
2. List the actions that the task force believes are essential for a successful transition.
3. Is your hypothetical SNF or HHA part of a larger health delivery system? If so, designate responsibility for each of these actions; will the individual SNF or HHA be responsible or will the system's home office take responsibility?
4. What types of financial costs will be required? Can the task force predict whether such costs will occur over time or all at once? Is there an example, such as EHR implementation, that would provide a model for this issue?
5. Produce an outline of essential subjects to be covered in the task force's draft implementation plan.

Assignment Exercise 29–2

Review the chapter text about public reporting requirements.

Required

1. Locate the *Nursing Home Compare* website as described in the chapter.
2. Review how the 5-Star Rating System composite scale works.
3. Pull up the website and locate nursing homes that are in your region. How many are listed? Review the 5-Star scores for the facilities in your region. Is there a big difference among the scores? Describe your region's overall scores.
4. All SNFs that accept Medicare should be represented on the website. Do you know of a facility in your area that is not on the list? If so, can you tell why that may be?
5. Would you find the website and the 5-Star system helpful in choosing a facility for a family member? If so, why? If not, why not?

CHAPTER 30

Practice Exercise 30–I

The Productivity Loss section of this chapter describes how the dollar amount of such loss was computed after determining that it took coders an extra 1.7 minutes per claim in the first month of ICD-10 transition.

Assume a hospital's coders are dealing with 1,500 claims within a certain period. What would the dollar amount of productivity loss be if the coders took an extra two minutes (instead of 1.7 minutes) per claim?

Assignment Exercise 30–1: Information About the ICD-10-CM and ICD-10-PCS Implementation.

Required

Locate some articles and/or government websites that describe the ICD-10-CM diagnosis codes and the ICD-10-PCS procedure codes and tools for their implementation over a period of years. Write a summary of whether the materials you have found fully explain the bradth and depth of the challenge for managers who must live through the implementation.

Assignment Exercise 30–2: Hospital Conversion to ICD-10

Try to locate sufficient detail about a healthcare organization – enough that you can perform a make-believe SWOT analysis about a conversion of electronic systems to ICD-10 as required. Write a description of theorganization's background, including its information system. (Add imaginary details if you need to.) This description will then lead into the ICD-10 implementation's situation analysis. Perform the make-believe SWOT analysis using the four-part format (internal Strengths and Weaknesses and external Opportunities and Threats).

As an alternative approach, you can use information from the Case Study about Sample General Hospital appearing in Appendix 33-B as your starting point. Use your personal experience and observations to fill out the rest of the details you would need in order to commence a make-believe SWOT analysis for this hospital's ICD-10 implementation.

Assignment Exercise 30–3: Hospital Costs To Implement

Refer to the Scenario For A Midwestern Community Hospital, appearing in Appendix 30–A.

Required

Part 1—Within this scenario the productivity loss for the six-month learning period is calculated to be $1,233. Beginning with month 1 at $353 ($1.41 times 250 equals $353), compute the cost of productivity loss for the remaining five months as explained in the scenario, to total an overall amount of $1,233. Be prepared to show and explain your computations.

Part 2—Later in the scenario, CMS states that the hospital's total cost amounts to $303,990. Study the explanation and summarize the totals of each type of cost discussed. When you are finished, your total should amount to $303,990. Be prepared to show and explain how you arrived at this total.

SUPPLEMENTARY MATERIALS: THE MECHANICS OF PERCENTAGE COMPUTATIONS

The Reason for This Explanation: Author's Note

I had just finished presenting a day-long finance seminar when the vice president of a bank who had been attending pulled me aside. After looking around to make sure no one was listening, he asked me to show him how to calculate a percentage.

As I didn't know him or anyone from the town he lived and worked in, he wasn't embarrassed to ask me. So we believe if the vice president of a bank can ask about how to figure a percentage, then that calculation deserves to be described within this Appendix, as follows.

The Fraction's Parts: Numerator and Denominator

Reminder: A fraction has two parts—the numerator is the top number and the denominator is the bottom number. Or, to be more precise, the numerator is the part of a fraction that is above the line and signifies the number of parts of the denominator taken.

The denominator is the part of a fraction that is below the line and signifies division and that in fractions with 1 as the numerator indicates into how many parts the unit is divided.

First Calculate the Fraction (Including the Decimal)

To calculate a fraction, the bottom number (denominator) is divided into the top number (numerator). For example, if the numerator is 90 and the denominator is 100, divide 100 into 90. The resulting answer is 0.90. (Note that the decimal point is to the left of the 0.90 answer.)

Next Convert the Fraction to a Percentage

To obtain the percentage, we need to convert the fraction. To do so, move the decimal two places to the right. Now the answer is 90, and the percentage answer is 90%.

Summary

We know that your computer or tablet will perform this computation automatically, but situations may still arise when you may need to calculate by hand. It's a good thing to know.

SOLUTIONS TO PRACTICE EXERCISES

Solution to Practice Exercise 4–I

Short-term assets: cash on hand; accounts receivable; inventory
Long-term assets: land; buildings
Short-term liabilities: payroll taxes due; accounts payable
Long-term liabilities: mortgage payable (noncurrent); note payable (due in 24 months)

Solution to Practice Exercise 6–I

	Intensive Care Unit	Laboratory	Laundry
Drugs requisitioned	X		
Pathology supplies		X	
Detergents and bleach			X
Nursing salaries	X		
Clerical salaries	X	X	X
Uniforms (for laundry aides)			X
Repairs (parts for microscopes)		X	

Note: If no clerical salaries are assigned to Laundry, this is an acceptable alternative solution.

SOLUTION TO PRACTICE EXERCISE 7–I

	Direct Cost	Indirect Cost
Managed care marketing expense	X	
Real estate taxes		X
Liability insurance		X
Clinic telephone expense	X	
Utilities (for the entire facility)		X
Emergency room medical supplies	X	

SOLUTION TO PRACTICE EXERCISE 7–II

In real life the solution to this exercise will depend upon factors unique to the particular organization. The following solution is a generic one.

	Responsibility Center	Support Center
Security	X	
Communications	X	
Ambulance services	X	
Medical records		X
Educational resources		X
Human resources		X

Reporting: Each responsibility center has a manager. All report to the director.

SOLUTION TO PRACTICE EXERCISE 8–I

Step 1. Find the highest volume of 1,100 packs at a cost of $7,150 in September and the lowest volume of 100 packs at a cost of $1,010 in August.

Step 2. Compute the variable rate per pack as:

	# of Packs	Training Pack Cost
Highest volume	1,100	$7,150
Lowest volume	100	1,010
Difference	1,000	$6,140

Step 3. Divide the difference in cost ($6,140) by the difference in # of packs (1,000) to arrive at the variable cost rate:

$6,140 divided by 1,000 packs equals $6.14 per pack

Step 4. Compute the fixed overhead rate as follows:

At the highest level:

Total cost	$7,150
Less: Variable portion	
[1,100 packs × $6.14]	(6,754)
Fixed Portion of Cost	$ 396

At the lowest level:

Total cost	$1,010
Less: Variable portion	
[100 packs × $6.14]	(614)
Fixed Portion of Cost	$ 396

Proof totals: $396 fixed portion at both levels.

SOLUTION TO PRACTICE EXERCISE 8–II

Step 1. Divide costs into variable and fixed portions. In this case $3,450,000 times 40% equals $1,380,000 variable cost and $3,450,000 times 60% equals $2,070,000 fixed cost.

Step 2. Compute the contribution margin:

	Amount
Revenue	$3,500,000
Less variable cost	(1,380,000)
Contribution margin	$2,120,000
Less fixed cost	2,070,000
Operating income	$ 50,000

SOLUTION TO PRACTICE EXERCISE 8–III

	Amount	%	
Revenue	$1,210,000	100.00	
Less variable cost	(205,000)	16.94	
Contribution margin	$1,005,000	83.06	= PV or CM Ratio
Less fixed cost	(1,100,000)	90.91	
Operating loss	$(95,000)	7.85	

SOLUTION TO PRACTICE EXERCISE 9–I

1. Straight-line depreciation would amount to $54,000 per year for 10 years. This amount is computed as follows:

Step 1. Compute the cost net of salvage or trade-in value: 600,000 less 10% salvage value or 60,000 equals 540,000.

Step 2. Divide the resulting figure by the expected life (also known as estimated useful life): 540,000 divided by 10 equals 54,000 depreciation per year for 10 years.

2. Double-declining depreciation is computed as follows:

Step 1. Compute the straight-line rate: 1 divided by 10 equals 10%.

Step 2. Now double the rate (as in "double-declining method"): 10% times 2 equals 20%.

Step 3. Compute the first year's depreciation expense: 600,000 times 20% = 120,000.

Step 4. Compute the carry-forward book value at the beginning of the second year: 600,000 book value beginning year 1 less year 1 depreciation of 120,000 equals book value at beginning of the second year of 480,000.

Step 5. Compute the second year's depreciation expense: 480,000 times 20% = 96,000.

Step 6. Compute the carry-forward book value at the beginning of the third year: 480,000 book value beginning year 2 less year 2 depreciation of 96,000 equals book value at beginning of the third year of 384,000.

Continue until the asset's salvage or trade-in value has been reached.

Book Value at Beginning of Year	Depreciation Expense	Book Value at End of Year
600,000	600,000 × 20% = 120,000	600,000 − 120,000 = 480,000
480,000	480,000 × 20% = 96,000	480,000 − 96,000 = 384,000
384,000	384,000 × 20% = 76,800	384,000 − 76,800 = 307,200
307,200	307,200 × 20% = 61,440	307,200 − 61,440 = 245,760
245,760	245,760 × 20% = 49,152	245,760 − 49,152 = 196,608
196,608	196,608 × 20% = 39,322	196,608 − 39,322 = 157,286
157,286	157,286 × 20% = 31,457	157,286 − 31,457 = 125,829
125,829	125,829 × 20% = 25,166	125,829 − 25,166 = 100,663
100,663	100,663 × 20% = 20,132	100,663 − 20,132 = 80,531
80,531	80,561 at 10th year	80,561 − 20,561 = 60,000

Balance remaining at end of 10th year represents the salvage or trade-in value.

Note: Under the double-declining balance method, book value never reaches zero. Therefore, a company typically adopts the straight-line method at the point where straight line would exceed the double-declining balance.

SOLUTION TO PRACTICE EXERCISE 9–II

Straight-line depreciation would amount to $9,000 per year for five years. This amount is computed as follows:

Step 1. Compute the cost of salvage or trade-in value: 50,000 less 10% salvage value or 5,000 equals 45,000.

Step 2. Divide the resulting figure by the expected life (also known as the estimated useful life): 45,000 divided by 5 equals 9,000 depreciation per year for 5 years.

SOLUTION TO PRACTICE EXERCISE 10–I

1. Compute Net Paid Days Worked

Total days in business year		364
Less two days off per week		104
# Paid days per year		260
Less paid days not worked		
Holidays	8	
Sick days	5	
Education day	1	
Vacation days	5	
		19
Net paid days worked		241

2. Convert Net Paid Days Worked to a Factor

Total days in business year divided by net paid days worked equals factor

$$364/241 = 1.510373$$

SOLUTION TO PRACTICE EXERCISE 10–II

	Shift 1 Day	Shift 2 Evening	Shift 3 Night	=	24-Hour Scheduling Total
Position: Admissions officer	2	1	1		four 8-hour shifts
FTEs—to cover position					
7 days/week equals	2.8	1.4	1.4		5.6 FTEs
Position: Clerical	1	0	0		one 8-hour shift
FTEs—to cover position					
7 days/week equals	1.4	0	0		1.4 FTEs

SOLUTION TO PRACTICE EXERCISE 11–I

Current Liabilities	30,000
Total Assets	1,000,000
Income from Operations	80,000
Accumulated Depreciation	480,000
Total Operating Revenue	180,000
Current Portion of Long-Term Debt	10,000
Interest Income	-0-
Inventories	5,000

SOLUTION TO PRACTICE EXERCISE 11–II

No, Doctors Smith and Brown's patient accounts receivable does not appear to be net of an allowance for bad debts, because we cannot find an equivalent bad debt expense on their statement of net income. Do you think the doctors should have an allowance for bad debts on their statement? Why do you think they do not?

SOLUTION TO PRACTICE EXERCISE 11–III

As mentioned in the chapter text, land is not stated at "net" because land is never depreciated.

SOLUTION TO PRACTICE EXERCISE 12–I

Current Ratio

The current ratio is represented as Current Ratio equals Current Assets divided by Current Liabilities. This ratio is considered to be a measure of short-term debt-paying ability. However, it must be carefully interpreted.

Current Ratio Computation

$$\frac{\text{Current Assets}}{\text{Current Liabilities}} = \frac{\$70,000}{\$30,000} = 2.33 \text{ to } 1$$

Quick Ratio

The quick ratio is represented as Quick Ratio equals Cash and Short-Term Investments plus Net Receivables, divided by Current Liabilities. This ratio is considered to be an even more severe test of short-term debt-paying ability (even more severe than the current ratio). The quick ratio is also known as the acid-test ratio, for obvious reasons.

$$\frac{\text{Cash and Short-Term Investments} + \text{Net Receivables}}{\text{Current Liabilities}} = \frac{\$65,000}{30,000} = 2.167 \text{ to } 1$$

SOLUTION TO PRACTICE EXERCISE 12–II

Solvency Ratios

Debt Service Coverage Ratio (DSCR)

The Debt Service Coverage Ratio (DSCR) is represented as change in unrestricted net assets (net income) plus interest, depreciation, and amortization, divided by maximum annual debt service. This ratio is universally used in credit analysis.

$$\frac{\substack{\text{Change in Unrestricted Net Assets (net income)} \\ \text{plus Interest, Depreciation, Amortization}}}{\text{Maximum Annual Debt Service}} = \frac{\$113,100}{\$22,200} = 5.1$$

Note: $80,000 + $3,100 + $30,000 = $113,100.

Liabilities to Fund Balance (or Debt to Net Worth)

The liabilities to fund balance or net worth computation is represented as total liabilities divided by unrestricted net assets (fund balances or net worth) equals total debt divided by tangible net worth. This figure is a quick indicator of debt load.

$$\frac{\text{Total Liabilities}}{\text{Unrestricted (Fund Balance)}} = \frac{\$200,000}{\$800,000} = 2.5$$

SOLUTION TO PRACTICE EXERCISE 12–III

Profitability Ratios

Operating Margin

The operating margin, which is generally expressed as a percentage, is represented as operating income (loss) divided by total operating revenues. This ratio is used for a number of managerial purposes and also sometimes enters into credit analysis. It is therefore a multi-purpose measure.

$$\frac{\text{Operating Income (Loss)}}{\text{Total Operating Revenues}} = \frac{\$80,000}{\$180,000} = 44.4\%$$

Return on Total Assets

The return on total assets is represented as earnings before interest and taxes (EBIT) divided by total assets. This is a broad measure in common use.

$$\frac{\text{EBIT (Earnings before Interest and Taxes)}}{\text{Total Assets}} = \frac{\$83,100}{\$1,000,000} = 8.3\%$$

Note: $80,000 + $3,100 = $83,100.

SOLUTION TO PRACTICE EXERCISE 13–I: UNADJUSTED RATE OF RETURN

1. Calculation using original investment amount:

$$\frac{\$100,000}{\$500,000} = 20\% \text{ Unadjusted Rate of Return}$$

2. Calculation using average investment amount:
   Step 1. Compute average investment amount for total unrecovered asset cost:

At beginning of estimated useful life	=	$500,000
At end of estimated useful life	=	$ 50,000
Sum		$550,000

   Divided by 2 = $275,000 average investment amount

   Step 2. Calculate unadjusted rate of return:

$$\frac{\$100,000}{\$275,000} = 36.4\% \text{ Unadjusted Rate of Return}$$

SOLUTION TO PRACTICE EXERCISE 13–II: FINDING THE FUTURE VALUE (WITH A COMPOUND INTEREST TABLE)

Step 1. Refer to the Compound Interest Table found in Appendix 13–B at the back of this chapter. Reading across, or horizontally, find the 7% column. Reading down, or vertically, find Year 6. Trace across the Year 6 line item to the 7% column. The factor is 1.501.

Step 2. Multiply the current savings account balance of $11,000 times the factor of 1.501 to find the future value of $16,511. In six years at compound interest of 7%, the college fund will have a balance of $16,511.

SOLUTION TO PRACTICE EXERCISE 13–III: FINDING THE PRESENT VALUE

Step 1. Refer to the Present-Value Table appearing in Appendix 13–A at the back of this chapter. Reading across, or horizontally, find the 7% column. Reading down, or vertically, find Year 15. Trace across the Year 15 line item to the 7% column. The factor is 0.3624.

Step 2. Multiply $150,000 times the factor of 0.3624 to find the present value of $54,360.

SOLUTION TO PRACTICE EXERCISE 13–IV

Assemble the assumptions in an orderly manner:

Assumption 1: Initial cost of the investment = $16,950.
Assumption 2: Estimated annual net cash inflow the investment will generate = $3,000.
Assumption 3: Useful life of the asset = 10 years.

Perform calculation:

Step 1. Divide the initial cost of the investment ($16,950) by the estimated annual net cash inflow it will generate ($3,000). The answer is a ratio amounting to 5.650.

Step 2. Now use the abbreviated look-up table for the Present Value of an Annuity of $1 appearing in Appendix 13–C. Find the line item for the number of periods that matches the useful life of the asset (10 years in this case).

Step 3. Look across the 10-year line on the table and find the column that approximates the ratio of 5.650 (as computed in Step 1). That column contains the interest rate representing the rate of return. In this case the rate of return is 12%.

SOLUTION TO PRACTICE EXERCISE 13–V

Assemble assumptions in an orderly manner:

Assumption 1: Purchase price of the equipment = $500,000.
Assumption 2: Useful life of the equipment = 10 years.
Assumption 3: Revenue the machine will generate per year = $84,000.
Assumption 4: Direct operating costs associated with earning the revenue = $21,000.
Assumption 5: Depreciation expense per year (computed as purchase price per assumption 1 divided by useful life per assumption 2) = $50,000.

Perform computation:

Step 1. Find the machine's expected net income after taxes:

Revenue (Assumption 3)	$84,000
Less	
Direct operating costs (Assumption 4)	$21,000
Depreciation (Assumption 5)	50,000
	71,000
Net income	$13,000

Note: No income taxes for this hospital.

Step 2. Find the net annual cash inflow the machine is expected to generate (in other words, convert the net income to a cash basis).

Net income	$13,000
Add back depreciation (a noncash expenditure)	50,000
Annual net cash inflow after taxes	$63,000

Step 3. Compute the payback period:

$$\frac{Investment}{Net\ Annual\ Cash\ Inflow} = \frac{\$500,000\ Machine\ Cost^*}{\$63,000^{**}} = 7.9\ Year\ Payback\ Period$$

*Assumption 1 above.
**Per Step 2 above.

The machine will pay back its investment under these assumptions in 7.9 years.

SOLUTION TO PRACTICE EXERCISE 14–I

Common sizing for the assets of the two hospitals appears on the worksheet below. Note that their gross numbers are very different, yet the proportionate relationships of the percentages (20%, 75%, and 5%) are the same for both hospitals.

	Same Year for Both Hospitals			
	Hospital A		Hospital B	
Current assets	$ 2,000,000	20%	$ 8,000,000	20%
Property, plant, and equipment	7,500,000	75%	30,000,000	75%
Other assets	500,000	5%	2,000,000	5%
Total assets	$10,000,000	100%	$40,000,000	100%

SOLUTION TO PRACTICE EXERCISE 14–II

	Hospital A			
	Year 1	Year 2	Difference	
Current assets	$1,600,000	$ 2,000,000	$ 400,000	25%
Property, plant, and equipment	6,000,000	7,500,000	1,500,000	25%
Other assets	400,000	500,000	100,000	25%
Total assets	$8,000,000	$10,000,000	$2,000,000	—

Note: The worksheet below shows Hospital A with both common sizing and trend analysis:

	Hospital A					
	Year 1		Year 2		Difference	
Current assets	$1,600,000	20%	$2,000,000	20%	$ 400,000	25%
Property, plant, and equipment	6,000,000	75%	7,500,000	75%	1,500,000	25%
Other assets	400,000	5%	500,000	5%	100,000	25%
Total assets	$8,000,000	100%	$10,000,000	100%	$2,000,000	—

SOLUTION TO PRACTICE EXERCISE 14–III

Q: How many procedures has your unit recorded for the period to date?

Solution: The unit has recorded 2,000 procedures ($200,000 divided by $100 apiece equals 2,000 procedures).

Q: Of these, how many procedures are attributed to each payer?

Solution: At 25% of the volume per payer, each payer accounts for 500 procedures (2,000 times 25% equals 500 procedures). Proof total: 500 procedures apiece times four payers equals 2,000 procedures.

Q: How much is the net revenue per procedure for each payer, and how much is the contractual allowance per procedure for each payer?

Solution: The computation is as follows:

Payer #	Gross Charges	% Paid by Each Payer	Net Revenue per Procedure	Contractual Allowance per Procedure
1	$100.00	90%	$90.00	$10.00
2	$100.00	80%	$80.00	$20.00
3	$100.00	70%	$70.00	$30.00
4	$100.00	50%	$50.00	$50.00

SOLUTION TO PRACTICE EXERCISE 16–I

Your initial budget assumptions were as follows:

Assume the budget anticipated 30,000 inpatient days this year at an average of $650 revenue per day, or $19,500,000. Further assume that inpatient expenses were budgeted at $600 per patient day, or $18,000,000. Also assume the budget anticipated 10,000 outpatient visits this year at an average of $400 revenue per visit, or $4,000,000. Further assume that outpatient expenses were budgeted at $380 per visit, or $3,800,000. The budget worksheet would look like this:

	As Budgeted
Revenue—Inpatient	$19,500,000
Revenue—Outpatient	4,000,000
Subtotal	$23,500,000
Expenses—Inpatient	$18,000,000
Expenses—Outpatient	3,800,000
Subtotal	$21,800,000
Excess of revenue over expenses	$1,700,000

Now assume that only 27,000, or 90%, of the patient days are going to actually be achieved for the year. The average revenue of $650 per day will be achieved for these 27,000 days (thus 27,000 times 650 equals 17,550,000). Also assume that outpatient visits will actually amount to 110%, or 11,000 for the year. The average revenue of $400 per visit will be achieved for these 11,000 visits (thus 11,000 times 400 equals 4,400,000). Further assume that, due to the heroic efforts of the Chief Financial Officer, the actual inpatient expenses will amount to $11,600,000 and the actual outpatient expenses will amount to $4,000,000. The actual results would look like this:

	Actual
Revenue—Inpatient	$17,550,000
Revenue—Outpatient	4,400,000
Subtotal	$21,950,000
Expenses—Inpatient	16,100,000
Expenses—Outpatient	4,000,000
Subtotal	$20,100,000
Excess of revenue over expenses	$1,850,000

Since the budgeted revenues and expenses still reflect the original expectations of 30,000 inpatient days and 10,000 outpatient visits, the budget report would look like this:

	Actual	Budget	Static Budget Variance
Revenue—Inpatient	$17,550,000	$19,500,000	$(1,950,000)
Revenue—Outpatient	4,400,000	4,000,000	400,000
Subtotal	$21,950,000	$23,500,000	$(1,550,000)
Expenses—Inpatient	$16,100,000	$18,000,000	$(1,900,000)
Expenses—Outpatient	4,000,000	3,800,000	200,000
Subtotal	$20,100,000	$21,800,000	$(1,700,000)
Excess of revenue over expenses	$ 1,850,000	$ 1,700,000	$ 150,000

Note: The negative effect of the $1,550,000 net drop in revenue is offset by the greater effect of the $1,700,000 net drop in expenses, resulting in a positive net effect of $150,000.

SOLUTION TO PRACTICE EXERCISE 17–I

Because there is no one right answer, students will approach this exercise in different ways.

SOLUTION TO PRACTICE EXERCISE 18–1

Required Solution to Practice Exercise 18–1

The Price Variance is $100,000 (favorable).
The Quantity Variance is $120,000 (unfavorable).
The Net Variance is $20,000 (unfavorable).

Actual Cost	$950,000
Less: Flexible Budget	1,050,000
Price Variance (favorable)	$100,000
Budgeted Cost	$930,000
Less: Flexible Budget	1,050,000
Quantity Variance (unfavorable)	−$120,000
Net Variance (favorable)	−$ 20,000

Assumptions

	Overhead Cost	divided by	# Therapy Minutes (Activity Level)	equals	Cost per Therapy Minute
Actual	(1) $950,000		(3) 350,000		(5) $2.71
Budgeted	(2) $930,000		(4) 310,000		(6) $3.00

Optional Solution to Practice Exercise 18–I

The $950,000 actual overhead cost represents 350,000 therapy minutes times $2.71 per therapy minute.

The $930,000 budgeted overhead cost represents 310,000 therapy minutes times $3.00 per therapy minute.

SOLUTION TO PRACTICE EXERCISE 18–II

The required revenue to achieve a target operating income of $20,000 amounts to revenue of $75,000.

The contribution income statement to prove the formula results is as follows:

Revenue $500/unit × 150 units =	$75,000
Variable costs $300/unit × 150 units =	45,000
Contribution margin	$30,000
Fixed costs	10,000
Desire (Target) Operating Income =	$20,000

SOLUTION TO PRACTICE EXERCISE 22–I

With beginning principal of $60,000, the monthly payment is $1,936.03 and the remaining principal balance at the end of six payments is $51,202.30.

SOLUTION TO PRACTICE EXERCISE 23–I

The present-value cost of leasing for Suburban Clinic amounts to $49,116.

SOLUTION TO PRACTICE EXERCISE 25–I

The retail pharmacy case study appearing in Chapter 33-C contains all of the assumption items listed in Example 25A.

SOLUTION TO PRACTICE EXERCISE 26–I

$50 per hour divided by 60 minutes equals $0.8333; thus 2 minutes equals $1.6667. If a hospital's coders are dealing with 1,500 claims, then the dollar amount of productivity loss is $2,499 (1.6667 per claim times 1,500 claims equals $2,499).

Index

Note: Page numbers followed with *f* and *t* refer to figures and tables.